THE PSYCHOLOGY OF EATING AND DRINKING

An Introduction
Second Edition

A. W. LOGUE
State University of
New York at Stony Brook

W. H. Freeman and Company
New York

To my parents,
Camille Woods Logue and
James Gibson Logue, Jr.

Library of Congress Cataloging in Publication Data

Logue, A. W. (Alexandra W.)
  The psychology of eating and drinking : an introduction /
A. W. Logue. — 2nd ed.
    p. cm. — (A series of books in psychology)
  Includes index.
  ISBN 0-7167-2232-1. — ISBN 0-7167-2197-X (pbk.)
  1. Food habits—Psychological aspects. 2. Nutrition—
Psychological aspects. 3. Drinking behavior. 4. Food
preferences.
  I. Title. II. Series.
TX357.L66 1991
613.2′ 01′9--dc20
                                              91-6812
                                                  CIP

  2 3 4 5 6 7 8 9 0   VB   9 9 8 7 6 5 4 3 2

Contents

Contents

Contents

Preface

When I was a year old I stopped eating everything except bread and milk. For years my diet showed little improvement, and by 15 I was eating mostly meat, milk, potatoes, bread, orange juice, and desserts. I did *not* eat pizza, spaghetti, or any other food that I considered "foreign." I avoided soda, fresh fruit except bananas, vegetables except peas, carrots, and beets, and cheese except grilled cheese sandwiches. Fish I regarded as poison.

My parents were not alarmed; I come from a long line of people with unusual food preferences. My mother, by choice, rarely serves fresh fruit or fish at home. She never serves liver, which she hates, although my father loves it. He always eats first the food he dislikes most, and many times I have seen him finish salad and string beans before touching baked potato and steak. My mother has frequently recounted to me how her grandfather would eat chocolate cupcakes but not cake made from the same batter; he said that the cake gave him indigestion.

At home my parents gave me vitamin pills and basically let me eat whatever I wanted. But everywhere else I had to contend with sticky social occasions in which I was served what I abhorred eating.

One of the worst situations occurred during my college years when I visited the Rappaport family on Martha's Vineyard. I did not know this family well then, and they certainly did not know about my peculiar eating habits. In honor of my visit they had specially cooked lobster. The lobsters were so expensive and so much fuss was made over them that there seemed to be no way out for me: I had to eat lobster. Luckily, with lobster it is easy to disguise how little you have really eaten and somehow I got down a respectable portion. But having eaten it I could not get the lobster taste out of my mouth. At bedtime I brushed my teeth, but the taste stayed with me and I could not sleep. Eventually I got up and put large globs of toothpaste into my mouth so that I could finally fall asleep.

Food aversions were not the only troubles of my youth. Food preferences also gave me problems. Although I disliked many things, when I did like a food I could eat it at any hour of the day or night. My Southern grandmother was happy to feed me fried chicken, mashed potatoes, and hot biscuits dripping with butter whenever I wished. I constantly had to fight to keep my weight at a reasonable level. One of the most dangerous places for me was the farm of my great-aunt and great-uncle in South Carolina, where the dinner table groaned with everything that I most loved to eat. One exception was the milk from their cows. Although I relished it when it came back from the packager, I found milk totally unacceptable when it came straight from the cow (even though my great-uncle had pasteurized it).

Two things saved me from an unhealthy preoccupation with eating certain foods: my husband and my study of experimental psychology.

My husband, Ian Shrank (known in childhood as the HGP, or human garbage pail, because of his voracious and indiscriminate eating habits), was directly responsible for the most successful diet I ever undertook. In 1974, when we were engaged and I was very poor, he paid me $5 for every pound I lost. In three weeks I was 10 pounds lighter and $50 richer, a fortune for a poor student at that time. By example, pleading, and occasional bullying over the 17 years of our marriage, he now has me regularly eating (and sometimes even liking) vegetables, fruits, and ethnic food. (No one, under any circumstances, will ever get me to eat fish.)

Becoming an experimental psychologist, the other saving factor, channeled my former embarrassment into research enthusiasm. As a graduate student, I was continually drawn to research on eating and drinking behavior. Sometimes I conducted studies that grew out of hypotheses I had about the origins of my own eating peculiarities. Only much later did I realize that a great deal of psychology focuses on eating and drinking.

As a graduate student at Harvard I was encouraged to pursue my interests wherever they led, a strategy that prepared me well for writing this book. As part of my studies I taught a small seminar for sophomore psychology majors. I was expected to come up with a topic for a year-long tutorial that would integrate material from many areas of psychology. I chose eating and drinking.

Later, as an assistant professor at the State University of New York at Stony Brook, I proposed a new lecture course: The Psychology of Eating and Drinking. With the support of the chair of the undergraduate program, Marvin Levine, the course was created, and although it is an advanced, nonrequired course, it has grown in popularity every year. In the first years of the course, the students read only original articles; the only textbooks that were at all relevant covered isolated topics such as hunger or alcoholism. The lack of a suitable text for my course and the enthusiasm of my teaching assistants and students finally convinced me that I should write this book.

The story of my path to writing this book would be incomplete without mention of Paul Rozin, the ultimate food psychologist. I met Paul in 1977 at the University of Pennsylvania, where he was pursuing research on why people eat chili pepper. That first meeting with Paul and his wife, Elisabeth, cookbook writer and culinary historian, and the time we spent in their kitchen, catalyzed my interest in the psychology of eating and drinking, and the effect has not yet worn off. Liz's cookbook, *Ethnic Cuisine: The Flavor-Principle Cookbook,* has always been my favorite, and I doubt if that will ever change.

In later years, after I was working at Stony Brook, Paul organized The Cuisine Group, a small collection of anthropologists, folklorists, culinary historians, psychologists, and others with an interest in food, who would meet occasionally in Manhattan on a Saturday for lunch, lectures (with snacks), and then dinner. As the only member of the group who had become interested in food primarily due to food *aversions,* I have been the constant object of discussion and experimentation by other group members. At one meeting, Linda Bartoshuk of Yale University, a specialist in the psychology of taste, tested me and discovered that I was unusually sensitive to the taste of the chemical PTC (see Chapter 4, "Taste and Smell"). Linda stated that this sensitivity could explain at least some of my food aversions. I have been eternally grateful to her for helping to educate me about PTC and other intricacies of taste perception, particularly when I use her information to explain why I do not have to try some strange food that someone is insisting that I eat.

My book describes scientific inquiries into eating and drinking behavior. I have elected to cover only those aspects of the psychology of eating and drinking that seem well researched and interesting, and I have had to cover some of these only briefly. Complete coverage of the psychology of eating and drinking would require many, many volumes. This book is meant only as an introduction. Nevertheless, I describe how the research was conducted—not just the results—so that readers may judge the implications for themselves. Readers who want further detail may turn to the reference notes, listed by chapter, at the end of the book.

This book covers the major eating and drinking disorders, but it will not tell you precisely how to diagnose or treat your own or someone else's eating and drinking problems. Some of the principles for doing so are described, but practical problem solving requires professional help. The section on Clinics and Self-Help Organizations at the back of the book can be useful in obtaining that professional help.

The Psychology of Eating and Drinking is intended for readers who may or may not have had courses in psychology. It can be used as a supplementary or main text in psychology courses, or, for a psychologist, it can serve as an introduction to eating and drinking behavior. It is also written for educated laypeople. The only requirement for reading and enjoying this book is that the reader be willing to approach psychology as a science. One of my goals in writing this book, as well as in my teaching, has been to show how much can be learned by applying scientific methods to the study of behavior.

The second edition offers a number of improvements over the first. All of the chapters have been extensively revised and updated with new and exciting research findings. In addition, three new chapters have been added describing the applications of the psychology of eating and drinking to everyday issues and problems. More specifically, Chapter 12 is concerned with female reproduction, Chapter 13 with the weight loss and weight gain associated with cigarette smoking, and Chapter 14 with cuisine and wine tasting. These chapters demonstrate some of the benefits of taking a unified, scientific approach to the psychology of eating and drinking.

ACKNOWLEDGMENTS

Many people and organizations assisted me in preparing this book. For the first edition, James Hassett gave me a great deal of valuable, general advice on how to write a psychology book. My library research assistants, Lawrence Epstein, Pilar Pena-Correal, Telmo Pena-Correal, and Michael Smith were always ready to run to the library to find source material for me. Herbert Terrace and Columbia University kindly provided me with space and library privileges that helped me finish the book during my sabbatical. Conversations with Alex Kacelnik on foraging and Nori Geary on hunger were also very helpful. Invaluable comments were made on the manuscript by Lorraine Collins, Howard Rachlin, Monica Rodriguez, Elisabeth Rozin, Paul Rozin, Diane Shrank, Ian Shrank, Michael Smith, and Richard Thompson. Their help is greatly appreciated. In particular I thank Camille M. Logue, whose hours of insightful and witty taped comments kept me company in the lonely hours of revision; she went far beyond the requirements of sibling duty.

In preparing the second edition, the comments made in the many reviews of the first edition were extremely helpful. Several reviewers (Leann L. Birch, John P. Foreyt, Bonnie Spring, and Rudy E. Vuchinich) made many insightful, useful suggestions regarding a previous draft of the second edition. Many researchers put up with my seemingly endless questions about this or that aspect of eating and drinking. In particular, Kelly Brownell provided much information regarding overeating and obesity, Jasper Brener helped me to identify research on metabolic rate, and The Cuisine Group (most notably Linda Bartoshuk, Barbara Kirschenblatt-Gimblet, Rudolph Grewe, Solomon Katz, Elisabeth Rozin, and Paul Rozin) were a constant source of inspiration. I also thank James Allison for sending me the Warm Feet. (Will the wonders of capsicum never cease?) Lori Bonvino exceeded all possible standards in word processing and organizing the seemingly endless lists of references. John Chelonis willingly and ably stepped in at the eleventh hour to finish the name index.

Ann Streissguth, at the University of Washington, generously supplied the photographs for Figure 12.2 (the children with fetal alcohol syndrome). Twentieth Century Fox provided the photograph of Marilyn Monroe from the movie *Monkey Business* for Figure 9.3a and Columbia Pictures provided the photograph of Jamie Lee Curtis from the movie *Perfect* for Figure 9.3b. Phototeque, in New York City, was of great assistance in locating these latter two photographs. Jacob Steiner, of Hebrew University in Jerusalem, Israel, kindly provided the photograph of newborn infants tasting various solutions (Figure 5.2).

The editorial staff at W. H. Freeman should also be lauded. The first edition was signed by W. Hayward (Buck) Rogers, and ably shepherded through the production process by Stephen Wagley. The second edition has been enthusiastically and effectively supported by Jonathan Cobb (who is far more fascinated with food than he will admit), and has proceeded through production ahead of schedule thanks to the calm, intelligent, and extremely thorough efforts of Sonia DiVittorio; she made a potentially painful process quite bearable.

Throughout it all, the Long Island Railroad provided many, many hours of uninterrupted work time. Harvard University, the United States Public Health Services Biomedical Research Support Grants, the National Institute of Mental Health, the National Science Foundation, and the State University of New York all provided funds for research of my own that is reported here. Many ideas and much inspiration have been provided by the students and teaching assistants in my undergraduate and graduate courses on the psychology of eating and drinking. One such student, Victoria Thode, provided material used in Chapters 10 and 11. Particular thanks are also owed to my graduate students, Lori Bonvino, Adolfo Chavarro, George King, Telmo Pena-Correal, Monica Rodriguez, and Henry Tobin, for their enthusiasm, and for never doubting the worth of this project. Finally, I want to express my deepest appreciation to my husband, Ian Shrank, and my son, Samuel Logue Shrank, for their constant, unquestioning encouragement and support.

CHAPTER

1

❦

Introduction

Consider the following quotations:

No animal can live without food. Let us then pursue the corollary of
this: namely, food is about the most important influence in determining the organization of the brain and the behavior that the brain organization dictates. *J. Z. Young (1968)* [1]

Almost every animal or plant is accessible as food to an animal with
the right feeding strategy. . . . [F]eeding is simply the means of acquiring the materials for building, maintaining and powering the
vehicle that carries the next generation, and for nourishing its early
stages. . . . Organisms must feed to survive, but survival of the individual is relevant only for its contribution to the next generation.
All life processes are ultimately adapted to ensure reproduction and
the only measure of the success of survival strategies is in terms of
breeding success. *Jennifer Owen (1980)* [2]

It is self-evident that nutrition is the main requirement of all living
systems. . . . Active feeding, that is to say feeding preceded by food-

seeking behavior, is a necessity of animal life. . . . It was and still is the most powerful agent in the evolution of species. *Jacques Le Magnen (1985)* [3]

Why is food important in the larger scheme of things? From the first efforts to explain human biological and cultural evolution, subsistence has been causally implicated. The very origin of the species is thought to have been related to changes in primate subsistence. *Anna Roosevelt (1987)* [4]

It seems unbelievable that primitive man could have invented such a curious, complicated instrument, but hunters on various continents did: the *atlatl* it would be named after the example the Europeans encountered in Mexico, but all versions were similar. Somehow, men with no knowledge of engineering or dynamics deduced that their harpoons would be trebly effective if they were loaded into their atlatls and slung forward instead of being thrown. . . . [O]ne must remember that for a hundred thousand years men spent most of their waking hours trying to kill animals for food; they had no occupation more important. *James Michener (1988)* [5]

SIR TOBY—
Does not our life consist of the four elements
[earth, air, fire, and water]?
SIR ANDREW—
Faith, so they say; but I think it rather consists
of eating and drinking.
SIR TOBY—
Thou'rt a scholar; let us therefore eat and drink.
William Shakespeare (1623/1936) [6]

These quotations clearly show that fiction writers, as well as psychologists, value the study of eating and drinking. All animals, including humans, have to eat and drink in order to survive. Consequently a large part of their behavior must be directed at obtaining and consuming foods and liquids. Similarly, understanding the eating and drinking behavior of a particular species is essential for anyone who wishes to acquire a full understanding of the behavior of that species.

THE STUDY OF EATING AND DRINKING

Psychology is the science of behavior, the science of "how and why organisms do what they do."[7] A psychological study of eating and drinking can proceed on many levels of analysis. These can include, for example, investigations of the neuronal basis of taste sensitivity to sweet (physiological studies), of the effect of illness on the preference for sweet (learning studies), and of the effect of widely available, inexpensive sweet foods on sugar consumption (group studies).

Traditionally, psychologists align themselves with one particular level of analysis and address issues only from that level. For example, physiological psychologists explore physiological determinants of behaviors such as eating, drinking, mating, aggression, and parenting. This book takes a different tack and explores one type of behavior—eating and drinking—using many different levels of analysis. This approach sheds light on the relationships between the different areas of psychology and makes it easy to see what each specialty contributes to our understanding.

The only orientation consistently espoused here is a natural science orientation, which assumes that natural laws govern behavior and that behavior is entirely the result of genetic and environmental influences. Further, a natural science orientation holds that there is no separation, no essential difference, between mind and body, and that what some refer to as mind consists entirely of physiological reactions. Only with this orientation is it possible to conduct experiments to determine the causes of behavior. If the mind were not a physiological entity, if it were not governed by traditional physical laws, then an experimenter could never assume that manipulation of an experimental variable was the cause of a subsequent change in behavior.

EVOLUTION AND EATING AND DRINKING

According to evolutionary theory, organisms behave so as to maximize the survival of their genes, their *inclusive fitness* (the probability that their biological relatives will survive).[8] In this way natural selection—survival and reproduction of the fittest individuals—occurs. Because survival and eating and drinking are so intertwined, evolution has undoubtedly played a role in the origins of the eating and drinking behavior of current species. Therefore evolutionary theory can serve as a useful overall framework for understanding eating and drinking. Evolutionary explanations will appear repeatedly throughout this book. However, just because natural selection is and has been in operation does not mean that all species' behaviors will be adaptive. For example, a species might have evolved in an environment different from the one in which it currently resides, genetic mutation or drift might have occurred, or behaving in the way so as to best ensure survival might require more information than the organism can acquire or retain. For all of these reasons, although there is widespread agreement that organisms' behavior is guided by evolutionary processes, organisms sometimes do very unadaptive things. There will be many examples of such unadaptive behaviors in this book.

OUTLINE OF THE BOOK

The material in this book has been divided into five parts such that basic information about eating and drinking is presented first (Parts I, II, and III). More specifically, Part I covers motivation for amount of eating and drinking; Part II, learning and motivation for selection of particular foods and drinks; and Part III, the effects of food consumption on behavior. Then the information from Parts I, II, and III is expanded in order to describe and explain eating and drinking disorders (Part IV). Finally, Part V covers additional special interest topics, including female reproduction and food and drink consumption, smoking and weight gain and loss, and cuisine and wine tasting.

Many of the data presented in this book have been collected from nonhuman subjects. Therefore it is necessary to confront immediately the problems of, first, the usefulness of nonhuman animal experimentation in psychology and, second, which species provide good models of human eating and drinking behavior. In addition, this material on the use of different species in studying the psychology of eating and drinking will provide a quick survey of many of the themes to come in later chapters.

SPECIES DIFFERENCES AND SIMILARITIES

Although psychology is the science of what *all* organisms do, it centers on human behavior. Given that focus, why study nonhuman eating and drinking behavior?

First, experiments usually require controlled conditions that are difficult to maintain with human subjects. For example, in order to discover to what degree the environment can affect behavior, an experiment may require that all of the subjects have identical genetic backgrounds, a requirement impossible to satisfy with human subjects. Second, an experiment may involve watching the life-long development of particular individuals, or observing several generations of subjects. This is much more difficult with humans because the time from their birth to maturity is quite long. Third, studies with nonhuman subjects, particularly long studies, are often less expensive. People expect to be paid well for the time they spend in an experiment. Finally, certain experiments require manipulations that cannot be done safely or ethically with humans. For example, an experiment that calls for depriving a subject of food until it loses 20 percent of its free-feeding weight is usually considered unethical for human subjects.

Which species, if used in an experiment, would yield results likely to apply to humans? To a certain extent the behavior of most species must be governed by similar rules, because all species live in a world governed by the same physical laws. An example of such a law is the following (see also Chapter 6): An event that causes an illness must occur prior to the illness. Accordingly, all species tend to associate an event with an illness more readily if the event precedes, rather than follows, the illness.[9] However, the particular ecological niche that a species inhabits also influences its eating and drinking behavior, and this accounts for many differences between the eating and drinking behavior of different species. The sections that follow describe the eating and drinking behavior of several different species and assess which nonhuman animals may be helpful as models of human eating and drinking behavior.

Invertebrates

THE BLACK BLOWFLY. We would expect the eating and drinking behavior of the common black blowfly to differ in many ways from human eating and drinking behavior. But consider the following episode:

> A fly is sitting on a lamp in a living room. Several hours have passed since it last ate. It is two o'clock in the afternoon. The fly takes wing and makes its way around the room. Gradually it heads toward the kitchen. It goes through the open kitchen door and lands on a jar of honey that has been left on the table. It walks about on the jar until it comes to a drip down the side of the jar. It uncurls its proboscis and begins to suck up the honey. Eventually the sucking stops, and the fly departs.

This behavior can be likened to that of a human who becomes hungry, goes looking for food, finds food, eats, and once satisfied, leaves. But the mechanisms responsible for the fly's behavior are actually quite different.

Given the presence of light and an empty gut, the fly takes wing, as shown in Figure 1.1. If it encounters the odor of sugar while it is flying, it flies upwind in the direction of that odor and eventually lands on the substance giving off the odor. When it steps on the sugar, sensory hairs in the fly's legs are stimulated. These stimulated sensory hairs cause the fly's proboscis to uncoil. When the proboscis comes into contact with the sugar, sensory cells in the proboscis cause the fly to suck in sugar through the proboscis. Finally the gut is full, and the fly stops sucking and departs.[10]

The fly's eating behavior is extremely adaptive. It searches for food when its gut has just emptied and its blood sugar level is still high, before it has

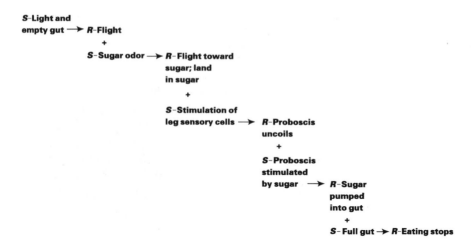

FIGURE 1.1   *A model of the reflexes involved in the black blowfly's feeding behavior.*
S represents a stimulus, and *R* a response. Each sequence showing a stimulus joined
with an arrow to a response is a reflex.

become completely depleted of nourishment. This protects the fly from
going without food for a dangerously long time and is known as *anticipatory
feeding*. The fly is able to find food, and it eats until it is full. But the fly's behavior is governed completely by innate *reflexes*, specific responses that
occur reliably following exposure to specific stimuli. No learning is involved.[11] The fly will perform this sequence of behaviors the first time that
the appropriate conditions arise, and the behaviors will be very similar each
time it performs them.

Human behavior is not so limited. Although in many respects it may appear similar to the fly's behavior, human behavior depends heavily on
learning. Consequently, human behavior is more variable, changing from
one time to the next and from one situation to another. In humans, one particular behavior can occur as a result of a number of different causes. In the
fly, a given set of reflexes is responsible for what appears to be voluntary,
purposeful behavior. Although the fly may not be a good model for studying human eating and drinking, studying its eating and drinking behavior
does provide a caution for work with humans. Behavior that appears voluntary and purposeful may actually be due to reflexes.

PLEUROBRANCHAEA.   Certain marine molluscs, for example *Pleurobranchaea* (see Figure 1.2), can be quite useful in the study of the psychology
of eating and drinking. This sea slug is carnivorous. Its neuronal system is
relatively simple, and therefore its neurons are easily identified and

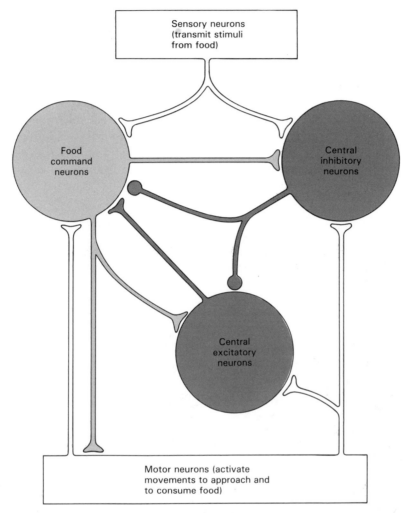

FIGURE 1.2   *Simplified diagram of the neuronal feeding command system of* Pleurobranchaea. If this sea slug has not been fed recently, the food command neurons fire at a high rate when stimulated by food sensory inputs. As a result, *Pleurobranchaea* will approach food. On the other hand, if this sea slug has been fed recently, the food command neurons fire at a low rate due to suppression from the central inhibitory neurons. Then *Pleurobranchaea* will not approach food. If *Pleurobranchaea* has been given a small shock each time it extends its feeding proboscis toward food, it will also approach food infrequently. However, this decrease in frequency of food approach is now a result of both increased suppression from the central inhibitory neurons and decreases in the efficacy of the central excitatory neurons in stimulating the food command neurons. (Adapted from W. J. Davis, "Motivation and Learning: Neurophysiological Mechanisms in a 'Model' System," *Learning and Motivation* 15[1984]: 377–393.)

manipulated. *Pleurobranchaea's* tendency to eat, its *motivation*, can be influenced by its nutritional history. Such motivational changes are represented by changes in the degree to which the central inhibitory neurons inhibit the activity of the food command neurons. The food command neurons are those that connect *Pleurobranchaea's* sensory neurons (which detect the presence of food) with its motor neurons (which induce movement). This mollusc's tendency to eat can also be affected by *learning*, its acquisition of knowledge about which stimuli and responses are and are not associated. If shock is paired with food consumption, *Pleurobranchaea* will be less likely to approach and consume food. Such an instance of learning is represented both by increases in the activity of the central inhibitory neurons and by decreases in the activity of the central excitatory neurons.[12] Nevertheless, despite this model system's usefulness in investigations of the neurobiology of the motivation and learning of feeding behavior, this usefulness is limited due to molluscs' limited behavioral repertoire, including that with respect to feeding.

Birds

Birds are a popular choice for studies of food consumption under natural conditions. They are abundant and active during the day, as well as being large enough to be observed easily. They also have a high metabolic rate that demands frequent consumption of food. A substantial number of studies with birds exist, thus providing much background information for any new study, as well as permitting cross-study comparisons. Finally, birds (in particular, Harris' hawks) have been observed engaging in cooperative hunting, a type of behavior for which previously there was only good evidence in a few species of mammalian carnivores. More specifically, during the nonbreeding season, Harris' hawks hunt in groups of two to six birds. This group hunting behavior, as compared with individual hunting, results in a greater probability of the hawks' capturing their prey, a greater net calorie gain, and an increased likelihood of the hawks' being able to capture larger prey.[13] Thus complex social behavior in these birds appears to be tied to the caloric, and therefore survival, benefits of this behavior. Chapter 14 describes how maximization of obtained calories may also play a role in complex human social behavior. Yet much of humans' eating and drinking behavior is not represented in birds.

Mammals

All infant mammals suckle, a behavior that has substantial genetic determination. In fact, suckling is the only behavior common to all mammals.[14]

Because humans are mammals, other mammalian species would seem the most likely choices as nonhuman animal models for understanding human eating and drinking behavior.

PRIMATES.   Primates are our closest evolutionary relatives. Like humans, they are *omnivores:* Although most primates consume mainly fruit, they also eat leaves, insects, and sometimes meat. In addition, similar to humans, some chimpanzees find it difficult to taste the chemical *phenylthiocarbamide* (PTC, see Chapter 4).[15]

Some species of primates are capable of a great deal of focused attention and can manipulate objects with precision, particularly when they eat insects. Focused attention and manipulation have parallels in human eating and drinking behavior.[16] Jane Goodall studied chimpanzees in the wild and observed that they stripped twigs of their leaves and utilized them to obtain termites. The chimps would poke a stripped twig into a termite hill, the termites would cling to the twig, and the chimps would pull out the twig and lick the termites off (Figure 1.3). This was the first recorded example of tool construction by nonhumans. Goodall recorded another example of tool construction associated with food consumption when she saw chimps chew up leaves and use them to sponge water from tree hollows.[17]

Food manipulation in the form of "seasoning," similar to humans' seasoning of their food, has been observed in a group of Japanese monkeys living on a small island called Kashima, where they were first studied by Japanese scientists in 1948.[18] In 1952 the scientists began giving the monkeys sweet potatoes to eat. In 1953, a female monkey named Imo became the first monkey to exhibit what the scientists called sweet-potato washing behavior. The sweet potatoes were frequently covered with sand. Imo would dip the sweet potato into the water with one hand and then brush off the sand with her other hand. By 1958 approximately 80 percent of the monkeys were exhibiting sweet-potato washing behavior. During the period that most of the monkeys were acquiring the sweet-potato washing behavior, that behavior began to change. At first the sweet potatoes had been dipped only in fresh water. By 1961 the potatoes were being dipped primarily in salt water. Further, the monkeys would take a bite of a sweet potato, dip it, and then take another bite, "seasoning" the sweet potato.

Goodall has also described instances of hunting and meat eating among chimpanzees. She found that the males usually engaged in the hunting and that the hunters demonstrated basic elements of cooperative hunting behavior. One chimp would creep toward the prey, usually a young baboon or other small animal, while other chimps positioned themselves to block the prey's routes of escape. After the hunters caught and killed the prey, they often shared the food among themselves, as well as with other chimps. It is

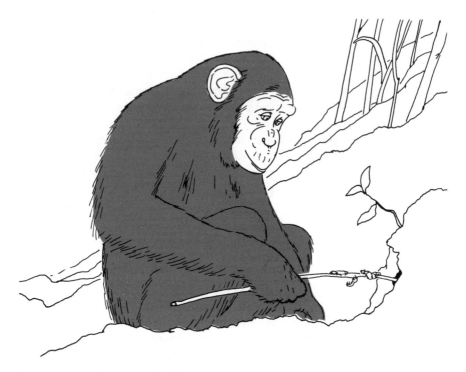

FIGURE 1.3   *Chimpanzee obtaining termites from a termite nest.*

possible, however, that the extreme proximity of Goodall's chimps to other animals, particularly baboons, increased the frequency of their hunting and meat eating. To attract the chimps, and thus facilitate their observation, Goodall put out large piles of bananas. Unfortunately, these piles of bananas drew baboons to the area as well, and ordinarily chimpanzees and baboons stay away from each other.[19] Nevertheless, when food lures are absent, chimpanzees' social structure is very similar to that of humans.[20]

Overall, chimpanzees' eating and drinking behavior shows many similarities to human eating and drinking behavior. Primates eat almost the same foods as do humans. Primates also sometimes make tools to help them obtain food. They may also hunt cooperatively. For all of these reasons, they seem good candidates for a model of human eating and drinking behavior. There are several practical disadvantages to using primates in experiments, however. They are very expensive to purchase and maintain, they can be difficult to handle, and they take a long time to produce sexually mature progeny (as do humans). Because they are similar to humans, ethical constraints that would apply to using humans in experiments might also apply to using primates. For all of these reasons, psychologists usually have not worked with primates in the investigation of eating and drinking behavior.

PIGS.   Some researchers have suggested that the pig may be the perfect animal for eating and drinking experiments. Pigs and humans have similar body sizes, growth rates, alimentary canals, diets, and food preferences (for example, pigs prefer sweet foods).[21]

But pigs have not become the most favored experimental subject for research on eating and drinking. The fact that their size does approximate that of humans makes them hard to handle and expensive to maintain; full-grown pigs eat quite a lot. And although pigs may produce sexually mature progeny more rapidly than do some primates, the time between conception and sexual maturity for pigs is still fairly long (approximately 1 year) compared with many other animals.[22]

RATS.   Perhaps the best alternative is the rat. The rat's diet is diverse and very similar to that of humans, which accounts for its ability to flourish so widely through centuries of human civilization. Although they cannot vomit, rats' individual and social behaviors with regard to avoiding poisons and identifying beneficial foods are in many ways similar to those of humans (see Chapters 6 and 14). Further, laboratory rats, bred for docility, are easy to handle.[23] They are inexpensive to buy and maintain. For the rat, the time between birth and sexual maturity is only about 2 months.[24] Because of these advantages, rats have become by far the most popular non-human animal for research on the psychology of eating and drinking, and for a great deal of other psychological research as well. This means that there is an extensive data base on all aspects of rat behavior and physiology, which allows results from new experiments to fit into a preexisting, extensive research framework.[25]

CONCLUSION

When financial, ethical, or methodological concerns make experiments with humans inadvisable, psychologists can do experiments with nonhumans. Even if the goal is to understand human eating and drinking behavior, experimental research with nonhuman animals can provide valuable insights. Rats are the animals most often used for these investigations because of the similarities between the ways that they and humans eat and because they are easy to work with. Experiments with rats play a large part in the next chapter, "Hunger."

Part I

THE AMOUNT CONSUMED

The two chapters that follow, "Hunger" and "Thirst," are concerned with how much organisms consume. Specifically, the chapter on hunger concerns the consumption of solid and liquid foods containing a variety of nutrients, and the chapter on thirst deals with the consumption of water. The central features of these chapters, making up Part I, are the factors that initiate and terminate eating and drinking. How organisms come to choose particular foods and drinks is the focus of Part II.

CHAPTER
2
❧

Hunger

The typical American eats not only breakfast, lunch, and dinner, but many snacks as well. The midnight raid on the refrigerator and the midmorning coffee break are virtual customs. It appears that at least some of us are eating almost all of the time. Despite the frequency of their contacts with food during the day, however, people eat not continually, but in *bouts*. Periods of continuous contact with food alternate with periods of minimal or no contact with food. Meals and snacks are eating bouts. Many species consume food in this way.

When a person begins an eating bout, we usually describe him or her as hungry. Without further elaboration, this statement means little. Someone is hungry if he or she eats; someone eats if he or she is hungry. Such a circular definition does not advance our understanding of the phenomena involved, and it provides us with little ability to predict future eating bouts. The concept of hunger is useful to psychologists when it allows them to group together many similar instances of behavior, all behaviors that involve initiating or terminating eating bouts. By examining and grouping together many different cases of initiation and termination of eating, psychologists can construct general rules for describing these cases as well as predicting new ones. They can also try to determine the mechanisms on which the rules are based.

Consider the following hypothetical example. A psychologist observes that adult humans almost always eat within 30 minutes following the setting of the sun. The psychologist could then generalize that people are hungry for 30 minutes after sunset. This principle not only describes what the psychologist has observed but allows him or her to predict that any human adult will have a high probability of consuming food for the 30 minutes following sunset. In addition, the psychologist can then begin to find out why there is this relationship between hunger and the disappearance of the sun. Is it due to changes in light levels, air temperature, or simply the number of hours since the sun first rose?

Understanding hunger means constructing principles that enable us to predict when an organism will start eating and when it will stop, including in new situations. The essential concern with regard to hunger is how much an organism eats, that is, how it regulates the amount of food that it ingests.

Organisms must regulate their food intake on both a short- and a long-term basis, and this complicates our understanding of hunger. Animals, including humans, need to regulate food intake, not only according to their daily needs but also according to their long-term average body weight. For humans, an addition to body fat that is equivalent to the calories in just one extra pat of butter or margarine a day results in a weight gain of 5 pounds per year. It is striking that most of us maintain our weights as well as we do, for this suggests an exquisitely sensitive system for long-term regulation of weight. To understand hunger, it is crucial to have an awareness of the distinction between short-term and long-term energy regulation, because different mechanisms may be responsible for each.

HOMEOSTASIS

When psychologists speak about organisms regulating their food intake according to short- and long-term energy needs, they are speaking about *homeostasis*—the maintenance of a constant, optimal, internal environment. This concept developed from Claude Bernard's ideas about the *milieu intérieur*.[1] Bernard, a French physiologist of the nineteenth century, stressed the necessity of an organism's keeping its internal environment at a constant, optimal level if it is to thrive. "It is the fixity of the 'milieu intérieur' which is the condition of free and independent life. . . . [A]ll the vital mechanisms, however varied they may be, have only one object, that of preserving constant the conditions of life in the internal environment."[2] The actual term *homeostasis* was coined by Walter B. Cannon, an American physiologist, in 1929.[3]

Homeostasis can be seen at work outside as well as inside our bodies. An example that will help illustrate the concept of homeostasis is the thermostat. After a household thermostat is set at a certain temperature, it reacts to deviations from that temperature (the *set point*) by changing the environment in ways that decrease or eliminate those deviations. If the temperature is too high, air conditioning may be turned on or heat turned off. If the temperature is too low, heat may be turned on or air conditioning turned off. This process by which deviations from a set point result in actions designed to reinstate the set point is called *negative feedback*. Deviations from a set point induce reactions that decrease those deviations. As the deviations diminish, so do the reactions to them, until a stable state is reached and maintained.

Most theories of hunger are based on the concept of homeostasis through negative feedback. The theme of homeostasis recurs frequently in the discussions that follow.

PERIPHERAL CUES

Peripheral cues of hunger and satiety are cues involving parts of the body's physiology other than the *central nervous system* (the *CNS*, the brain and the spinal cord). Especially in the early years of scientific psychology, when not much was known about the CNS, scientists turned to peripheral factors as explanations of hunger.

Stomach Contractions

To most people, a contracting, growling stomach is synonymous with hunger. When our stomachs growl we have positive proof that we are hungry. The reverse is also often true; if our stomachs do not feel empty and rumbling, we are likely to say that we are not hungry. Perhaps initiation and termination of eating can be predicted on the basis of stomach contractions: Someone whose stomach has been contracting might be more likely to eat, and vice versa.

Cannon, in addition to coining the term homeostasis, is also known for his investigations of the stomach contraction theory of hunger. In fact, his 1912 work on this problem with A. L. Washburn was one of the first experimental studies of hunger.[4]

To perform this study it was necessary to measure stomach contractions and reports of hunger simultaneously. Cannon and Washburn had to develop a technique for measuring stomach contractions. The strategy they settled on is shown in Figure 2.1. The subjects first had to become accustomed to having a small tube inserted down the esophagus into the stomach and left there for several hours each day. The experiment involved partially inflating a balloon inside the stomach with air passed through the tube. A manometer, which translates changes in air pressure into a graphic record, was connected to the tube to measure any stomach contractions. The subject pressed a key whenever he or she experienced sensations of hunger.

The first subject to undergo this procedure was Washburn, and the findings appeared to be clear-cut. Stomach contractions, as measured by the manometer, were closely associated with Washburn's own reports of

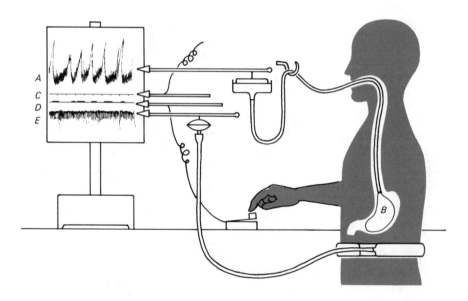

FIGURE 2.1   *Cannon and Washburn's method for measuring stomach contractions. A* records the increases and decreases in the volume of the stomach balloon, *B*. Time in minutes is shown by *C*. The subject's own reports of hunger are shown in *D*. *E* records the movements of the abdominal wall, to demonstrate that these movements are not responsible for the changes in stomach volume, *A*, or the subject's reports of hunger, *D*. (Adapted from W. B. Cannon, "Hunger and Thirst," in *The Foundations of Experimental Psychology*, ed. C. Murchison, Worcester, MA: Clark University Press, 1929.)

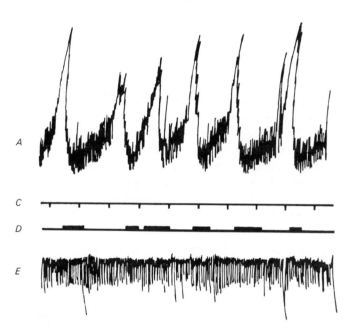

FIGURE 2.2   *Results from one of Cannon and Washburn's experiments (see Figure 2.1 for explanation of symbols).* (Adapted from W. B. Cannon, "Hunger and Thirst," in *The Foundations of Experimental Psychology,* ed. C. Murchison, Worcester, MA: Clark University Press, 1929.)

hunger. Apparently Washburn would report hunger at the height of a contraction, not at the beginning, which suggests that the stomach contractions caused the feelings of hunger and not the other way around. Figure 2.2 diagrams these results. When Washburn was not hungry there were no contractions. Follow-up studies with additional subjects obtained similar results.[5] The stomach contraction theory was the first peripheral theory of hunger to receive experimental support, and it was the dominant peripheral theory for many years.

However, criticisms of Cannon's peripheral theory of hunger have pointed to the fact that neither stomach contractions nor even a stomach are necessary prerequisites for reports of hunger.[6] In fact, more recent research than Cannon's, employing improved methods such as a catheter rather than a balloon to measure stomach contractions, has found the relationship between hunger and stomach contractions to be extremely weak.[7] The stomach contraction theory of hunger now appears to be of little more than historical interest.

Stomach Distention and Oral Stimulation

⌈When food is consumed, there is stimulation of the entire gastrointestinal tract, from the mouth down to the large intestine. Two specific aspects of this stimulation—the pleasantness of the taste of the food and the distention of the stomach—have received particular attention with regard to the initiation and termination of hunger. People often say that the taste of food becomes less and less appealing during the course of its consumption. Perhaps continued oral stimulation helps to terminate feeding. Researchers have found both that food is initially eaten at a higher rate when the food has a pleasant taste and that the rate of food consumption decreases during a meal.[8] ⌉

Similarly, people describe themselves as feeling "empty" prior to a meal and "full" after a meal.[9] Many dieters load themselves with glasses of water or large amounts of fibrous, noncaloric foods such as carrots and lettuce. This decreases the amount of heavily caloric food they feel they can consume. Perhaps stomach distention is a precursor to the cessation of eating; in fact, stomach distention might be the actual cause that terminates an eating bout.

To study oral stimulation and stomach distention experimentally, scientists needed a way to control whether or not their subjects' stomachs were distended (see Table 2.1). One common method is called an *esophagostomy*. This involves first bringing the subject's esophagus out through the neck. The esophagus is then cut, forming an upper and a lower piece. If an animal that has had this operation eats, the food consumed passes out through the animal's neck instead of continuing to its stomach. This is known as *sham feeding*. An animal that is sham fed experiences all the usual oral stimuli that accompany feeding but none of the stimuli that originate in the stomach. The subject tastes, chews, and swallows the food, but the stomach never receives it.

It is also possible to bypass the mouth and feed the subject by injecting semisolid or liquid food into the lower cut portion of the esophagus. This is called *intragastric feeding*. It results in the subject's experiencing the gastric (stomach) stimuli of feeding but not the oral stimuli. Variations on this method include using a *gastric fistula* (a hole by which substances can be inserted in the stomach) instead of an esophagostomy and inserting food or inert substances such as gum arabic or an inflated balloon into the stomach. Used singly and in combination, these procedures permit oral and gastrointestinal factors to be studied separately in experiments.

Among the first experiments done using these techniques were a series of studies reported by Henry D. Janowitz and M. I. Grossman in 1949.[10] These

TABLE 2.1

Anatomical Methods for Investigating the Separate Contributions of Oral and Gastrointestinal Factors in the Control of Eating

| Procedure | Delivery of Stimuli | PRESENCE OF STIMULI | | Results |
		Oral	Gastro-intestinal	
Esophagostomy with sham feeding	Food ingested through mouth passes out through the neck	Yes	No	More food consumed than usual; oral factors by themselves do not precisely regulate food intake
Esophagostomy with intragastric feeding	Liquid or semisolid food ingested by way of the lower cut portion of the esophagus passes into the stomach	No	Yes	By itself, gastric distention has little effect on feeding
Gastric fistula	Food or inert substances placed in stomach	No	Yes	Gastric distention caused by food is rewarding and terminates eating

researchers showed, first, that sham fed dogs eventually stop eating but before they stop they consume much more food than usual. In addition, sham feeding 1 hour or more before a subsequent sham feeding does not affect the amount of food consumed in the later sham feeding. In other words, oral factors can contribute to the cessation of eating, but by themselves oral factors do not precisely regulate food intake. The studies bore this out particularly well when they were continued for long periods of time.

Janowitz and Grossman also gave their dogs intragastric feedings. These feedings only decreased sham feeding when they were large and given at the same time as the sham feeding. When a balloon was used instead of food, there was no effect on sham feeding until the balloon was inflated so much as to cause nausea and retching. Janowitz and Grossman therefore concluded that stomach distention has very little to do with terminating a bout of eating.

However, a few sessions under experimental conditions may not fully test an organism's ability to regulate food intake; animals learn to regulate their food intake over a long period of time. Subsequent studies[11] discovered that dogs with gastric fistulas or esophagostomies would adjust their oral intake in accord with gastric feedings if they were exposed to the procedure for several months. Yet research continued to find that placing an inflated balloon in the stomach had little effect on oral feedings.

In 1952 Neal E. Miller and Marion L. Kessen studied rats with gastric fistulas and found that they could learn to go to one arm of a T maze for stomach injections of milk.[12] In 1983 J. A. Deutsch reported on a number of experiments in which rats were fed milk. The nutrients in the milk, but not stomach distention by itself (unless the distention was extreme), played a role in the cessation of eating.[13] Findings such as these clarified the conclusions from Janowitz and Grossman's studies: Gastric distention by itself is not very influential in terminating eating except when the distention is extreme. Gastric distention caused by food, however, is rewarding and effective in terminating eating. This is true even when oral factors have been eliminated, if the animal is allowed some time to adjust to the procedure. Oral factors are also important in terminating eating, but they have less effect in isolation than they do when accompanied by stomach distention.

Another way to look at the separate effects of oral and postingestive stimuli on feeding is to give subjects four different types of foods: each possible combination of low and high calories and of low and high sweetness (Figure 2.3a). An example of a food of type A, a food that is both sweet and high in calories, would be a muffin made with lots of sugar and butter. An example of a food of type B, a food that is sweet but low in calories, would be a muffin made with an artificial sweetener and very little butter. A food of type C, high in calories but not sweet, could be a muffin made with a relatively high percentage of butter but no sugar or artificial sweetener. Finally, a food of type D, low in calories and not sweet, could be a muffin made without much sugar, artificial sweetener, or butter. Subjects could be fed each of these four types of foods as a regular meal or as a preload prior to a regular meal on 4 separate days. Amount of the regular meal consumed on each of the 4 days could then be compared. If the oral factor of sweetness alone affects amount of food consumed, then intake of the regular meal would be relatively low only with foods A and B; if the gastrointestinal factor of calories alone affects amount of food consumed, then intake of the regular meal would be relatively low only with foods A and C; if amount of food consumed is decreased only when calories and a sweet taste are present, then lower food intake would be found with food A; and so on.

Experiments using these types of designs have found that decreasing the caloric content of a food does not result in a subject's eating a greater volume of food. Therefore total ingested calories decrease.[14] Subjects do, however, consume more sweet than nonsweet foods, whether the sweet

CALORIES

	High or present	Low or absent
Present	A	B
Absent	C	D

SWEETNESS

(a)

CALORIES

	High or present	Low or absent
Present	Increased consumption	Increased consumption
Absent	No effect	No effect

SWEETNESS

(b)

FIGURE 2.3   *The separate contributions of sweetness and calories to the control of eating.*
(a) Experimental design. (b) Results. ([a] Adapted from J. E. Blundell, P. J. Rogers, and
A. J. Hill, "Uncoupling Sweetness and Calories: Methodological Aspects of
Laboratory Studies on Appetite Control," *Appetite* 11 Supplement [1988]: 54–61.)

taste results from a caloric or a noncaloric sweetener (Figure 2.3b). This latter result may occur because the consumption of sweet food causes increased release of insulin (and a consequent lowering of blood sugar)
and/or because it causes increased storage of (and a consequent decrease in
easy availability of) metabolic fuel.[15]

Through this series of experiments, and the experiments on stomach contractions already described, a picture of how the body regulates its food intake begins to emerge. There is no single, perfect mechanism; a regulatory
system malfunctions more readily if it has only one way of collecting and
using information. Instead, the body uses several ways of determining how
much has been eaten and how much should be eaten. All of this information, including oral factors and stomach distention, plays a part in initiating
and terminating eating. Another important factor in this process is environmental temperature.

Chapter 2

Temperature Regulation

An easy way to quell appetites at a summer dinner party is to turn off the air conditioning. Likewise, the reaction of many people to a cold house is to eat an extra large meal or some highly caloric food such as chocolate cake. Most people probably are aware that on the average they eat more when their environment is colder than when it is warmer.

One explanation for this influence of environmental temperature on the amount eaten is that in cold weather the body needs more fuel to keep itself heated to 98.6°F. Such a mechanism has been proposed as a peripheral theory of hunger.

Because a major source of heat for any organism is the food it consumes, perhaps initiation and termination of feeding are related to the maintenance of a specific, optimally efficient body temperature by means of a homeostatic mechanism. Thus a lower environmental temperature would require a person to eat more, and a higher environmental temperature would require a person to eat less. This theory was proposed by John R. Brobeck in the late 1940s.[16] He supported his hypothesis by doing some experiments with rats in which he showed that rats ate more when they were in a 65°F environment than when they were in a 97°F environment.

Many observations have now shown that several different species, including human beings, consume more in cold environments. A number of different mechanisms have been proposed to explain why this is so. Recent experiments have shown that exposure to the cold speeds the movement of food from the stomach into the intestine. Such a process, of course, would decrease the gastric stimulation, such as stomach distention, that normally inhibits feeding.

If environmental temperature affects the rate of stomach clearance, meal patterns, as well as total amount consumed, should be affected. As environmental temperature decreases and rate of stomach clearance increases, the signals for meal termination should dissipate more quickly, and therefore meals should be initiated more frequently. Consistent with this hypothesis, rats exposed to the cold eat more, not by increasing meal size but by increasing meal frequency. There appears, however, to be some additional effect of the cold on feeding that is independent of stomach clearance. Rats will work harder for food in the cold and will consume more unpalatable food than they would ordinarily.[17] Such studies are beginning to identify what appear to be many complex effects of environmental temperature on feeding.

Energy Commitment

Theories of hunger based on energy commitment propose that an organism eats when it has committed (used up) some energy and stops eating when it has gained back that energy. Body fat, the body's means of storing energy, may be included in these models. In all energy commitment models an organism adjusts its energy intake according to its energy needs, an efficient homeostatic method of food intake regulation.

Theories such as this one assume that the body has some sort of signal or signals that tell it just how much energy it has available at any moment. It is generally agreed that this signal must be carried in the blood, because of results from research involving *parabiotic rats,* pairs of rats that have been surgically joined side to side so that blood circulates between the two animals where the incision heals together. In general, the members of a pair eat and grow normally. Their appearance is simply that of two normal rats, joined together at the side.

Researchers have taken advantage of this unusual preparation to study the regulation of feeding. One series of experiments reported by David G. Fleming in 1969 involved feeding the members of a parabiotic pair separately to determine what effects feeding one member could have on the feeding of the other.[18] Fleming would feed one member of a pair and then, after a delay, feed the other. He varied the feeding times for each member as well as the delay between their feeding times. Fleming was able to show that something was being passed from the blood of one member of the parabiotic pair to the other. When one member of a pair was fed for 3 hours, beginning 2 hours before the start of the other member's 3-hour-long feeding, over a period of weeks the second rat came to eat significantly less than the first. Clearly some information about what was being consumed was being passed between the parabiotic pairs of rats.

One theory, the *glucostatic theory of hunger,* postulates that the information is passed through the level of sugar in the blood. Jean Mayer, the internationally known physiologist and nutritionist, proposed this theory in 1952.[19] Mayer concluded that circulating sugar levels act as a signal to the brain, indicating the amount of immediately available or needed energy. Blood sugar increases quickly following feeding and slowly decreases with time until the next feeding. Blood sugar is also known to be the primary energy source for the CNS.

The glucostatic theory, however, is not a sufficient explanation for at least some special cases of food regulation. Mayer was aware that diabetics may still crave sweets even when their blood sugar level is very high due to inadequate insulin production. Mayer got around this problem by specifying that the glucostatic theory referred to the body's effective blood sugar, as measured by the difference between the blood sugar concentration in the arteries and the veins, known as the *arteriovenous difference*, or *A-V difference.* If that difference is high, it indicates that sugar is being removed from the blood as it passes from the arteries, through other tissues, and then into the veins (Figure 2.4). The body is therefore receiving a fair amount of sugar. If that difference is low, then the body is not receiving much sugar. For example, this may happen when there is very little blood sugar in the arterial blood supply or when the body does not produce enough insulin to metabolize the blood sugar (as in uncontrolled diabetes). To support this theory

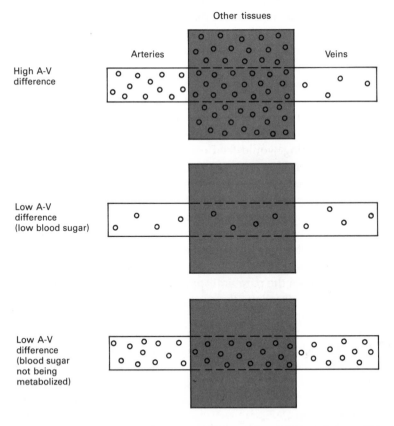

FIGURE 2.4   *Diagram depicting the origins of high and low A-V (arteriovenous) blood sugar differences.* The number of dots per unit area represents the concentration of sugar. Only with high A-V differences is a large amount of sugar being removed from the blood as it passes from the arteries to the veins.

Mayer performed some experiments in which he measured the A-V glucose difference in humans. He found that this difference correlated well with the subjects' own reports of hunger, both in normal subjects and in subjects with diabetes mellitus.[20]

Mayer realized that his glucostatic mechanism would make errors on a daily basis and that some long-term mechanism would be needed to correct them. A mechanism related to the fat stores in the body was the obvious choice. Excess energy is stored as fat. One pound of fat is equivalent to 3500 *calories* (the common term calories will be used in this book, although the correct technical term is *kilocalories*). In order to take advantage of this storage system, the body must have a way of detecting the extent of its energy store. *Lipostatic theories* propose that a circulating metabolite of the body's stored fat is responsible for long-term regulation of stored fat. Mayer was among the the first to propose a lipostatic theory of long-term regulation.[21]

The specific metabolites of stored fat are known as *free fatty acids.* When circulating levels of free fatty acids are high, as a result of the breaking down of stored fat, the organism increases its food consumption. When they are low, indicating that fat is being stored rather than utilized, the organism consumes less. The fat stores are thus implicated as determinants of the organism's *set point*, the weight at which the organism stabilizes.[22] In this way the glucostatic and lipostatic mechanisms could work together to regulate the body's food intake on both a daily and a long-term basis.

Nevertheless, extensive evidence supporting the A-V glucose difference as a primary determinant of hunger has not been forthcoming.[23] In addition, recent experimental results have necessitated the proposal of various alternatives to both Mayer's glucostatic theory and his lipostatic theory. For example, because blood glucose level is sometimes too variable to predict feeding behavior reliably, *glycogen* level (a form in which carbohydrate is stored in cells, particularly in the liver and muscles[24]) has been proposed as an alternative to blood glucose level in the glucostatic theory. Because amount of glycogen in the body reflects changes in levels of both glucose and fat, this theory can be viewed as integrating the glucostatic and lipostatic mechanisms.[25] Some of the other areas of recent investigation that call into question Mayer's glucostatic and lipostatic theories involve: the study of cells particularly sensitive to the presence of glucose (i.e., *glucoreceptors*) in the liver, cells that appear to be involved in satiety; the study of the oxidation of fat that occurs during metabolism, another factor involved in satiety; and the study of short-term decreases in blood glucose and their role in initiating food seeking and food consumption.[26] Mayer's original glucostatic and lipostatic theories have spawned a huge and complex literature on the role of glucose and fat in meal initiation and termination. A theory involving a single, simple mechanism is inadequate to describe the roles of blood sugar and body fat in the consumption of food.

Gut Peptides

The effects of certain *gut peptides* involved in the metabolism of nutrients have also been strongly implicated as factors in satiety. Relatively high circulating levels of these peptides, such as the pancreatic peptide *glucagon* or the small intestine peptide *cholecystokinin* (CCK), decrease the amount of food that an animal takes in a meal.[27] Apparently, when these peptides are released during digestion they may help to terminate feeding. The case is particularly strong for cholecystokinin.

In one recent experiment, rat pups were first administered a chemical that causes the release of CCK from the small intestine. These experimental rats subsequently ate less than untreated rats. However, if the experimental rats were initially given another chemical that blocks the detection of CCK by receptor cells, there was no decrease in food consumption. Together, these results suggest that CCK plays a role in rat pups' satiety, and that this effect is dependent on CCK receptor cells.[28]

Other Peripheral Factors

Stomach contractions, oral stimulation, stomach distention, temperature regulation, glucostatic, lipostatic, and gut hormone mechanisms have been the major peripheral factors postulated as determinants of hunger, some with more success than others. However, many parts of the body are involved in the ingestion and metabolism of food, and just about all of them have been proposed at one time or another as factors important in the regulation, and not just the process, of feeding. Blood amino acid levels and the food–water ratio in the stomach and small intestine also have a peripheral influence on initiating and terminating eating, according to some studies. The many peripheral theories of hunger reflect the complexity of the feeding system.[29]

CNS INTEGRATING MECHANISMS

Studies of CNS integrating mechanisms have sought to determine whether or not there are particular locations in the brain that control hunger and satiety, the initiation and termination of eating. Such brain regions could collect information about the organism's energy state using sensory pathways and, based on that information, could initiate or terminate eating through motor nerve pathways. The existence of such brain locations would greatly simplify explanations of what controls eating behavior.

Satiety

The search for a particular part of the brain that controls satiety began in earnest around 1940, when A. W. Hetherington and S. W. Ranson published the first detailed physiological study of the brain and the control of feeding.[30] Previous studies had suggested that the hypothalamus (Figure 2.5a) was a likely place to look. For example, in 1901 a now famous case of obesity was reported in an adolescent boy with a large tumor of the pituitary gland (Box 2.1). Functionally and anatomically the pituitary is closely related to the hypothalamus (Figure 2.5b), and it therefore seemed possible that the hypothalamus was involved in eating behavior.

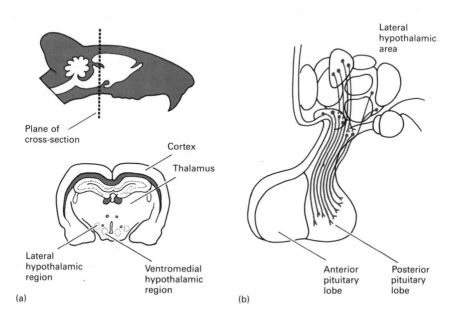

FIGURE 2.5   (a) Rat brain showing location of hypothalamus. (b) Anatomical relationship of the hypothalamus with the pituitary gland; major neural pathways are shown.
([a] Adapted from H. Gleitman, *Psychology*, New York: W. W. Norton, 1981. [b] Adapted from E. L. House and B. Pansky, *Neuroanatomy*, New York: McGraw-Hill,

---

BOX 2.1

Description of a Boy with Frölich's Syndrome

R. D., a boy, was born in 1887. . . . Since March 1899 the patient, who previously had been slim, had been rapidly gaining weight. In January 1901 he complained about diminishing eyesight on the left. . . . Later, vision in the right eye also began to fail. . . . Since the patient suffered from severe headaches and his eyesight was rapidly decreasing, an operative procedure appeared justified. The operation by the nasal route was performed by von Eiselsberg on June 21 [1907]. In the depth of the sphenoid sinus the whitish membrane of a cyst the size of a hazelnut was encountered. After incision in the midline, several spoonfuls of a fluid resembling old blood drained out. By measuring with the finger and comparison with the roentgenogram, it could be ascertained that the cyst which contined this fluid corresponded to the hypophysis [pituitary gland, connected to and near the hypothalamus]. The walls of the cavity were cut away as far as could be done without damaging the optic chiasm and the carotid arteries. . . . The postoperative course was favorable. . . . There was considerable improvement in the general condition.

From H. Bruch, "The Frölich Syndrome: Report of the Original Case," American Journal of diseases of children *58(1939):1282, 1283, 1285.*

Hetherington and Ranson's experiments involved inserting small electrodes into the brains of anesthetized rats. When the electrode was in the proper place in a rat's brain, electrical current was passed through the electrode, thereby destroying the cells surrounding the electrode. Several such small lesions were made in each rat's brain. The rats subjected to this procedure usually recovered after the operation and appeared fairly normal. However, they ate excessively and became obese (*hyperphagia*). Despite the fact that the procedure caused larger lesions than intended, Hetherington and Ranson were able to point to the *ventromedial hypothalamus (VMH)* as the most likely place that, if lesioned, would result in obesity. Because the rats overate after their VMHs were destroyed, the researchers thought that the VMH was involved in the control of satiety.

A follow-up study published in 1942 provided further information about rats with VMH lesions.[31] First, their activity level is much lower than that of nonlesioned rats. Second, VMH-lesioned rats only eat enough to become obese if the available food is palatable; if the food is not palatable, they eat neither more nor less than control rats. For this reason VMH-lesioned rats have been called finicky. Third, VMH-lesioned rats are less willing to work for food. Fourth, the overeating that leads to weight gain, the *dynamic phase,* is only temporary; later the rat stabilizes its intake and weight, the *static phase.*[32] Fifth, experiments showed that stimulation of the VMH (activating the cells with an electrical current, rather than destroying them with lesions) inhibits eating.[33]

Further, brain injections of toxic glucose analogs caused rats to behave like VMH-lesioned rats. *Glucose analogs* are absorbed by cells that use glucose, and toxic glucose analogs destroy the cells that absorb them. The injection experiments suggested that some cells in the VMH are particularly sensitive to glucose and that destruction of these glucoreceptors results in the VMH syndrome. Through the glucoreceptors the VMH might receive information about blood sugar levels.[34] The VMH results therefore seemed to fit within the glucostatic peripheral theory of hunger and suggested a central integrating mechanism.

Hunger

Scientists reasoned that if there were a location in the VMH that controls satiety, a location involved in the inhibition of feeding, there might also be a location in the hypothalamus that is involved in the excitation of feeding, that is, hunger. Bal K. Anand and John R. Brobeck's 1951 report[35] identified such a location as the *lateral hypothalamus (LH).* Their study seemed to show that destruction of this specific area of the hypothalamus resulted in rats that never would eat again, rats that eventually would die of starvation.

Death by starvation is not a necessary consequence of an LH lesion, however. LH-lesioned rats at first refuse to eat any food or drink any water (*aphagia* and *adipsia*). But if the rats are carefully handled, after several weeks they will eat wet palatable foods, then dry foods, and finally drink water. Apparently the tissue surrounding the lesion aids in this recovery. If recovered LH-lesioned rats are lesioned again in the areas surrounding the original LH lesion, the aphagia and adipsia return.[36]

Rats with LH damage also show sensorimotor and arousal deficits. For example, they have difficulty coordinating their limbs when climbing in the cage. But as with appropriate eating and drinking behavior, they eventually recover their cage-climbing ability.[37]

TABLE 2.2
Summary of Findings with Hypothalamus in the Mid-1950s

Area of Hypothalamus	Lesion	Stimulation
Ventromedial hypothalmus	Increases eating	Decreases eating
Lateral hypothalamus	Decreases eating	Increases eating

The Hunger and Satiety Centers Hypothesis

All of these results, plus the finding that stimulation of the LH induced rats to eat,[38] seemed to form a tidy package for those wishing to understand the initiation and termination of eating (see Table 2.2 for a summary of these data). In 1954 Eliot Stellar formally proposed that the VMH is the brain's satiety center and the LH its hunger center.[39] According to Stellar, these centers, essentially small brains within the larger brain, gather information through glucoreceptors and other sensory receptors in the hypothalamus, synthesize this information, and then may effect some action. Stellar saw brain centers as major locations in the brain that integrate information. However, he stated specifically that areas of the brain other than the hypothalamus are probably involved in the initiation and termination of feeding.

Peripheral theories by themselves had been inadequate to explain completely the initiation and termination of feeding. Stellar's concept of brain centers did not eliminate the peripheral theories but integrated them with central theories of hunger. Stellar saw the peripheral theories as describing the kinds of information that are synthesized in the hypothalamus: temperature, blood sugar level, and other peripheral stimuli. The brain centers theory dominated motivational theory of the initiation and termination of feeding for many years.

Problems with the Hunger and Satiety Centers Hypothesis

In the 35 years since Stellar proposed the hunger and satiety centers hypothesis, a number of research findings have pointed to problems with this hypothesis.

RESULTS NOT PREDICTED BY THE THEORY.   First, the VMH syndrome does not always develop as the theory says it should. For example, recent evidence has shown that if a VMH-lesioned rat in the static phase is forced to eat small meals, it will continue to overeat and get fatter instead of stabilizing its weight. As another example, even if a VMH-lesioned rat in the dynamic phase is prevented from overeating, it will still become fat. The theory also does not predict the finickiness of the rats after destruction of the satiety center. Finally, various sorts of peripheral manipulations (for example, manipulations involving stomach distention or injections of nutrients) affect hunger in VMH-lesioned rats just as they do in nonlesioned rats. These and other results are difficult to reconcile with the hypothesis that destruction of the VMH is simply the destruction of a satiety center.[40]

Further, recent research has identified the *neurotransmitters* responsible for the initiation and termination of feeding. Neurotransmitters are the chemical substances released in the small gaps (the *synapses*) between two adjoining neurons, and these substances are responsible for the occurrence of the electrical impulses by which neurons communicate. Neurotransmitters that stimulate feeding include *catecholamines* such as *norepinephrine*. Neurotransmitters that inhibit feeding include *dopamine* and *serotonin*.[41] The hunger and satiety centers hypothesis is silent about these sorts of underlying mechanisms. (See Chapter 8 for further discussion of the relationships between food intake and neurotransmitters.)

BEHAVIORAL SPECIFICITY.   Another difficulty for Stellar's theory sprang from a problem with the methodology of many of the experiments on which the theory was based. More specifically, experimental manipulations of the brain may result in unspecified, general changes in behavior. For example, suppose a psychologist makes a lesion in a particular part of the brain of an experimental animal. After the operation the animal can no longer perform a certain task. A control animal, which has undergone a sham operation in which anesthesia is administered but no surgery performed, shows no such impairment. The psychologist then concludes that the part of the brain that was destroyed is essential to the performance of the given task. Alternatively, some part of an experimental animal's brain is stimulated; whatever the animal subsequently does, the psychologist then concludes that the particular part of the brain that was stimulated has resulted in the performance of that behavior. Physiological psychologists have used these types of strategies for many years to map the brain and determine which areas are responsible for which functions.

It is very difficult, however, to be precisely certain about what particular behavior has been affected by lesions or stimulation. Every action consists of many component actions. The seemingly simple act of picking up a ball in response to a command involves hearing and understanding the instructions given by the experimenter, seeing the ball, bending the knees, maintaining balance, reaching for the ball, maintaining eye–hand coordination, clasping the ball, standing up, and, in addition, finding this act in some way rewarding. A physiological intervention that affected ball retrieval might affect one or more of these components. Psychologists are now aware that interfering with what seems to be a very small part of the brain can have profound effects on general arousal or on complex sensory functions.[42]

These criticisms can be applied to the brain centers theory of hunger. Hyperphagia following lesions of the VMH, or eating following stimulation of the LH, may occur because of a metabolic disorder, a hormonal disorder, or a change in the subject's sensitivity to the environment. Similarly, changes in the brain activity of an animal that follow exposing the animal to food may result from a change in the subject's sensitivity to the environment, rather than from the exposure to food.

SPECIFICITY OF THE MANIPULATION.   The specific locations of lesions, of stimulation, and of the measured electrical activity in the brain have also been criticized in studies of the brain centers theory. Physiological psychologists have sometimes assumed incorrectly that only the brain cells originating at the location of the electrode have been destroyed, stimulated, or measured. In fact, such manipulations may affect not the actual cell body of a neuron but rather a neuronal fiber whose origin may be many millimeters distant. Therefore neuronal pathways, and not neuronal centers, could regulate initiation and termination of eating.

These points can be illustrated using examples based on both the VMH satiety center and the LH hunger center. Lesions of the VMH are not the only lesions that can induce hyperphagia. Lesions in other nearby locations can also cause all of the symptoms of the VMH syndrome. In fact, it appears that lesions strictly confined to the VMH are less effective at inducing the VMH syndrome than lesions not strictly confined to the VMH. Lesions of the *paraventricular nucleus*, which is located just ahead of the ventromedial nucleus in the hypothalamus, may be more effective in eliminating satiety than are lesions of the VMH.[43] Previous demonstrations of the VMH syndrome using VMH lesions may have been due to unsophisticated techniques that destroyed a greater proportion of the brain than was intended. In addition, there are many ascending and descending neuronal pathways (connecting neural fibers) that are interrupted by these lesions. Although interrupting only these pathways is not enough to induce all of the symptoms of the VMH syndrome, interruption of these pathways is clearly important in inducing that syndrome.

The LH syndrome appears to be based on two mechanisms. The decrease in eating and drinking following LH lesions can be caused solely by destruction of cell bodies in the LH.[44] However, the sensory and arousal deficits that are also part of the LH syndrome are apparently caused by the destruction of certain (dopaminergic) neuronal fibers passing through the LH region. The stages of recovery following LH lesions, already described, seem due to subjects' becoming increasingly reactive to low levels of stimulation as they recover from damage to the dopaminergic fibers that pass through the LH.[45] Damage to these fibers alone interferes with eating and drinking behavior because of the resulting sensory and arousal deficits.[46]

CONCLUSION. Not all of the results obtained in the past 35 years have been critical of Stellar's theory. For example, one experiment[47] showed that if specific sites in the rat's hypothalamus were given localized injections of a chemical substance that inhibits neuronal activity, either spontaneous feeding or no feeding would result. In accordance with Stellar's theory, the injection sites that increased feeding were in the VMH, while those that decreased feeding were in the LH. Next, a nutrient substance was infused into the *duodenum*, the part of the small intestine connected to the stomach. In response, the LH sites (Stellar's hunger center) showed suppressed activity, while the VMH sites (Stellar's satiety center) showed increased activity, probably by means of activity in the *vagus nerve*, which projects between the intestine and the part of the brain containing the hypothalamus. This experiment showed not only that the LH and VMH do vary in activity according to hunger and satiety (just as Stellar's theory would predict) but also that information on the amount of food consumed could be passed quickly from a rat's stomach to the LH and VMH.

Nevertheless a great deal of evidence now shows that neither the VMH nor the LH syndromes are expressed only by neurons originating in these locations.[48] A host of interconnecting neuronal pathways is responsible for these syndromes. The hypothalamus is one of the major integrators of external sensory stimuli, internal sensory stimuli, and activity from higher and lower brain structures.[49] However, the little brains within a brain that would have so neatly explained the initiation and termination of eating do not exist.

The Cephalic Phase Hypothesis

During investigations of the effects of the hypothalamus on feeding, it became apparent that lesions of the VMH affect certain metabolic functions of the body, which in turn affect feeding behavior.[50] These findings resulted in the formulation of the *cephalic phase hypothesis* (CPH). This hypothesis is based on the *cephalic phase reflexes*, stimulus–response sequences that are related to the ingestion and digestion of food and that occur immediately upon a subject's direct contact with food.[51] These reflexes include the secretion of insulin in response to food intake and the gag and vomiting reflexes. When Ivan Pavlov investigated the salivation reflex that dogs show in response to food, he was studying one of the cephalic phase reflexes.

The CPH begins with the assumption that VMH destruction results in an exaggeration of the cephalic reflex responses. The CPH further assumes that these heightened responses disrupt the energy balance of the organism. The VMH lesion increases insulin secretion and disrupts the *sympathetic* and *parasympathetic nervous system* balance responsible for storing and metabolizing fat, so that increased fat is stored.[52] The organism attempts to compensate for this decrease in food immediately available for energy needs by increasing its food intake.[53] This hypothesis appears to explain many of the behavioral changes following VMH lesions.

For example, the finickiness caused by VMH lesions can be explained by the CPH in the following way. In a normal animal the cephalic reflex responses, such as salivation, will be larger the more palatable the food. Suppose VMH lesions increase all cephalic phase reflexes by the same proportion. Then the responses to some foods would be very great cephalic phase reflexes, and the organism would eat a great deal of those foods, thus showing hyperphagia. However, the responses to other less palatable foods still might not reach the threshold for consumption. At the same time, the rejection reflexes (gagging and vomiting) to unpalatable foods would also be exaggerated. Thus, the organism would appear to have an increased preference for its favorite foods and an increased dislike for unpalatable foods (finickiness).[54]

If the CPH provides an accurate description of the origins of the VMH syndrome, then elimination of the cephalic phase reflexes in a VMH-lesioned rat should also eliminate the rat's hyperphagia. The cephalic phase reflexes can be removed by cutting or by pharmacologically blocking the vagus nerve. Several (although not all) experiments have confirmed that such manipulations decrease VMH-lesioned subjects' eating,[55] providing some support for the CPH and casting some doubt on the hypothesis of the VMH as a satiety center.

It should be emphasized that the CPH does not exclude the possibility that VMH lesions may affect responses other than cephalic ones.[56] Many different aspects of motivational behavior are affected by such lesions, including sexual behavior, circadian rhythms, and learning ability. In addition, predictions of the CPH have not always been confirmed. For example, quite problematic for the CPH is the fact that VMH-lesioned rats fed intragastrically gain weight just as do rats fed orally. This finding is contrary to the CPH because, without oral stimulation, there can be no excess cephalic phase reflexes, the mechanism by which the CPH postulates the weight gain in VMH-lesioned rats to occur.[57] The CPH is a working hypothesis designed to organize the data in a way that affords increased understanding of the VMH syndrome.

PHYSIOLOGICAL MODELS OF INGESTION

There is now a great deal of information concerning peripheral and central physiological mechanisms of hunger. In order to synthesize this information, one strategy adopted by some researchers has been to construct elaborate models of hunger that incorporate many of these mechanisms. For example, D. A. Booth, F. M. Toates, and S. V. Platt[58] have described a physiological model of feeding that attempts to deal with some of the multitude of physiological influences on hunger (Figure 2.6). This model includes many variables, such as gut clearance rate, the energy density of food, the

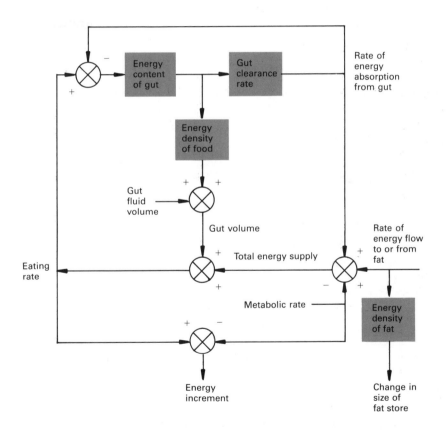

FIGURE 2.6   *Simplified diagram of Booth, Toates, and Platt's feeding model.* (Adapted from D. A. Booth, F. M. Toates, and S. V. Platt, "Control System for Hunger and Its Implications in Animals and Man," in *Hunger: Basic Mechanisms and Clinical Implications,* eds. D. Novin, W. Wyrwicka, and G. A. Bray, New York: Raven Press, 1976.)

energy density of stored fat, the energy content of the gut, and so on. With this model, knowledge of all variables except one makes it possible to determine what value the one remaining variable must have. Booth and his colleagues claim that this model successfully predicts "temporal patterns of feeding bouts, gut contents, actual or virtual inhibition or facilitation of feeding by energy supply, [and] change in total body energy."[59] All variables and all transformations from one part of the system to another (such as from the energy content of the gut to the rate of energy absorption from the gut) are measured physiologically. Note, however, that these are all peripheral measurements. At no time do Booth and his colleagues refer to central mechanisms of feeding. They assume that the sole function of central mechanisms is to integrate peripheral information. Booth and his colleagues do not cope with the tricky problem of exactly where in the body the integration is taking place; for these researchers, the integration takes place in their model.

Models are abstract representations of the available information. No model has an exclusive hold on the truth. For any given set of data, there are always at least two models that can predict those data. Very successful models tend to inspire confidence that a physiological representation of the model will be found, but such a representation may not exist.

NONPHYSIOLOGICAL MODELS

All the theories and models of hunger discussed so far involve only physiological mechanisms; the explanations they give about the initiation and termination of eating are based entirely on physiological factors. Criticisms of this general approach point out that it is impossible to describe any behavior completely by referring only to an organism's physiology.[60] Physiological studies have no meaning unless they address the environmental stimuli that cause the physiological reactions in the organism's body and the behavioral responses that the physiological reactions cause.

The Effects of Learning on Feeding

The effects of environmental stimuli on the initiation and termination of feeding are shown clearly by the many experiments demonstrating the effects of learning on subjects' tendency to eat. For example, repeated experiences in which sham feeding is associated with food of flavor A, but real feeding with food of flavor B, result in subjects' consuming more food of flavor A even if sham feeding is no longer occurring.[61] The subjects have learned that food of flavor A usually results in the ingestion of few calories, so they increase the size of meals with flavor A.

As another example, if rats have learned to associate flavor A with a caloric solution, and flavor B with a noncaloric solution, CCK will suppress their drinking of any solution containing flavor A, but not flavor B.[62] In other words, CCK induces satiety only when the rat expects to (though does not necessarily) consume calories.

As a final example, Leann Birch and her colleagues first repeatedly gave preschool children snacks in a specific location and in the presence of certain distinctive visual and auditory stimuli, but not in another location with other visual and auditory stimuli. Even when the children had been recently fed, they were more likely to eat in the presence of cues that had been associated with eating in the past than in the presence of cues that had not.[63]

Behavioral Homeostasis

In all of the preceding examples of the effects of learning on feeding, meal initiation and termination were no longer determined solely by the body's acting to return itself to an optimal physiological, internal state, that is, homeostasis. Consistent with these findings, Jerry A. Hogan[64] has argued that it is not reasonable to conceive of homeostasis as a system solely influenced by physiological factors. He has pointed out that the body's internal environment is always being affected by reactions within the body as well as by occurrences in the body's external environment. Animals deprived of food will not always eat, even when they have the opportunity to do so. For example, the food intake of a hen incubating eggs is 20 percent less than its usual intake. According to most definitions, hunger in incubating hens would have to be classified as nonhomeostatic.

The mechanisms involved in the maintenance of an optimal internal environment are very complex. In addition to negative feedback mechanisms, animals' behavior may be maintained by *positive feedback* mechanisms in which a deviation from a set point results in reactions that increase the deviation, as well as by mechanisms in which feedback does not function at all. Further, a system that always regulates itself according to the same set point cannot be the criterion for a homeostatic system; there are few, if any, systems that fall within this definition.[65]

The concept of homeostasis must be made very broad or abandoned. For Hogan, there are so many problems with the concept of homeostasis when applied to motivational processes that he would abandon this term altogether. He maintains that one can only specify the optimal internal state for an organism and the mechanisms that lead to that state given knowledge of the organism's particular situation.[66]

Chapter 2

The Psychodynamic Approach

Psychodynamic theorists adopted a combined physiological–environmental approach to hunger many years ago. For these theorists, hunger has a physiological base but is immediately affected by learning. From its early feeding experiences an organism learns how to regulate its intake properly according to its energy needs.[67]

With learning, feeding can become associated in early life with experiences that usually accompany feeding, such as a mother's attention and warmth. Harry F. Harlow's experiments on infant monkeys help illustrate how this learning process might occur. In one typical experiment Harlow gave infant monkeys the opportunity to choose between two "pseudo-mothers." One mother was made out of wire but contained a milk bottle. The other mother had no milk bottle, but the wire frame was wrapped in soft cloth (see Figure 2.7). The infant monkeys would feed from the wire mother but spent most of their time in close contact with the cloth mother. By this research Harlow showed that the softness of the mother is extremely

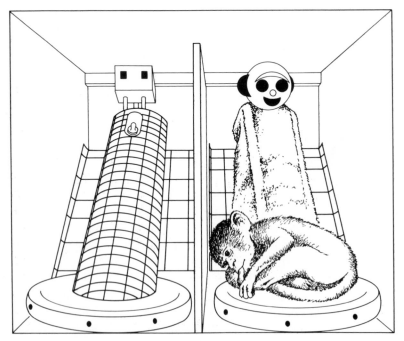

FIGURE 2.7   *The infant monkey's wire and cloth mothers.* Only the wire mother has a bottle and delivers milk. (Adapted from H. F. Harlow, "The Nature of Love," *American Psychologist* 13[1958]:673–685.)

rewarding by itself to an infant monkey, independent of the feeding experience. He called this attraction of the infant monkey to the cloth mother "love."[68] Usually the soft mother and the milk-giving mother are one and the same. It is therefore easy to see how "love" could become associated with food, although they might have originally been independent.

By such mechanisms psychodynamic theorists postulate that feeding can come to stand for many things and thus can occur inappropriately. Alternatively, if early caretakers are wise in feeding a child and respond well to its biological needs, they can teach the child to consume food only when it is really needed.[69]

This may be difficult for the caretakers because infants differ a great deal, and it is therefore easy to misinterpret the signals the child is sending.[70] Whatever occurs, psychodynamic theorists believe that learning is so intimately tied to the physiological regulation of hunger that it is virtually impossible to separate the two. According to psychodynamic theory, it is easy to see how a child might come to eat when frightened or lonely, since he or she has associated feeding with security and a mother's love.[71]

Although the psychodynamic approach seems an eminently reasonable one, in general it has lacked the research findings to make its conclusions significant for experimental psychologists. However, alternative approaches have been proposed that go beyond a strictly physiological account of hunger.

Behavioral Models of Feeding

Behavioral models of feeding attempt to explain hunger without reference to any internal physiological variables. Instead, principles for explaining and predicting hunger are based primarily on behavior, especially *operant behavior*, so-called voluntary behavior that results from actions of the skeletal muscle system. For example, Gary A. Lucas and William Timberlake have developed a model in which meal size is determined by two factors.[72] The first factor consists of an increase in meal size due to positive gustatory stimulation (a positive feedback mechanism). The second factor consists of a decrease in meal size as a function of total amount consumed (a negative feedback mechanism). These two factors combine to determine meal size.

J. E. R. Staddon postulates four factors in his model: "body weight (the size of the energy store), metabolic level (energy expenditure), eating frequency (energy income), and taste (the evolutionary predictor of food quality)."[73] Staddon's model focuses on energy economics, but instead of looking for a physiological focus for energy input and output within the organism, he considers the whole organism as an energy package and looks at the organism's observable behavior. Staddon's model, like the physiological models, includes feedback mechanisms, but these mechanisms are expressed entirely in terms of operant behavior. Three assumptions about the feedback functions characterize the model. First, eating rate is maintained at an optimal level by operant behavior. Second, the effect of taste is to increase or decrease the eating rate. Third, organisms tend to eat at higher rates when their body weight is low.

Although neither of these models accounts for some of the more subtle points of initiation and termination of feeding, they are simple enough and general enough to explain easily a great many instances of feeding behavior.

Lucas and Timberlake's and Staddon's work on the regulation of feeding are only two examples of how nonphysiological psychologists have tried to account for feeding behavior. In part, their reasons for abandoning physiological explanations involve the increasing complexity of what we already know about the physiological determinants of hunger, combined with the fact that much is still not known. Building physiological models can appear hopeless in this circumstance. But perhaps more importantly, these psychologists are among many who believe that an organism interacts with its world at the level of behavior, not at the neuronal level. They therefore reason that explanations of behavior should be constructed on a behavioral basis.

CONCLUSION

Researchers began investigating hunger by considering peripheral cues involved in the initiation and termination of feeding bouts. The stomach contraction, stomach distention, environmental temperature, glucostatic, and lipostatic theories have been studied over the years and have advanced our understanding of feeding regulation. Theories involving such peripheral factors as oral stimulation and the gut peptides have been proposed and tested more recently. The variety and extent of these theories have made it clear that a multitude of factors are involved in hunger. For this reason many researchers searched for particular locations in the brain that might coordinate and synthesize the peripheral information. The ventromedial hypothalamus and the lateral hypothalamus seemed likely candidates as locations involved in satiety and hunger, respectively.

Recent evidence has shown that small, circumscribed areas that are exclusively responsible for affecting hunger and satiation behavior, in other words, hunger and satiety brain centers, do not exist. Although the hypothalamus serves a major integrating role for sensory inputs and motor outputs relevant to feeding, neural control of feeding seems generalized throughout the brain. Recent attempts to understand hunger and feeding have therefore involved constructing elaborate behavioral or physiological models that eliminate any reference to central determinants of feeding.

CHAPTER
3
❧
Thirst

Thirst and hunger are not independent of each other. Deprived of food, an animal consumes less water.[1] Likewise, an animal deprived of water consumes less food.[2] Both of these occurrences may be related to the ratio of the weight of food to the weight of water that the animal tends to keep in its stomach. In the rat, this ratio is always approximately 1 to 1. The rat also tends to maintain a balance of food and water in its intestine, and the ratio there is approximately 1 part food to 3 parts water.[3] Rats, and perhaps other species, apparently need to maintain a certain ratio of food to water in their gastrointestinal tracts for optimal digestion and absorption of nutrients. This suggests that the more an animal eats, the more it will drink. Further, if the animal is not perspiring or losing water in some other way, water will have little appeal unless food is available.

Thirst and hunger also interact because many foods contain at least some water and many liquids contain at least some nutrients. Thus eating can help satisfy thirst and drinking can help satisfy hunger. For example, a person is unlikely to feel hungry after drinking a large chocolate milkshake, and he or she is unlikely to feel thirsty after eating large amounts of lettuce (lettuce is 96 percent water).[4]

TYPES OF DRINKING BEHAVIORS

In some ways thirst is easier to study than hunger because it involves the intake of only one nutrient, water. Despite this simplicity, an astonishing number of different types of drinking behaviors can be observed. These behaviors divide into two major categories: homeostatic and nonhomeostatic. Homeostatic drinking restores an organism's water balance following fluid deprivation or depletion. Nonhomeostatic drinking encompasses all other types of drinking. Both basic types occur frequently. To be comprehensive, a theory of thirst needs to address both homeostatic and nonhomeostatic drinking.

Homeostatic Drinking

The overall goal of homeostatic drinking is to maintain, within fairly narrow limits, the concentration of solutes in the blood plasma, as well as the overall volume of the blood plasma.[5] There are two kinds of homeostatic drinking: drinking following extracellular fluid loss and drinking following intracellular fluid loss. The term *intracellular fluid compartment* refers to the water inside cells. *Extracellular fluid compartment* refers to the water outside cells, including the water between the cells and in the blood plasma. These two fluid compartments interact across the cell boundaries. If the concentration of *ions* (charged particles such as *sodium* and *potassium*) is higher on one side of a cell boundary than on the other, water tends to move across the boundary in a process called *osmosis* until the ion concentration on the two sides is equal.[6]

It is possible to decrease the size of the extracellular compartment without affecting the intracellular compartment by simply removing some of the extracellular fluid. This changes neither the concentration of the extracellular fluid that remains nor the concentration of the intracellular fluid. A typical example of this kind of extracellular fluid loss occurs during a hemorrhage, such as the sudden loss of blood following a car accident. Medical personnel generally administer fluids intravenously when this has happened. But if the extracellular fluid level is not restored, the person who has lost blood will become thirsty.[7] This kind of fluid loss is known as *hypovolemia*.

Intracellular fluid loss can occur when ions attain a high concentration in the plasma, such as due to an injection of saline. This causes water to be drawn out of the cells by osmosis.[8] A person who suffers this kind of fluid loss becomes thirsty.[9] Another way of losing intracellular fluid is water deprivation, which causes extracellular fluid loss as well. Once again, the water loss brings on thirst.[10]

In all of these instances the set point for the fluid content in one or both of the fluid compartments is disturbed. The optimal internal environment no longer prevails. Drinking reduces these deviations from the optimal state, through negative feedback, until the optimal state is restored. Like water deprivation, water consumption affects both compartments. It increases the amount of water in the extracellular compartment, thereby decreasing the ionic concentration of that compartment. Consequently, osmosis occurs: water moves from outside to inside the cell boundary and equalizes the ionic concentration on both sides of the boundary.[11] Water consumption following water deprivation is a homeostatic drinking behavior.

Nonhomeostatic Drinking

Much of the drinking that animals and humans do replenishes no water deficit. For example, rats exhibit *circadian rhythms* in their drinking behavior (i.e., patterns of drinking behavior dependent on the time of day). They consume about 75 percent of their water during the 12 dark hours of the 24-hour day, even when their meals are scheduled at 2.4-hour intervals around the clock.[12]

As another example of nonhomeostatic drinking, consider the fact that most of the drinking that you do occurs while you are eating a meal.[13] If asked what the physiological reasons are for your drinking, you might say that you need the water to help digest your food, or that you need the water because the food is salty and you want to replenish the water that the salt draws out of your cells. Both reasons, however, are only partly correct. You do not actually need the water until several hours after you consume the food. You are anticipating a need for water and taking advantage of available water to prevent a deficit. This is known as anticipatory drinking.[14] *Anticipatory drinking* is comparable to the anticipatory feeding described for the blowfly in Chapter 1. Animals drink as well as eat before there is any actual need for doing so.

Anticipatory drinking might represent learned drinking behavior. Perhaps organisms learn to associate eating with subsequent fluid deficits and so come to drink while eating. Alternatively, organisms may have evolved in such a way that anticipatory drinking occurs automatically. The extent to which anticipatory drinking is learned or inherited is not yet known.

There are other aspects of nonhomeostatic drinking behavior that are clearly and strongly influenced by learning. Humans traveling in the desert with no means of carrying water will consume as much water as possible at each waterhole before moving on. In general, when water is scarce, organisms learn to drink when it is available. This has been shown in the laboratory by giving animals stimuli that normally elicit no response but, after having been paired with a subsequent need for water, come to elicit drinking.[15]

Another example of nonhomeostatic drinking is *hysteresis,* a Greek word that means lagging behind. This word is used scientifically for cases in which the effect of a manipulation on a response persists even after the manipulation has been terminated. Organisms demonstrate hysteresis when they continue to drink (or not drink) after the causes for doing so have been removed. Consider the following example. An animal that eats a high-carbohydrate diet needs less water than one that eats a high-protein diet. If a rat is switched from a high-protein diet to a high-carbohydrate diet, we might expect that its water intake would immediately decrease. In fact, this decrease takes several days to occur.[16]

One example of nonhomeostatic drinking has puzzled researchers of motivation for many years. Why would a rat that has been deprived of food but not water consume a huge amount of water during a 3-hour daily experimental session in a cage in which food is available for a lever press every 60 seconds but water is available continuously? Why would the rat consume half its body weight in water while consuming an amount of food appropriate for a 24-hour period?[17] Such behavior is relatively easy to demonstrate in the laboratory. Not only is this behavior nonhomeostatic, it contradicts the previous statement that food deprivation decreases water consumption. This behavior is known as *schedule-induced polydipsia* (*SIP*).

Demonstrations of SIP are not confined to the laboratory. In an arcade in New York City's Chinatown there are some unusual games in which the action is provided by a chicken rather than electronics. One of these is a game of tic-tac-toe. A customer puts money in and then selects a square for the first X. The chicken pecks at a board to place its O. As the game continues the chicken receives food after each of its pecks. In the back of the chicken's cage is a cup of water (Figure 3.1). Each time the chicken receives food, it runs over to the cup and drinks copiously. People in the arcade often comment that the chicken must be very thirsty, that the poor chicken usually must not get enough to drink. But the chicken is not water deprived; it is merely showing SIP. (By the way, the customer never wins.)

Demonstrations of SIP are also not confined to nonhuman subjects. When human subjects in the laboratory were given monetary rewards from a slot machine every 90 seconds, they consumed an average of 285 milliliters

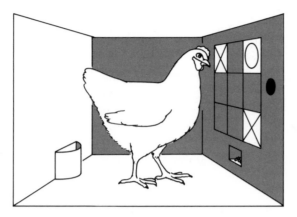

FIGURE 3.1   *Diagram of a tic-tac-toe game played by a chicken inside a chamber.* The chicken pecks at the round button on the right wall of the chamber each time a human opponent (outside) makes a mark on an outside tic-tac-toe grid. One of the chicken's marks then appears in a square of its grid, and the chicken receives a reward of food through the opening at the bottom of the chamber's right wall. Water is continuously available in the cup on the left of the chamber.

(about 1.2 cups) of water in a 30-minute session, despite not having any food available and not being water deprived.[18]

THEORIES OF THIRST

A good theory of thirst must explain all of these variations in drinking behavior. As is true of the theories of hunger, theories of thirst developed by focusing first on peripheral physiological cues, later on central physiological mechanisms; some recent theories of thirst have been built on nonhomeostatic models. The remainder of this chapter considers each of these kinds of theories and discusses their advantages and disadvantages.

The Dry Mouth Theory

The peripheral theory of thirst that dominated research on thirst following 1919 is Walter B. Cannon's dry mouth theory.[19] According to Cannon, organisms drink when their mouths feel dry and do not drink when their mouths feel wet. In the years prior to and following the conception of this theory, a great deal of evidence has been amassed both supporting and attacking it.

Probably the strongest evidence in support of the dry mouth theory is the fact that salivary flow does correlate well with water deprivation. If a human is increasingly deprived of water, the salivary flow decreases correspondingly.[20]

There is additional evidence supporting the dry mouth theory. For example, various ways of removing the sensation of dryness in the mouth also remove thirst. The thirst of hospital patients awaiting surgery, who are not permitted to drink, can be assuaged if they simply rinse their mouths with a liquid. This does not increase the fluid supply in their bodies, but it does lessen their thirst. Applying cocaine to the mouth of a person or a dog anesthetizes the mouth and also decreases thirst. Still another example is provided by people in the desert, who sometimes decrease their thirst by increasing their salivation. They increase salivation by putting small amounts of acidic fruit juices or insoluble objects such as rocks in their mouths.[21]

One last piece of evidence supporting the dry mouth theory concerns the small decrease in thirst that follows infusion of water directly into the stomach. If rats deprived of water are infused with 14 milliliters of water, they subsequently drink almost as much as rats that have not had an infusion. Rats that have been allowed first to drink 14 milliliters normally, however, subsequently drink much less than rats that have had an infusion or rats that have had no pretreatment.[22]

Probably the strongest evidence against the dry mouth theory comes from experiments on *sham drinking*. In a sham drinking procedure the water consumed by the subject is prevented from reaching the subject's stomach, for example by means of an esophagostomy. These experiments typically find that sham drinking is not very effective in suppressing future drinking. The subjects drink much larger quantities of water than they would ordinarily, given the same water deficit.[23] Even though the mouth is continually moistened, thirst is not satisfied.

Other evidence against the dry mouth theory comes from experiments in which the salivary glands are removed. Animals subjected to this procedure still consume relatively normal amounts of water. This has been demonstrated in experiments with dogs and in studies of humans who have had no salivary glands since infancy.[24] In all these cases the mouth is never moistened, but thirst functions fairly normally.

The general consensus has been that a dry mouth is a signal of thirst but not a cause. When the mouth is moistened, there is an immediate but temporary diminution in thirst. For lasting satisfaction of thirst, it is necessary to drink fluids that reach the stomach.[25] Further, initiation of thirst by a dry mouth or termination of thirst by a moistened one would apply mainly to homeostatic drinking. The dry mouth theory has little to say about non-homeostatic drinking.

The Lateral Hypothalamus

Because the dry mouth theory has proved unsatisfactory, researchers have sought more central, neural mechanisms as the causes of thirst. Using a strategy similar to that used in the research on hunger, researchers have looked for a particular location in the brain that satisfies two criteria. The first criterion is that the location should integrate bodily information on fluid supplies. The second criterion is that, using the integreated information, the location should then initiate or terminate drinking or make no change. This search has focused on the lateral hypothalamus.

The hypothalamus first attracted attention because of the work of B. Andersson in the early 1950s. Andersson showed that injections of sodium chloride into the hypothalamus initiated drinking in goats.[26] His work suggested that there are cells in the hypothalamus that, when exposed to substances that prompt intracellular fluid loss, cause the organism to begin drinking. These cells have been called *osmoreceptors.*

Andersson later showed that electrical stimulation of cells in the same region also elicited drinking.[27] Other researchers have shown that lesions in the area of the hypothalamus disturb drinking behavior. This research, discussed in the previous chapter on hunger, pointed out that lesions in the lateral hypothalamus cause not only aphagia but also adipsia.[28]

A further indication that the hypothalamus is the central link for water regulation is its role in the release of *antidiuretic hormone* (*ADH*, also known as *vasopressin*). When this hormone is released by the hypothalamus, water is retained by the kidneys. The hypothalamus releases ADH both when the hypothalamic osmoreceptors indicate an intracellular fluid loss and when the plasma pressure receptors (*baroreceptors*) in the blood vessels indicate an extracellular fluid loss.[29]

These results all seemed to suggest that a location within the hypothalamus is responsible for thirst and water regulation. This conclusion, however, is subject to many of the same criticisms that have been made of the brain centers theory of hunger and satiety, discussed in the previous chapter. These criticisms have pointed to the possibility that neither the experimental manipulations of the brain nor the modified behavior that results from them are specific enough to prove the theory. In other words, a lesion in the hypothalamus may appear to affect drinking but may actually affect some other aspect of motivation or behavior. For example, if the procedure interferes with the animal's ability to move its tongue, eating and drinking behaviors could also change. The electrical current used to create these lesions may destroy not only the neurons close to the electrodes but also the neuronal fibers passing through that area.

Angiotensin

A theory that recently has been gaining acceptance postulates that *angiotensin* is the cause of thirst (Figure 3.2). Water deprivation causes peripheral physiological changes, such as decreased arterial blood pressure and increased sodium concentration in the blood. These changes in the extracellular fluid compartment are detected by specialized cells in the kidney, which then secretes the enzyme *renin*. When renin comes into contact with blood, angiotensin is produced. Consequently, the concentration of angiotensin in the blood is greater under conditions of greater water deprivation.[30] Experiments have shown that angiotensin injected intravenously or applied directly to the brain increases drinking.[31] Similar to the way blood sugar affects eating, the level of angiotensin in the blood may increase drinking by acting on centrally located receptors. Angiotensin may function as the link between peripheral indicators of water deprivation and a central control of drinking. Angiotensin also compensates for fluid loss using three additional physiological mechanisms: (1) it causes constriction of the blood vessels, which raises blood pressure; (2) it causes increased release of *aldosterone*, a hormone important in the regulation of sodium reabsorption by the kidney; and (3) it causes increased release of ADH.[32] The renin–anigiotensin system appears to be quite similar across all mammalian species. This may reflect the fact that all species need water and that need is relatively independent of individual species' particular diets.[33]

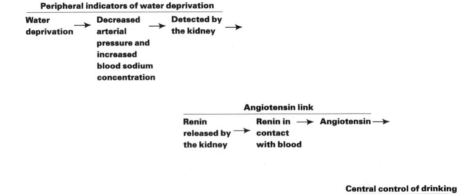

FIGURE 3.2   *A model of the way in which angiotensin may link peripheral indicators of water deprivation with central control of drinking.*

Nonhomeostatic Theories of Drinking

At best, the theories of thirst discussed above can account only for homeostatic drinking behavior. The hypothalamic theory, for example, proposes that thirst is caused when a specific part of the brain detects inadequate fluid levels in the body. Because much of the drinking that animals and humans do is nonhomeostatic, and is not in response to any water deficit, a purely homeostatic theory of thirst is inadequate. This section discusses some of the alternative theories.

A strong argument for a nonhomeostatic model of drinking has been presented by F. M. Toates.[34] Toates, a motivational theorist, became dissatisfied with explanations of thirst and hunger based on homeostasis. Like other such theorists described in the previous chapter, Toates noted that a great deal of eating and drinking behavior is nonhomeostatic and much of it is determined by the environment and by learning (rather than by peripheral physiological stimuli), so that there is little point in retaining the traditional definition of homeostasis. Toates has proposed that future efforts to explain drinking eliminate the concept of homeostasis and focus on creating models that include the many different physiological and environmental factors that influence drinking.

Certainly it is difficult to conceive of a homeostatic model that could explain SIP. One explanation that has gained wide acceptance makes no reference whatsoever to physiological factors. John L. Falk[35] has classified SIP, along with other schedule-induced behaviors, as *adjunctive behaviors*. These are behaviors that increase in response to reinforcers that ordinarily do not motivate these types of behavior. The adjunctive behavior, in this case drinking, occurs as an adjunct to a different motivational system, in this case food consumption. In schedule-induced polydipsia, animals drink even though the reinforcer in the experiment is food; despite the fact that a desire to eat is motivating the animals, the probability that they will drink increases. According to Falk, animals exhibit SIP when they are motivated to eat but cannot do so. Their motivation to eat is displaced to another drive whose satisfaction is available, in this case thirst. Falk hypothesizes that such displacement increases the probability that animals in the wild will take advantage of whatever reinforcers are available. However, under the particular conditions by which SIP is demonstrated in the laboratory, quite unadaptive behavior (i.e., excessive drinking) does result.

Most nonhomeostatic drinking consists of drinking around mealtimes, before the food consumed during the meal has had time to create a need for water. The physiological bases for this type of drinking are now being elucidated. When eating commences, and beforehand, a great variety of neuroendocrine events occur—many have been implicated in eliciting drinking. In particular, during mealtimes but prior to food's being absorbed or even entering the stomach, the vagus nerve causes *histamine* to be released, which in turn elicits drinking.[36] This is an adaptive mechanism because, similar to the blowfly's feeding system described in the previous chapter, a substance (here, water) is acquired by the organism before the need for this substance becomes critical. Thus physiological mechanisms can provide a basis for understanding anticipatory eating and drinking.

THIRST AND AGING

Research on thirst is of more than laboratory interest. Determination of the causes of the initiation and termination of drinking can have direct clinical applications. For example, such research can help to identify methods for the prevention and treatment of potentially dangerous water deficits in the elderly. Such deficits can occur even in apparently healthy elderly persons following water deprivation or exposure to heat. Many elderly persons do not drink sufficient amounts of water to compensate for the amounts lost due to these environmental challenges. Although the precise causes of these thirst deficits are not yet known, they may be related to the elderly's decreased homeostatic capacity, including a decreased ability to excrete excess water. Further research on fluid homeostasis and excretion will benefit basic theories of thirst as well as the health of the elderly.[37]

CONCLUSION

Using an approach similar to that taken in investigating hunger, scientists began by trying to explain thirst according to, first, peripheral and then more central physiological factors. While these factors clearly are influential in the initiation and termination of drinking, much of drinking is nonhomeostatic and therefore is not fully explained by this type of approach. More recently, researchers have turned to nonhomeostatic models to explain thirst, models that focus on the many different factors that influence drinking behavior, including the animal's interaction with its environment.

Continuing investigations of the physiological bases of thirst will enrich the interpretations based on learned behavior that have previously been used to explain drinking.[38]

Part II

THE KIND OF SUBSTANCE CONSUMED

I began by considering the question of how organisms regulate the amount of what they eat and drink. Part II considers a related question: Given that an organism is hungry or thirsty, how does it choose what to eat or drink? The chapters that follow examine this question at the sensory level and then proceed to behavioral measures of preference. The concluding chapter in this part discusses formal models that psychologists have devised to describe how organisms choose what they eat or drink.

CHAPTER
4

❦

Taste and Smell

The two senses most involved in eating and drinking are taste and smell. Both taste and smell are chemical senses: They operate by detecting molecules of chemical substances. The sense of taste, *gustation*, operates by detecting molecules in solution on the tongue, and the sense of smell, *olfaction*, by detecting molecules in the air as they come in contact with the olfactory epithelium in the nose.

In humans, both taste and smell are exquisitely sensitive. The average person can detect the presence of sodium saccharin in a solution at a molar concentration of only .000023 (grams of saccharin divided by the molecular weight of saccharin, per liter of total solution).[1] People, on the average, can also detect the scent of perfume when as little as one drop is diffused into the air of an average house. Our ability to detect low concentrations of odors compares well with the sensitivity of artificial detectors, such as smoke alarms.[2]

Gustation and olfaction are not necessarily independent. Chemical stimulation that affects one can also affect the other. Everyone has experienced the tastelessness of food that comes with a stuffy nose. The tastes of foods and drinks seem less strong when they are not also accompanied by their odors. *Flavor* is actually a combination of a number of different sensations, including not only taste but also smell and touch, along with temperature sensations and any feelings of pain.[3]

An experiment by J. G. Beebe-Center illustrates the relatively small contribution of taste to flavor. Beebe-Center asked subjects to rate 14 foods and drinks for the presence of the four tastes: sweet, sour, salt, and bitter. The foods and drinks included such items as sour pickles, honey, Riesling wine, raspberry jam, and anchovy fillets. The subjects could rate these foods and drinks on a scale ranging from 0 to as high as 100 for each of the four tastes, but in only one instance, the sweetness of honey, did any of the subjects' ratings exceed 50.[4] The taste component of flavor is actually quite small for much of the food we eat.

THE IMPORTANCE OF THE SENSES OF TASTE AND SMELL

The senses of taste and smell are critical to an animal's survival, particularly animals that are omnivores. Omnivores have the difficult task of identifying which foods and drinks are which so that they can avoid poisonous substances and find the foods and drinks that nourish them best.

Once a food or drink has entered the stomach, removing it from the body may be difficult or impossible. Rats lack the musculature for vomiting.[5] Even for species that can vomit, some poisons act so quickly or take effect only after such a delay that vomiting may come too late. To be able to eject a poisonous food from the mouth before it has been swallowed is clearly an advantage.

The location of the taste receptors on the tongue helps prevent any undesirable items from reaching the stomach. In addition, for most animals the sense of taste is linked to the gagging and vomiting reflexes.[6] A man who bites into a piece of bitter horseradish hidden in a dish of ice cream is likely to forcefully eject everything in his mouth without any thought whatsoever.

Taste sensations can also be rewarding. Some tastes, such as sweet, can be pleasant even though they may not be associated with positive consequences, such as an increase in available energy (calories). However, the sweet taste continues to be pleasurable only if the sweet substance is not swallowed. Swallowing a sweet substance apparently results in negative feedback from the stomach, leading to a decrease in the perceived pleasantness of that substance (a phenomenon known as *alliesthesia*).[7] Presumably, this happens because the body's need for a sweet substance decreases once a sweet substance has been swallowed.

Even better than preventing an undesirable substance from getting into the stomach is preventing it from getting into the mouth, and this is one of the functions of olfaction. Like gustation, olfaction is also linked to ejection reflexes and helps identify desirable foods and drinks.[8]

The body has evolved in such a way that a food or drink must pass several tests before an animal or a person judges it acceptable. The senses of taste and smell are essential to this process. While smell is more helpful than taste in rejecting a food or drink before it enters the body, these two senses interact in influencing acceptance or rejection of a food or drink.

TASTE AND SMELL CODING

Definition of Primaries

Much of the research on gustation and olfaction has explored the ways in which tastes and odors are perceived, that is, the ways in which chemical stimuli are coded by the body into specific subjective impressions of taste and odor. This research has not proceeded as quickly as has research on the coding of visual and auditory stimuli. In part, at least, this discrepancy has been due to the fact that taste and smell operate by chemical detection, which makes research on these two senses more difficult. For example, in experiments on olfaction it is difficult to deliver a particular odor without contamination by another odor occurring sometime during the procedure. In addition, one of the main problems for researchers has been to determine what aspects of the chemical stimuli are responsible for the tastes and odors they induce. Unlike the variations in wavelength that correspond with the perception of color and pitch, no single physical dimension can be varied to yield all possible tastes or odors.[9]

Serious investigation of taste and smell coding began at the beginning of the twentieth century, when little equipment was available and few sophisticated techniques were in use. Early scientists attempted to identify *taste* and *odor primaries*—the smallest number of tastes and odors that could be used to describe all other tastes and odors. If primaries could be found for gustation and olfaction, investigations of how chemical stimuli are physically coded could be limited to the features that distinguish the primaries.

It is important to keep in mind that the primaries for gustation and olfaction would not be those tastes and odors with which all tastes and odors could be made chemically, but those with which all tastes and odors could be *described*. For example, if the primaries for taste consisted of sweet, sour, salt, and bitter, it would not necessarily be possible to take sugar, table salt, lemon juice, and quinine and, by mixing them together in a bowl in various quantities, create the flavor of a hamburger. Chemical reactions among the ingredients could cause the mixture to taste like something quite different. Identifying the primaries would simply make it possible to describe the taste of a hamburger as a combination of a few tastes, for example, sweet, sour, salt, and bitter, in various proportions.[10]

Taste Primaries

FIRST DESCRIPTION.   H. Henning,[11] often identified as the first investigator of the taste primaries, proposed that the four primary tastes were sweet, sour, salt, and bitter. Using these four primaries, he set out to show

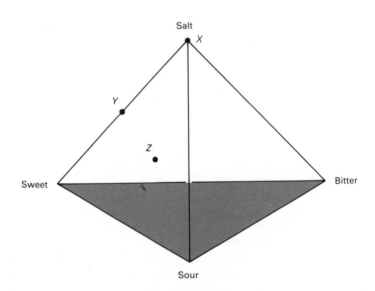

FIGURE 4.1   *Henning's tetrahedron representing tastes as a function of the four taste primaries: sweet, sour, salt, and bitter.* Point X, at the vertex of the tetrahedron labeled salt, represents a taste that would be described only as salty. Point Y, on the edge of the tetrahedron between the vertexes labeled salt and sweet, represents a taste that would be described as both salty and sweet. Point Z, inside the tetrahedron, represents a taste that would be described as sweet, sour, salty, and bitter. (Adapted from F. A. Geldard, *The Human Senses,* New York: John Wiley & Sons, 1972.)

that the description of any taste could be represented using his taste tetrahedron (Figure 4.1).

The composition of a particular taste is represented by a specific location on the tetrahedron. For example, each of the four corners of the tetrahedron represents maximal sensation of one of Henning's primary tastes, with no sensation of any of the other three tastes. Thus, if a taste were represented by a point located at the corner labeled salt, that taste would be entirely salty and nothing else. Tastes represented on the edges of the tetrahedron, the lines connecting two corners, are tastes described by various quantities of the two tastes at the corners, with more of one taste if the point is closer to one of the corners. A taste represented by a point on a plane of the tetrahedron is described by the three tastes whose corners define that plane, and a taste that can only be described using all four of the taste primaries would be located inside the tetrahedron.

PHYSIOLOGICAL BASIS FOR TASTE PRIMARIES. Because Henning's four taste primaries did appear to describe most tastes fairly well,[12] scientists reasoned that the physiological coding of taste must be organized in some way according to Henning's four primary tastes. Perhaps, scientists thought, there are four types of sensory cells on the tongue, and each type is maximally sensitive to one of the four taste primaries.

Evidence suggested that this was a likely possibility. It had long been known that the surface of the human tongue has four types of *taste papillae,* the small protuberances visible to the naked eye. Figure 4.2 shows these four types of papillae and their locations on the tongue. The filiform papillae, which look like little points, are distributed throughout the surface of the tongue. Foliate papillae, resembling ridges, are located mostly on the rear sides of the tongue. Circumvallate papillae, which look like enclosed circles, are located mostly on the back of the tongue. Finally, fungiform papillae, shaped like mushrooms, are located on the tip and edges of the tongue.[13] Further, many substances tasting mainly like one of the four taste primaries were known to have distinctive chemical properties.[14] For example, substances that taste sweet often contain a certain configuration of oxygen or nitrogen bonded to hydrogen, those that taste bitter are often soluble in lipids, those that taste salty usually ionize easily, and those that taste sour are often acids.[15]

Given all this evidence, obtained without recourse to microelectrode recording from gustatory neurons, it is easy to formulate a hypothesis about how tastes are coded. Perhaps each of the four taste primaries represents a general class of chemical stimuli, and each of these classes of chemical stimuli is best detected by one of the four types of taste papillae. Then, if the four types of papillae are connected to distinct neurons, the brain could dis-

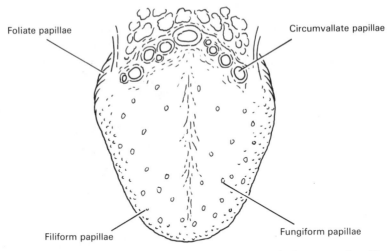

Foliate papillae

Circumvallate papillae

Filiform papillae

Fungiform papillae

FIGURE 4.2   *Diagram of the surface of the tongue, showing the four types of papillae and their locations.* (Adapted from P. L. Williams and R. Warwick, *Gray's Anatomy,* Philadelphia: W. B. Saunders, 1980.)

tinguish different tastes by determining which of the four types of neurons is most active. A theory which postulates that there are specific sensory neurons whose activity indicates the detection of particular stimuli is known as a *labeled line theory.* The stimuli are categorized, and some neurons (the "lines") are presumed to respond well to certain categories but not to others; the lines are labeled for certain categories.

Carl Pfaffmann examined the labeled line theory for taste with his electrophysiological research, which he began publishing in 1941.[16] Pfaffmann was the first to investigate intensively the neuronal responses of a mammal (the cat) to taste stimuli placed on the tongue. First, he anesthetized the cats and surgically exposed the *chorda tympani nerve,* the nerve responsible for taste sensations from the front two-thirds of the tongue. This nerve consists of a bundle of many separate neuronal fibers. Next, Pfaffmann used microelectrodes to record electrical responses from individual fibers in the chorda tympani nerve while he placed various chemical stimuli on the cats' tongues.

Pfaffmann found no fibers in the cat that were sensitive to sweet, but he located several fibers that were sensitive to sour and salt, or to sour and bitter. He did further studies with rats and rabbits and concluded that the labeled line theory was incorrect. Instead, he thought, the different tastes must be coded by a complex pattern of firing that arises from many different fibers. The overall rate of firing of the neurons would indicate the concentration, or intensity, of the substance that was being tasted. Pfaffmann's theory is known as the *pattern theory* of taste perception.[17]

Other studies showed that the receptors are not the papillae or even necessarily cells within the papillae. The filiform papillae are not associated with taste receptors. Circumvallate papillae have taste receptors located in the trenches around their sides. Only the fungiform and the foliate papillae have taste receptors located on their top surfaces.[18]

Figure 4.3 shows a cross section of a taste receptor cell underneath a *taste pore,* an opening on the surface of the tongue. Fibers in the chorda tympani nerve can be connected to one or to several of these taste receptors.[19] This last finding was particularly destructive to the credibility of a labeled line theory for gustation; the chances that any single neuron would code for a particular taste appeared highly unlikely.

More recent research has shown, however, that individual fibers in the chorda tympani nerve are responsive to all of the taste primaries but are usually most responsive to one of those primaries. Further, receptors that are connected to the same fiber tend to have similar sensitivities to various tastes.[20]

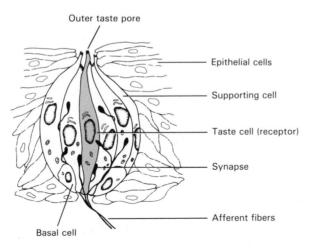

Outer taste pore

Epithelial cells

Supporting cell

Taste cell (receptor)

Synapse

Afferent fibers

Basal cell

FIGURE 4.3   *Anatomy of the area surrounding a taste receptor cell.* (Adapted from V. F. Castellucci, "The Chemical Senses: Taste and Smell," in *Principles of Neural Science,* 2nd ed., eds. E. R. Kandel and J. H. Schwartz, New York: Elsevier, 1985.)

An elegant experiment, published in 1980 by Kristina Arvidson and Ulf Friberg, helps illustrate these points. Arvidson and Friberg's procedure involved isolating fungiform papillae on the tongues of human subjects, using suction to draw single papillae into tiny tubes. The researchers could then stimulate the papillae, one at a time, with various chemical substances. The papillae were then excised and examined under a microscope to see how many taste receptors were located in each one. The results showed that a papilla containing a single taste receptor could be sensitive to more than one of the four primary tastes. Further, the number of primary tastes that a papilla could sense was greater in proportion to the number of receptors located in it.[21]

Taste appears to be coded by a system that operates in accord with elements of both the labeled line and pattern theories of taste perception.[22] The perception of taste resembles the perception of color: One neuron firing by itself is insufficient to convey a particular taste or color. A pattern of firing is needed. But certain neurons are more sensitive to certain tastes. These primary tastes, at least in humans, are sweet, sour, salt, and bitter.[23]

EVOLUTION AND THE TASTE PRIMARIES.   For people who have studied humans' evolutionary history, it is not surprising that the four taste primaries should be sweet, sour, salt, and bitter. At least three of these tastes help identify foods that are critical to the survival of omnivores. A sweet taste often indicates a good source of carbohydrates; in other words, foods that taste sweet usually are good sources of energy. Poisonous foods are sometimes bitter. Salt is necessary for maintaining cellular homeostasis;[24] an inability to taste salt could imperil an animal's survival.

TRANSDUCTION.   One piece of the coding puzzle is still missing: How do chemical stimuli in solution cause the receptor cells on the tongue to fire (i.e., how does transduction occur)? In other words, once the chemical stimulus in solution has entered the taste pore and come into contact with the parts of the receptor cell that project into the taste pore, how does that stimulus change the receptor cell membrane so that a neural signal occurs? The evidence here is not complete and is controversial. One popular theory was proposed by Lloyd M. Beidler.[25]

According to Beidler's model, the surface membrane of the receptor cells is made up of chains of fats and proteins linked together by several different kinds of chemical bonds. The bonding is imperfect and is affected by electrical charges on the membrane surface. The surface of the receptor cells therefore provides a number of sites for different kinds of chemical links with substances that happen to be in the vicinity. Various substances can bind in many places and in many different ways. Further, binding can inhibit, as well as excite, neuronal activity.[26] Recent investigations have been able to identify some of the specific physical chemistry that causes a taste stimulus to produce a change in receptor cell activity. For example, it appears that the saltiness of sodium chloride is detected when the positively charged sodium ions are attracted to, and subsequently neutralize, the negative charge of the surface of particular parts of the receptor cell membrane. This causes a change in the membrane's surface tension, such that ion channels that permit the passage only of sodium ions are opened. It is these sodium ions, admitted through the receptor cell membrane, that change the receptor cell activity level.[27]

More Evidence for Taste Receptors Sensitive to Particular Stimuli

CROSS-ADAPTATION STUDIES.   A general method for studying taste receptors sensitive to specific stimuli has been that of cross-adaptation. *Adaptation* is the decrease in a sensory response that occurs when a sensory stimulus is continuously present. The human tongue, for example, is usually adapted to the taste of sodium chloride in saliva. When that adaptation is removed—for example, by bathing the tongue in water—much lower concentrations of sodium chloride can be tasted.[28]

In *cross-adaptation* studies, the tongue is first adapted to a specific taste. Then, if the perceived intensity of a different taste decreases, cross-adaptation is said to have occurred. The assumption is that any tastes that cross-adapt must be detected by means of the same receptor mechanisms. Cross-adaptation studies have suggested that there may be more than one type of receptor mechanism for the taste of sweet and more than one type for the taste of bitter, but only one type for the taste of salt and only one type for the taste of sour.[29]

SWEET RECEPTORS.   Two substances found in nature produce unusual changes in taste perception that seem to confirm the existence of sweet receptors on the tongue. One of these substances is *gymnemic acid*, a chemical derived from the leaves of a plant native to India. When gymnemic acid is applied to the human tongue, the taste of sweet is depressed.[30] The chorda tympani nerve stops reacting to sweet substances on the tongue, although it continues to react to other tastes.[31] The fact that only the reactions to sweet substances are affected implies that the tongue has specialized receptors for sweet and that gymnemic acid somehow blocks these receptors.

The West African miracle fruit, a berry about the size of a small grape, causes the opposite effect. After this fruit has been eaten, sour substances taste sweet. The active substance in the miracle fruit is aptly named *miraculin*.[32] Again, the fact that a substance placed on the tongue can specifically affect the taste of sweet suggests that specialized receptors for sweet are located on the tongue.

BITTER RECEPTORS.   If people are given different concentrations of something to taste, a graph showing the lowest concentration that each person can taste yields a curve with a single peak; the lowest concentration tasted by different people tends to be similar, falling near a single concentration (Figure 4.4a). However, PTC yields a dual-peaked curve (Figure 4.4b). This means that instead of there being one average lowest concentration that a given group of people can taste, there are two. The subjects whose data fall near the left peak are able to taste a relatively low concentration of PTC; they are called "tasters." The subjects whose data fall near the right peak can only taste a relatively high concentration of PTC; they are called "nontasters." Although not necessarily chemically similar to PTC, some other bitter substances, such as caffeine and saccharin, produce similar results.[33]

Whether someone is a taster or a nontaster turns out to have a genetic basis, and the genes for being a taster or a nontaster vary among different ethnic groups. About one-third of Northern Europeans are nontasters. The proportion of nontasters in other groups is much smaller.[34]

All of this information suggests that there is a general class of mechanisms for tasting bitter substances. Whether these mechanisms involve bitter receptors on the tongue or some more central mechanism is not yet clear.

Odor Primaries

Investigations of odor detection have paralleled the studies of taste. Scientists have tried to identify the odor primaries as well as how the body detects them.

There is no general consensus about which odors are the primaries. For many years a set of seven primaries proposed by John E. Amoore received attention. Amoore[35] has identified ethereal, camphoraceous, musky, floral, minty, pungent, and putrid as the seven primary odors. The study of specific *anosmias* (a specific anosmia is the inability to detect

FIGURE 4.4   (a) Hypothetical diagram of the number of people for whom a given concentration of a typical taste stimulus is the lowest concentration tasted. (b) Number of people for whom a given concentration of PTC is the lowest concentration tasted. These data are from a sample of 855 people and are somewhat unusual in that, in this sample, there are more nontasters than tasters. (Adapted from H. Kalmus, "Inherited Sense Defects," Scientific American 186 [5][1952]:64–70.)

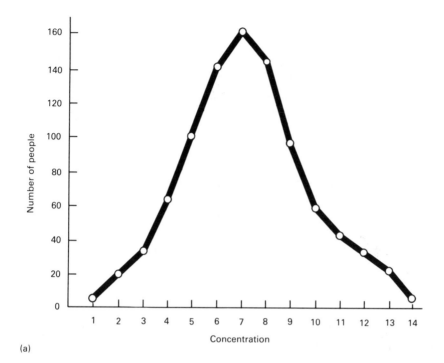

(a)

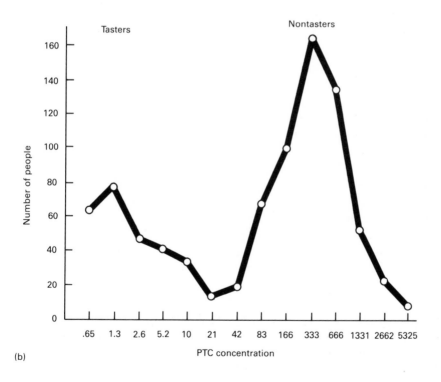

(b)

a particular smell) was helpful in the investigation of these odor primaries. The fact that specific anosmias are frequently inherited and that they frequently correspond to Amoore's specific odor primaries suggested that the ability to detect specific odors is genetically determined[36] and that Amoore's seven primary odors are indeed elements in the body's system of coding odors.

Based on this evidence, Amoore proposed a description of how the body might detect the seven odor primaries. His theory is known as the stereochemical theory of odor discrimination.[37] Similar to Beidler's theory of taste discrimination, Amoore's theory postulated that there are specific sites on the olfactory epithelium to which odor molecules with the appropriate shape can bind, and that the types of available sites would in general correspond to the odor primaries. If a molecule does fit a particular site, then that molecule acts as a "key" for that "lock" (Figure 4.5).[38]

It now appears that Amoore's seven odor primaries are insufficient to describe all odors. In addition, it has not been possible to identify types of sites on the olfactory epithelium that correspond to the shapes of his primaries. Recent research has proposed sets of as many as 146 primaries; however the issue of which odors are the primaries has by no means been settled.[39] In addition, although the olfactory receptors appear to consist of molecules of protein,[40] it is not precisely known how molecules on the olfactory epithelium cause the receptors to signal detection of an odor. It is also not known to what extent there are sites on the olfactory epithelium that are responsive to molecules of some shapes but not others, although shape does appear to have a role in odor coding. For all of these reasons Amoore's stereochemical theory has passed into disfavor.[41]

Some general information is available concerning the anatomy and the transduction process of the olfactory system. Figure 4.6 shows the cells present on the surface of the olfactory epithelium. Somehow, odors that come into contact with the olfactory cilia change the activity levels of the receptor neurons. The mucus covering the olfactory epithelium affects the transduction process. Only certain molecules can pass through the mucus, and some molecules change as a result of this passage.[42]

Further, similar to the gustatory system, there are indications that the olfactory system contains elements of both the labeled line and the pattern theories of sensory perception. Individual receptor cells are sensitive to not just one, but to a particular set of odors. Apparently no two cells, or very few cells, are sensitive to the same set.[43] Receptor cells at different locations on the olfactory epithelium are activated differently, depending on the particular odor that is present.[44] The receptor cells project to the *olfactory bulb*, a collection of neurons that is part of the CNS. Particular odors induce activity in particular regions of the olfactory bulb.[45] Thus, although individual cells

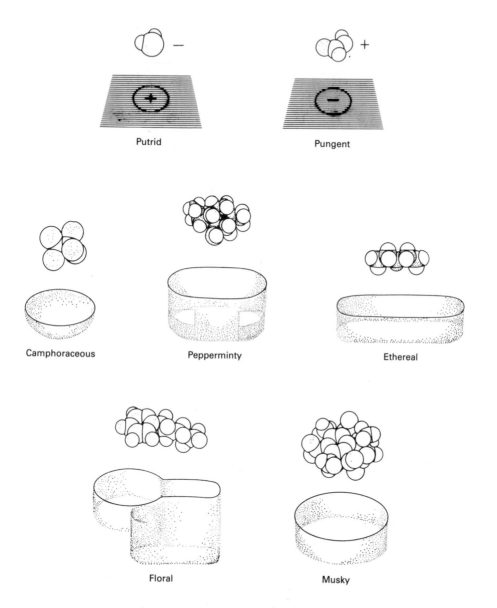

Putrid

Pungent

Camphoraceous

Pepperminty

Ethereal

Floral

Musky

FIGURE 4.5   *Hypothetical diagram of odor detection as postulated by Amoore, showing the "key" (the odor molecule) and the "lock" (the receptor site).* (Adapted from J. E. Amoore, J. W. Johnston, and M. Rubin, "The Stereochemical Theory of Odor," *Scientific American* 210[2][1964]:42–49.)

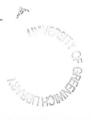

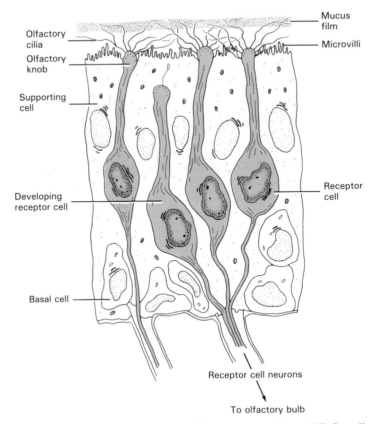

Olfactory cilia
Olfactory knob
Supporting cell
Developing receptor cell
Basal cell

Mucus film
Microvilli
Receptor cell

Receptor cell neurons

To olfactory bulb

FIGURE 4.6   *Anatomy of the olfactory epithelium.* (Adapted from V. F. Castellucci, "The Chemical Senses: Taste and Smell," in *Principles of Neural Science,* 2nd ed., eds. E. R. Kandel and J. H. Schwartz, New York: Elsevier, 1985.)

and parts of the olfactory bulb are sensitive to particular odors, patterns of activity also appear to play a role in olfactory coding.

INDIVIDUAL DIFFERENCES IN TASTE AND ODOR SENSITIVITY

Taste and odor sensitivity are not the same for all people all of the time. Different people are born with different abilities to taste and smell, and environmental influences, as well as the aging process, subsequently affect these abilities.

Taste

Although the evidence is not completely clear, *threshold sensitivity* to tastes (the lowest concentration of a substance that can be tasted) appears to decrease with age. For *suprathreshold sensitivity,* which is sensitivity to increases in stimulation above threshold, the evidence again seems to indicate that elderly people are less sensitive than young adults.[46] It is not known whether these decreases in taste sensitivity as a function of age are primarily due to genetically determined changes in the taste sensory system, or primarily due to changes in that system resulting from many years of exposure to tastes and other stimuli. The effect of the environment is clear, however, in the loss of the sense of taste over a particular part of the tongue that can occur following head trauma, upper respiratory infection, or bulimia nervosa (see Chapter 9).[47] On the other hand, variations in taste sensitivity between different people are to some extent inherited, as the research on PTC detection has shown.

Smell

There are also large individual differences in the ability to smell.[48] Both threshold olfactory sensitivity and the ability to discriminate between different odors decline with age.[49] After age 80, more than 75 percent of elderly people are significantly impaired in their ability to smell.[50] However, this means that almost 25 percent of people over the age of 80 do not show such impairment; the relationship between the ability to smell and age is heterogeneous.[51] Some of this heterogeneity may be due to the effects of disease on olfactory sensitivity; as with tastes, sensitivity to odors can decrease following head trauma or viral infection.[52] Further, at any point throughout the life span, environmental stimuli can temporarily affect odor sensitivity. For example, consumption of mild to moderate amounts of alcohol can temporarily increase odor sensitivity.[53]

A study by Helen B. Hubert, Richard R. Fabsitz, Manning Feinleib, and Kenneth S. Brown set out to investigate genetic determinants of olfactory sensitivity but instead concluded by emphasizing the effects of environmental factors.[54] Hubert and her colleagues tested the olfactory sensitivity to several substances in 97 pairs of adult male twins. Of these 97 pairs, 51 were *identical (monozygotic)* twins, and the rest were *fraternal (dizygotic)* twins. Monozygotic twins have identical sets of genes, while dizygotic twins on the average share half of their genes. Assuming that the environments for members of monozygotic twin pairs are no more similar than for members of dizygotic twin pairs (not always a correct assumption), if members of monozygotic twin pairs are more similar in showing a trait than are members of dizygotic twin pairs (see Figure 4.7), the trait is to at least some degree inherited. Hubert and her colleagues found no differences in the degree of similarity in odor sensitivity among the members of monozygotic as compared with dizygotic twin pairs, but they did find that if a subject smoked, he or she was less sensitive to some odors. Nevertheless, firm evidence on the importance of heredity in odor sensitivity is provided by the data on genetically based anosmias already described.

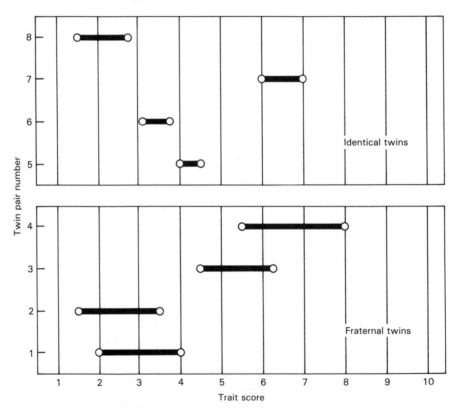

FIGURE 4.7   *Hypothetical results from an experiment comparing scores from identical and fraternal twins. The points indicate the scores of individual subjects. A line links the scores of each twin pair. In this hypothetical example, although there is considerable variation in the absolute values of the scores of both the identical and the fraternal twin pairs, the scores of the members of the identical twin pairs are more similar than those of the fraternal twin pairs. In other words, on the average, the lines linking the members of the identical twin pairs are shorter than those linking the members of the fraternal twin pairs. Therefore, in this hypothetical example, the trait being measured does seem to be at least partly a result of genetic factors.*

The environment, however, clearly affects the ability to *recognize* an odor or taste and to correctly identify its source. This ability depends on familiarity with the stimuli and their origins. For example, suppose human subjects are given the task of learning to identify the odors of many different chemicals, such as pyridine, butanol, and acetone. Suppose further that the subjects are given a great deal of practice and feedback while they are making their identifications. Experiments that have followed this strategy have found that subjects can learn to identify no more than 22 odors (the range was 6 to 22 odors).

William S. Cain obtained different results when he followed this procedure, but instead of using chemicals that had little daily significance for the subjects, he used substances whose odors were likely to occur frequently in the subjects' daily lives.[55] For example, he used chocolate, several different meats, Band-Aids, baby powder, and the like. On the average, Cain's subjects were able to identify 36 of these substances.[56]

The success of Cain's subjects in identifying odors suggests several principles of odor identification. First, it is easier to identify substances that are encountered frequently. Second, it is easier for a subject to identify an odor if he or she has associated it with a particular name for a long period of time. Third, subjects learn to identify odors more easily if they are given feedback following their attempts at identification.

These principles may help explain why we sometimes recognize an odor but cannot recall the circumstances in which we smelled it before. Such odors are usually ones for which we had no names when we smelled them previously. If you want to remember a particular odor, a good strategy would be to assign a name to that odor and then to review the circumstances associated with the odor of that name as much as possible. If you follow this procedure, then the next time you are in the supermarket or the subway and encounter that odor, you probably will not need to say "Where have I smelled that before?"

Both genetic disposition and the environment appear to be factors in the ability to detect specific odors; both heredity and environment play a role in odor sensitivity.

HEALTH IMPLICATIONS

Whether primarily due to genetic or environmental influences, the decreases in taste and odor sensitivity as a function of age have significant implications. Elderly people who cannot taste and smell well complain that their food lacks flavor; they are therefore less likely to consume a nutritionally adequate diet.[57] In addition, they are less likely to detect the odors of smoke and gas, making them more likely to succumb in a fire or when there is a gas leak.[58] Family members and health professionals need to be aware of these potential dangers so that they can take steps to help the elderly avoid them. For example, family members can ensure that their elderly relatives have working smoke alarms, and they can add extra flavorings to their elderly relatives' meals.

CONCLUSION

Our chemical senses of taste and smell are complex and subject to many different influences. Nevertheless, we must explore how these senses function if we want to understand the psychology of eating and drinking. An animal's ability to taste and smell is crucial because these senses help it determine which foods should be eaten or whether something should be eaten at all. Preference for different foods and drinks is the subject of the two chapters that follow.

CHAPTER
5

❡

Genetic Contributions to Food Preferences

"I used to drink milk all the time when I was young, but now I hardly ever do. Why did I change?"

"Why can my wife never seem to get enough sweet or salty snacks, even though she knows they are bad for her?"

"Five years ago I ate a hot dog and a few hours later got sick with the flu; I vomited several times. I still cannot stand even the thought of hot dogs. Will this ever go away?"

"Our son will not eat vegetables, but the rest of the family loves them. How did this happen? What can we do?"

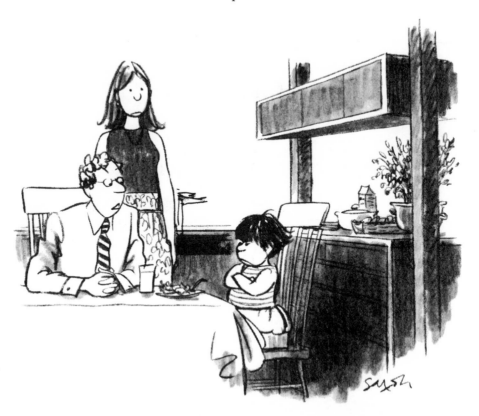

"Let's review the whole picture, Janine. You don't like milk. You don't like chicken. You don't like anything green. Now, you tell me, Janine—what does that leave us with?"

FIGURE 5.1   *Drawing by Saxon.* Copyright © 1981 The New Yorker Magazine, Inc. Reprinted by permission from *The New Yorker,* August 10, 1981,:p. 37.)

Questions such as these are frequently asked of psychologists who study eating and drinking. It seems that almost everyone, even President Bush with his well-known aversion to broccoli, has a food preference or aversion of mysterious origin, or one that he or she would like to change.[1] Parents worry about the food preferences and aversions of their children (Figure 5.1), and for good reason. Not only is a good diet synonymous with good nutrition, but diet is now known to influence the incidence and course of many diseases. For example, cutting down on saturated fats and increasing the proportion of fiber in our diets may decrease the risk of heart disease and some types of cancer.[2] Food preferences and aversions clearly have medical as well as social consequences.

To explain food preferences and aversions, information must be gathered from many sources. Therefore getting the most out of the available information on food preferences and aversions requires a willingness to look at research coming from many disparate areas of psychology.[3]

PREFERENCE, CHOICE, AND LIKING

This chapter and the next one are concerned with *food preferences,* the food selections that people and animals make when all foods are equally and simultaneously available. Food preference is not necessarily equivalent to *food choice,* because equal availability rarely exists except in the laboratory; a number of constraints affect the ease of obtaining many foods. For example, a particular food may be chosen because little work is required to obtain it. Chapter 7 discusses how people and animals make choices among foods affected by these types of constraints.

Food preference also does not necessarily correspond to *food liking.* For example, a dieter may prefer a carrot stick to a piece of chocolate cake. However, if the dieter could take a miraculous pill that prevented the absorption of calories, preference would probably reverse, revealing a liking for the chocolate cake. The consequences of consuming some foods may obscure the fact that animals and people *like* those foods. In these cases, food preference needs to be distinguished from food liking. Food preference, food choice, and food liking refer to overlapping, but not precisely equivalent, behaviors concerning which foods are consumed.

FOOD PREFERENCES: GENETIC AND ENVIRONMENTAL CONTRIBUTIONS

Because much of the research on food preferences comes from disparate sources, it will be helpful to begin with three particular food preferences and group a great deal of information around them: the preferences for sweet foods, for salty foods, and for milk and milk products. Describing them will introduce many of the themes and problems common to all studies of food preferences.

These three food preferences were chosen for the present chapter because, to at least some degree, most people prefer them at some point in their lives. The fact that these preferences are virtually universal, despite the varied circumstances in which people grow and mature, suggests that they are substantially genetically determined and that possession of these preferences has resulted in increased inclusive fitness.

Knowing the extent to which taste and food preferences are genetically determined can help us understand how to change undesirable food preferences. If a food preference or aversion is determined primarily by the genes, it will be difficult to change that preference by changing the environment. If a preference is primarily the result of learning, changing it by changing the environment will be less difficult. Following discussion of the origins of the preferences for sweet foods, salty foods, and milk and milk products, the remainder of this chapter will focus on more general evidence for food preferences that appear to be largely genetically determined. The next chapter will focus on evidence for food preferences that appear to be largely the result of learning.

It is important to remember that no trait is entirely determined by the genes or by the environment. For example, whether a fetus develops as a male or as a female is generally thought to depend on the genes. But if the necessary amount of male hormone is not present at the appropriate time during gestation, a genetic male can develop into an apparent female.[4] How to sing a particular song is learned. But without vocal cords and a mouth, which are genetically determined, singing that song would be impossible.

PREFERENCE FOR SWEET

Prevalence of the Preference for Sweet

Few people need to be convinced that there is a general preference among humans for sweet foods and drinks. Despite their diverse origins, almost everyone in the United States can find room for Jell-O, and many people can find room for anything sweet, even after a satisfying dinner.

People of any age are likely to pick sweet foods over others.[5] This is also frequently true of many other species, for example, horses, bears, and ants.[6] Common laboratory lore holds that if you are having trouble training your rat to press a lever in a Skinner box, smearing a little milk chocolate on the lever will solve the problem.

It is not surprising that many species have a preference for sweet foods and drinks. Sweet foods and drinks tend to have a high concentration of sugar, and therefore of calories. Calories provide energy for the body and are necessary for the body to function. In the natural environments of most species, digestible calories are not freely available and frequently are not available in sufficient amounts. Therefore a preference for a concentrated source of calories is likely to confer an evolutionary advantage on animals that have that preference.[7]

Like many other species, *Homo sapiens* first appeared in an environment in which available calories were often few and far between.[8] One concentrated source of sugar and therefore of calories was ripe fruit, which can be distinguished from unripe fruit by its sweetness. In addition to sugar, fruit provides many vitamins and minerals necessary for body function and growth. A preference for sweet foods and drinks that would encourage consumption of ripe fruit was probably advantageous to our early ancestors.[9]

Now, thanks to advanced technology, most people can count on having a variety of cheap foods and drinks readily available that contain sugar but very little else. From cupcakes to cola, candy to Cocoa Pebbles (46 percent sugar by dry weight), we are confronted at every turn with foods whose main nutritive value consists of the calories they provide.[10] Because sweet foods and drinks are so cheaply and easily available and are advertised so much, and because of our preference for sweet, we tend to consume these foods and drinks instead of others. The result in highly developed countries such as the United States is that we consume too much sugar and not enough of other nutrients. This not only degrades nutrition but also can increase the incidence of cavities, heart disease, and obesity, all of which are significant health problems.[11] It is essential for our health that we understand what causes our preference for sweet foods and drinks and what factors do affect and can affect that preference.

First Exposure to Sweet

J. A. Desor, Owen Maller, and Robert E. Turner[12] have studied newborn infants' preference for sweet fluids. The fluids were presented to the infants in bottles, and the researchers measured the amounts that the infants consumed. The infants preferred the sweet fluids to water, and they consumed more of the sweet fluids as the concentration of the sugar in those fluids was increased. Although it is not clear whether the prelacteal feeding influenced the sweet preference of these 1- to 3-day-old infants, the existence of a preference for sweet at such an early age suggests a strong genetic component in the determinants of the preference for sweet.

There have been several documented instances in which a culture that lacked sweet foods and drinks (with the exception of milk, which is slightly sweet) came into contact with a culture that regularly consumed sweet foods and drinks. In these cases none of the cultures previously without sugar rejected the sugar-containing foods and drinks of the other culture.[13] The Eskimos of northern Alaska are an example of such a sugar-adapting culture.[14] As in Desor, Maller, and Turner's research with newborns, these

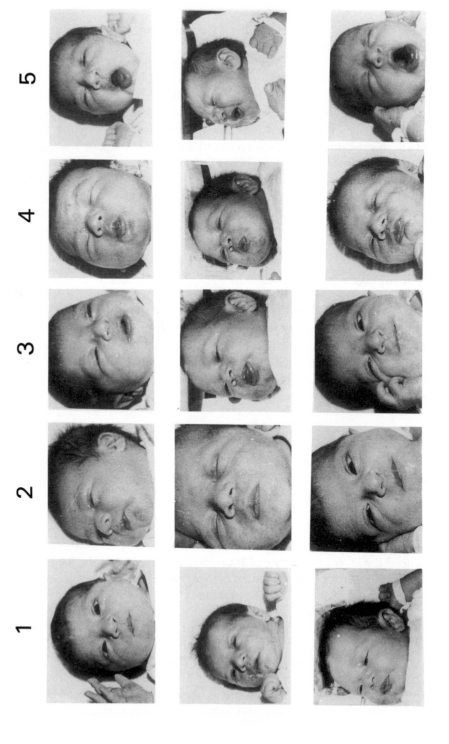

cases indicate that early experience is not a requirement for a person to prefer sweet tastes.

Facial Expression

Additional evidence supporting genetic determination of the preference for sweet comes from research on facial expressions accompanying taste stimuli. Jacob E. Steiner[15] has shown that human infants, tested prior to any breast or bottle feeding, show a facial expression very similar to that of adults when something sweet is tasted (see Figure 5.2):

> The sweet stimulus leads to a marked relaxation of the face, resembling an expression of "satisfaction." This expression is often accompanied by a slight smile and was almost always followed by an eager licking of the upper lip, and sucking movements. This licking and sucking is almost "aloud" sucking. The facial play elicited by the sucrose stimulus was labeled by the observers of the films and pictures as an expression of appreciation, liking or enjoyment.[16]

One might argue that these responses could be due to imitation of the facial expressions of the researcher presenting the taste stimuli; perhaps researchers unconsciously show an expression of satisfaction when delivering a sweet stimulus, and infants have been shown to imitate facial expressions as early as 36 hours after birth.[17] However, this argument cannot be made when rats are the subjects. In fact, rats also make a facial expression of satisfaction when a sweet stimulus is placed on their tongues, and both normal rats and rats missing the upper portions of their brains do this.[18] Note that these characteristic responses to a sweet taste, as described by Steiner, result in ingestion of the sweet substance. The acceptance of sweet substances in many cases appears to be a reflex, a reflex that can occur without conscious awareness.

FIGURE 5.2   *Facial expressions of newborn infants.* Typical features of the Gustofacial Response, recorded in neonate infants between birth and the first feeding. 1: Resting face. 2: Reaction to distilled water (control). 3: Response to sweet stimulus. 4: Lip-pursing, response to sour stimulus. 5: Response to bitter stimulus. (Reprinted with permission from J. E. Steiner, "Facial Expressions of the Neonate Infant Indicating the Hedonics of Food-Related Chemical Stimuli," in *Taste and Development*, ed. J. M. Weiffenbach, Bethesda, MD: U.S. Department of Health, Education, and Welfare, 1977.)

Chapter 5

Imprinting

The prevalence of *prelacteal feeding* in many cultures could be an environmental determinant of the preference for sweet. Infants are often given some sort of solution of sugar and water soon after birth. In the United States a solution of 5 percent glucose has frequently been given.[19] In comparison, breast milk and cow's milk are far less sweet; they contain 7 percent and 4.8 percent lactose, respectively, and lactose has only about one-fifth the sweetening power of glucose.[20] Whatever may be the medical reasons for this supplementary prelacteal feeding, the very first feeding of many infants has consisted of nothing but sugar and water. It is possible that this practice has resulted in a type of *imprinting* phenomenon, in which early exposure to a stimulus results in a long-term increased preference for that stimulus.[21]

Supporting this hypothesis, Gary K. Beauchamp and Marianne Moran[22] showed that 6-month-old infants who were being fed sweetened water preferred sweetened water more than 6-month-old infants who were not being fed sweetened water. It therefore seems possible that prelacteal feeding could influence later food preferences, although there is not yet definitive proof of this influence. The greater preference for sweet shown by the infants being fed sweetened water could have been due simply to greater familiarity with the taste of sweet (see Chapter 6).

For rats the evidence is clear: There is no imprinting involved in their preference for sweet. Judith J. Wurtman and Richard J. Wurtman exposed rat pups, 16 to 30 days of age, to one of three nutritionally equivalent diets containing either 0, 12, or 48 percent *sucrose* (table sugar). Between 31 and 63 days of age, the rats were switched from diet to diet, so that eventually each rat had access to all three diets. During this period of switching diets the rats' total consumption of sucrose from all three diets was unrelated to early diet exposure.[23]

Sweet Detection

An additonal line of evidence suggesting a significant genetic component in the preference for sweet concerns the existence and prevalence of physiological mechanisms specifically for detecting sweet tastes. As discussed in Chapter 4, the evidence for the existence of sweet receptors on the tongue is fairly substantial. Nevertheless, evidence that the genes impart a specific ability to taste sweet substances is not the same as evidence for a genetic preference for sweet substances.

However, additional physiological specialization for tasting sweet substances is found in the chorda tympani, the nerve that relays taste sensations from the tongue to the brain. In many species the chorda tympani contains more fibers maximally sensitive to the taste of sweet than fibers maximally sensitive to any other taste.[24] This suggests that the sweet taste is more important to the body than any other taste, again indicating that the preference for sweet has a substantial genetic component.

Conversely, early extensive experience with sugar could increase the sensitivity of chorda tympani fibers to sweet. In rats, early exposure to an odor has been shown to increase neural responses to that odor.[25] To eliminate this possibility for the taste of sweet, experiments are needed that use either neonates or subjects with no previous exposure to sweet.

Age Differences

Both humans and rats show a greater preference for the taste of sweet when they are young, and less preference for it when they are older. J. A. Desor, Lawrence S. Greene, and Owen Maller[26] demonstrated this by comparing people 9 to 15 years of age with adults, and Judith J. Wurtman and Richard J. Wurtman[27] obtained similar findings when they compared rats pre- and postpuberty. Both of these studies involved measuring actual consumption of sucrose. A. W. Logue and Michael E. Smith,[28] in a questionnaire study using human subjects between 14 and 68 years of age, found that older subjects tended to report lower preferences for sweet foods than did younger subjects. J. A. Desor and Gary K. Beauchamp[29] examined preferences for the taste of specific concentrations of sucrose in 11- to 15-year-old human subjects, and then again when these subjects were 19 to 25 years old. During the intervening time period, the subjects' preferred concentration of sucrose decreased. In general, adults consume less sugar than do children,[30] although this difference might be due to increased adult concern about weight gain and/or nutritious eating. Together, all of these findings support the hypothesis that, as a result of the usually greater caloric requirements of younger, prepubertal, growing organisms, some mechanism has evolved that automatically increases these subjects' preference for sweet,[31] independent of individuals' actual caloric needs. Consistent with this hypothesis, rats' gustatory neuronal activity has been shown to be a function of the blood glucose level, such that there is more activity when blood glucose level is low and when the need for glucose is therefore high.[32]

Gender Differences

One strategy for identifying possible genetic influences on the preference for sweet is to look for gender differences. For this strategy to yield meaningful information, the researchers need to study males and females who ingful information, the researchers need to study males and females who have been treated similarly following birth. One way to do this is simply to use newborns as subjects. A number of researchers have examined newborns to see if the preference for sweet fluids differed between male and female subjects. Unfortunately, the results have been inconclusive. Richard E. Nisbett and Sharon B. Gurwitz's results have indicated that female newborns prefer sweet fluids more than do male newborns,[33] while other experiments have shown no difference.[34] Because these studies used different methods (Nisbett and Gurwitz allowed the infants to consume as much as they wanted, but the other experimenters allowed consumption for only a brief period), it is difficult to come to any conclusions about differences between male and female newborns in their preference for sweet.

Findings from research with older subjects are also inconclusive due to noncomparable methodologies. Consistent with the results of the Nisbett and Gurwitz study, Logue and Smith's[35] questionnaire study of people between 14 and 68 years of age found that female subjects tended to report higher preferences for sweet foods than did male subjects. In contrast, when Greene, Desor, and Maller[36] gave 9- to 15-year-old subjects four different concentrations of sucrose, the male subjects preferred the higher concentrations more than did the female subjects. Other recent studies have also obtained conflicting results, some finding a greater preference for sweet foods in men, and others in women.[37] Because the methods of all these studies were so different, it is difficult to say whether or not their results are contradictory.

The only firm conclusion that can be drawn regarding gender differences in the preference for sweet is that, as yet, no consistent, striking differences have been demonstrated.

Fructose Intolerance

Fragmentary evidence supporting the idea that the environment contributes to sweet preference has come from research done with people who are fructose intolerant. People with fructose intolerance are unable to digest *fructose,* a sugar present in fruit and honey. If these people do consume fructose, they become nauseated and pale, they vomit, they develop diarrhea, and eventually they may lose consciousness. Because one of the products of sucrose during digestion is fructose, people who are fructose intolerant can consume neither sucrose nor fructose.

What is relevant here about the behavior of people who are fructose intolerant is that they learn to decrease their consumption of sucrose and fructose.[38] This would seem to suggest that the preference for sweet substances is modifiable by environmental contingencies, and therefore that the genetic contribution to the preference for sweet must not be very large. However, this may be a case of a discrepancy between food preference and food liking, as defined earlier in the chapter. A liking for a food and the frequency of consuming that food need not be related.[39] In fact, some fructose-intolerant individuals persist in eating small amounts of fructose and sucrose and risking the consequences.[40]

Environmental Contingencies

There is some evidence that food preferences can be affected by environmental contingencies. For example, rats learn to prefer the same foods that other rats they come in contact with prefer,[41] young children can come to prefer the same foods that the people they eat with prefer, and children develop an increased preference for foods that are given as rewards or that are accompanied by attention from adults.[42] However, none of the research responsible for these findings has been specifically directed at the preference for sweet. Here it is sufficient to say that there are known environmental mechanisms that can affect food preferences. Whether or not they are important in the preference for sweet is not clear.

Economic change (an environmental contingency) can affect the consumption of sweet foods and beverages. For example, per-capita consumption of sugar increases as the economy of a country develops.[43] However, food preference is not necessarily the same as food choice. If foods and beverages with a high sugar content become relatively less expensive as the economy of a country develops, those foods and drinks would probably be consumed more. But preference for those foods and drinks would not necessarily have increased in a situation in which price was irrelevant.

Customarily Sweetened Foods

Gary K. Beauchamp and Beverly J. Cowart[44] think that the greatest influence of the environment on the preference for sweet is not on the preference for sweet itself, but on the particular foods that we prefer to be sweetened. Adults do not wish a sugar coating to be added to pot roast or fried eggs, but they would often prefer to eat ice cream or cake rather than the pot roast or fried eggs. Our culinary experiences, which may be very different for different cultures (see Chapter 14), determine which foods we expect to be sweet. For example, in the United States chocolate is usually sweeted, but in traditional Mexican cuisine it is often not. As adults, it is by means of our preferences for commonly sweetened foods that we demonstrate our preference for sweet.

Chapter 5

Twin Studies

The traditional way of assessing the heritability of a trait has been through the use of twin studies. Lawrence S. Greene, J. A. Desor, and Owen Maller conducted a study with identical and fraternal twins that was designed to assess the extent of genetic contributions to certain taste preferences.[45] The members of each fraternal twin pair were of the same gender. Of both the identical and the fraternal twins, some pairs were male and some were female. In this type of study, if genes play a role in determining a trait, an identical twin pair will, on the average, be more similar with respect to that trait than will a fraternal twin pair (see Chapter 4 for additional explanation of twin studies).

Greene and his colleagues asked the twins in their study to rank their preference for four different concentrations of sucrose, *lactose* (the sugar that is present in milk), and *sodium chloride* (salt). The results showed that the preferences of the subjects correlated poorly with the preferences of their twin brothers or sisters, be they identical or fraternal twins. The members of a twin pair do not appear to have similar preferences for sucrose, lactose, and sodium chloride.

One way to interpret these findings is to say that the preferences for sucrose, lactose, and sodium chloride are not inherited; the preferences of the identical twin pairs were no more similar than the preferences of the fraternal twin pairs. However, if these taste preferences are not inherited, they must be environmentally determined. Because twins, both identical and fraternal, share much of the same environment, their taste preferences should therefore all be somewhat similar. But this was not found to be the case.

A possible explanation for this paradox, and the fact that other twin studies have also found low heritability for preference for sweet foods,[46] is that the reported ratings had limited range, and that this, not a lack of genetic determination, was responsible for the low correlations. Without sufficient range, it is difficult to determine statistically if some subjects are more alike than others. Some subjects must score high on a trait and some must score low for an analysis of this kind to succeed. In Green and his colleagues' study, subjects' ratings could vary only between 2.4 and 6.4. Further, the mean ratings for sucrose by the monozygotic and dizygotic twins were 4.8 and 4.7, respectively, virtually identical, with a standard error for each group of subjects of only 0.2 (a standard error is a measure of data variance). In other words, all of the subjects in this study tended to respond very similarly. Therefore the possibility that individuals are genetically predisposed to prefer similar concentrations of sucrose must be considered.

It is possible that all humans easily learn a preference for sweet, but even so, the ease of such learning and the virtual universality of the preference for sweet in cultures that have sweet foods and drinks available suggests a strong genetic component in the preference for sweet. Traits that are largely determined by the genes usually show some variability due to variations in their survival value for different breeding populations. However, all species need food, and the taste of sweet is often a good indicator of a food source. Therefore one would expect a genetically determined preference for sweet to show little variation as a result of natural selection.

Breeding Experiments

Rats, one of many species that show a preference for sweet foods and beverages, can be selectively bred to have a greater or lesser preference for sweet.[47] The fact that this is possible shows clearly that genes can play a role in the preference for sweet in rats. However, this does not, of course, necessarily mean that genes make a significant contribution to the preference for sweet in humans.

PREFERENCE FOR SALT

Prevalence of the Preference for Salt

Like calories, salt is essential for the body to function properly, in humans as well as many other species. Many physiological functions depend on the presence of salt and even on a particular concentration of salt.[48] For example, the concentration of salt in the blood must be kept at a specific level. Small amounts of salt are lost continually through sweat and through the action of the kidneys. If someone ceased to ingest salt, the body would excrete water in an attempt to keep the concentration of salt in the blood at the optimal level. Eventually that person would die of dehydration.[49]

Salt is necessary for the body to function properly, but unfortunately it is not easily available in the wild. Prior to industrialization, humans sometimes had great difficulty obtaining enough salt. Many species must constantly seek salt in order to have sufficient amounts. Therefore it would not be surprising that natural selection would result in an innate preference for salt and that this preference would be present in most species.[50]

The evidence strongly supports this suggestion. First, with the exception of newborn infants (see below), the preference for salt is ubiquitous, and it is one of the strongest preferences shown by humans and other species.[51] Many species, including humans, show a strong preference for salt the first time they taste it.[52] Rats will always drink a salt solution when it is presented in the absence of other fluids or food.[53]

Physiological Need

The appetite for salt depends, at least to some extent, on biological need independent of learning. The preference for salt increases following sodium deprivation, and the release of angiotensin and aldosterone (see Chapter 3) may be a factor in this preference increase.[54] Robert J. Contreras and Marion Frank have investigated one aspect of the physiological basis for this phenomenon.[55] First they deprived rats of sodium for 10 days. This amount of deprivation induced a behavioral preference for sodium. Then they measured the responses of various fibers in the chorda tympani nerve to various concentrations of sodium.

They found that while the lowest concentration of sodium that would induce a response in the nerve did not change, the slope of the function relating the stimulus concentration to the response of the nerve was less steep following sodium deprivation. In other words, following deprivation, a higher concentration of salt was necessary to make the nerve respond as vigorously as before. After deprivation the rat would therefore perceive a particular concentration of salt as equivalent to a lower concentration prior to deprivation, and would prefer saltier foods. This change appears to be automatically programmed by the rat's physiology, and not dependent on the rat's having had previous experience with sodium deprivation. However, despite these automatic physiological changes, experience can still modify the expression of a need-based sodium preference. A sodium-deficient rat will eat less of a sodium-enriched diet if it has recently interacted with other rats that are not sodium-deprived.[56]

Need-based preference for salt has also been documented in porcupines living in the Catskill Mountains in New York State.[57] These porcupines must maintain approximately equal amounts of potassium and sodium in their bodies in order to remain healthy. However, the summer vegetation in the Catskills generally contains at least a 300-to-1 ratio of potassium to sodium. As the porcupine's body works to remove the excess potassium, it also removes the sodium, and the porcupines cannot keep sufficient amounts of sodium in their bodies. Therefore the porcupines seek out sources of sodium (such as sodium chloride) that contain no potassium. The locations of two such sources are the salt left on the sides of roads from the previous winter and the wood on the sides of barns. Seeking out salt in either of these two locations is extremely dangerous for the porcupines, for in one case they are likely to get run over and in the other they are likely to get shot by an angry farmer. Yet the majority of porcupines are driven to areas of human habitation by their need for sodium.

Evidence for the influence of physiological state on the preference for salt is not limited to rats and porcupines. In 1940 L. Wilkins and C. P. Richter published a letter written to them by the parents of a boy who had an unusual preference for salt due to an adrenal tumor (see Box 5.1).[58] The boy had died in a hospital because the hospital diet did not give him the salt that he craved and his body needed.

Desor, Greene, and Maller[59] have shown that, similar to their results with the taste of sweet, 9- to 15-year-old human subjects prefer saltier solutions than do adults. Again, these findings may be related to the evolutionary history of humans. If, during this history there was generallly an increased need for sodium by younger, growing subjects, some automatic mechanism that generates relatively high salt preferences in these subjects, independent of actual sodium need, could have evolved.

Excess Consumption of Salt

Great physiological need is not a prerequisite for consumption of large amounts of salt. Like sweet foods, salty foods are more easily and inexpensively available now than when humans first evolved. Consequently, the preference for salt, like the preference for sweet, has resulted in consumption of salt in amounts far exceeding the body's needs: in the United States, an average of 4 to 6 grams per adult per day, as compared with the 1.1 to 3.3 grams per adult per day that have been found to be adequate and safe. This excess consumption may be a contributing factor to one of the major health problems in developed countries: hypertension.[60] Not only can excess salt consumption by adults lead to increased blood pressure; consumption of large amounts of salt by children may lead to hypertension in adulthood. However, ingestion of large amounts of potassium may help prevent the development of sodium-induced hypertension.[61]

Because the preference for salt is so strong, so prevalent, and so affected by physiological need, it has been described as *sodium hunger.*[62] Nevertheless, learning can also affect the preference for salt, as described in more detail in the next section.

Development of the Preference for Salty Foods

Gary K. Beauchamp and his colleagues, similar to their work on the development of preference for sweet foods, have examined the development of preference for salty foods when there is no specific physiological

BOX 5.1

Excessive Preference for Salt in a Boy with an Adrenal Tumor

When he was around a year old he started licking all the salt off the crackers and always asked for more. He didn't say any words at this time, but he had a certain sound for everything and a way of letting us know what he wanted. . . . [H]e started chewing the crackers; but he only chewed them until he got the salt off, then he would spit them out. He did the same with bacon, but he didn't swallow the pieces. . . . In an effort to try to find a food that he would like well enough to chew up and swallow, we gave him a taste of practically everything. So, one evening during supper, when he was about eighteen months old, we used some salt out of the shaker on some food. He wanted some, too. We gave him just a few grains to taste, thinking he wouldn't like it; but he ate it and asked for more. . . . [T]his one time was all it took for him to learn what was in the shaker. For a few days after that, when I would feed him his dinner alone at noon, he would keep crying for something that wasn't on the table and always

pointed to the cupboard. I didn't think of the salt, so I held him up in front of the cupboard to see what he wanted. He picked out the salt at once; and in order to see what he would do with it, I let him have it. He poured some out and ate it by dipping his finger in it. After this he wouldn't eat any food without the salt, too. I would purposely let it off the table and even hide it from him until I could ask the doctor about it. . . . But when I asked Dr. _____ about it, he said, "Let him have it. It won't hurt him." So we gave it to him and never tried to stop it altogether. . . . [B]ut he wouldn't eat his breakfast or supper without it. He really cried for it and acted like he had to have it. . . . At eighteen months he was just starting to say a few words, and salt was among the first ones. We had found that practically everything he liked real well was salty, such as crackers, pretzels, potato chips, olives, pickles, fresh fish, salt mackerel, crisp bacon and most foods and vegetables if I added more salt.

From L. Wilkins and C. P. Richter, "A Great Craving for Salt by a Child with Cortico-Adrenal Insufficiency," Journal of the American Medical Association 114(1940):866–867. *Copyright 1940, American Medical Association.*

need for salt.[63] They have found that at birth, human infants show no preference between water and a salt solution. This lack of preference is probably a lack of discrimination; newborn humans may not be able to taste salt well. Apparently, at around 4 months of age, the ability to taste salt increases and infants now prefer a salt solution to plain water. Another change occurs after about 24 months of age; now children have learned which foods are supposed to be salty and reject foods that do not contain the customary degree of saltiness. As people get older, it is possible to decrease their need-free preference for salt to some extent by giving them weeks of experience only with foods with relatively low salt content.

Consistent with these findings, several researchers have found that when the usual salt content of foods is reduced, and people are allowed free access to a salt shaker, they do not add as much salt as has been removed from the food. In fact, they add only about 20 percent of the salt that has been removed. One possible explanation for these findings is based on the fact that food tastes saltier when the salt is concentrated on its surface than when the salt is dispersed throughout the food's entire contents. Perhaps the saltiness the mouth experiences, not the amount of sodium actually ingested, is responsible for how much someone prefers a salty food.[64] Thus it appears that reduced-salt diets should be successful not only in decreasing salt consumption but also in decreasing salt preference. Beauchamp and his colleagues have described a universal taste preference, initially largely under genetic control, whose expression is subsequently modified by environmental experience.

PREFERENCE FOR MILK AND MILK PRODUCTS

Group Differences in Milk Consumption and Lactose Intolerance

At birth virtually every human infant avidly consumes milk (perhaps not surprising given that milk contains a type of sugar, lactose). However, milk and milk products are not consumed equally often by all groups of adult humans. Some groups, such as Northern Europeans, not only drink a great deal of milk but also eat a great deal of milk products, such as cheese. Other groups, such as the Chinese, consume neither milk nor its products. Still other groups, such as the Hausa-Fulani of Nigeria, consume yogurt but do not drink milk.

In addition to differences in milk consumption, these groups show differences in what is called *lactose intolerance*, the inability to digest the sugar present in milk. An individual's lactose intolerance is determined by the amount of *lactase*, the enzyme that breaks down lactose, he or she has. In people who have sufficient amounts of lactase, lactose is broken down into glucose and other products. In people who have insufficient amounts of lactase, the lactose passes undigested into the colon. There, the molecules of lactose create osmotic pressure that causes water to be drawn into the intestine. At the same time, bacteria living in the gastrointestinal tract ferment the lactose. If substantial amounts of milk have been drunk, the result is sufficient diarrhea, with organic acids and carbon dioxide gas to be unpleasant for both the person lacking the lactase and for those nearby. This intolerance of lactose can cause death in infants.

Groups that tend to drink milk are made up of people who tend to have amounts of lactase sufficient to digest large amounts of milk. Groups that tend not to drink milk are made up of people who tend to have amounts of lactase insufficient to digest large amounts of milk. Most groups are of the latter type. The known exceptions are Northern Europeans, of whom approximately 90 percent are lactose tolerant, and a few African tribes, of whom approximately 80 percent are lactose tolerant (Figure 5.3). Groups that consume cheese and yogurt but do not drink milk are made up of people who tend not to have large amounts of lactase.[65] Cheese and yogurt are milk products that have already been fermented by bacteria, and they possess relatively small amounts of lactose. Therefore lactase is not needed to digest these foods.

Origins of Group Differences

At birth virtually all humans are lactose tolerant; they are able to digest milk, their primary food. However, by $1\frac{1}{2}$ to 3 years of age, most humans have become largely unable to manufacture lactase, a loss that is shared with all adults of all other species. Adult humans who can digest milk are the exception in the adult animal world.[66] The question is, how did this exception arise?

One possibility is that humans who continue to drink milk throughout their lifetimes simply maintain their ability to manufacture lactase.[67] The offspring of all mammals are weaned early in life to allow more nutrition for the mother or for her subsequent offspring. Humans are able to continue drinking milk into adulthood because of their domestication of other species that produce milk. Nevertheless, experiments have shown that even if lactose-intolerant adult humans or rats are fed large amounts of lactose for long periods, there are only slight increases in lactase activity, if any.[68]

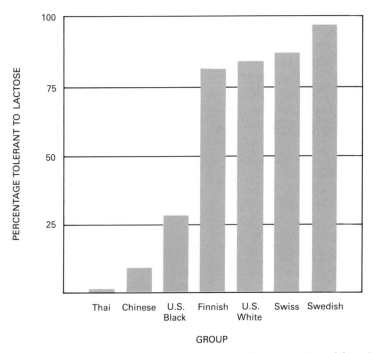

FIGURE 5.3   *Percentage of various groups tolerant to lactose.* (Adapted from N. Kretchmer, "Lactose and Lactase," in *Human Nutrition,* San Francisco: W. H. Freeman and Company, 1978.)

It now appears that lactase manufacture is genetically determined. Further, the genes for lactase secretion in maturity are dominant. If someone who is unable to digest lactose conceives a child with someone who can digest lactose, the child is likely to be lactose tolerant.[69] Therefore the answer to the question of why some groups of individuals tend to possess lactase and to drink milk and some groups of individuals tend not to possess lactase and not to drink milk may lie in some evolutionary advantage for one or the other group.

The most popular hypothesis is that humans first domesticated cattle for their meat and/or for the work they can do. During humans' evolutionary history, those adult humans who could digest the milk of these livestock in times of famine would have had a selective advantage over those who could not, and so the frequency of the genes for producing lactase would have increased in future generations. This selective advantage would have been particularly helpful to those adult humans living far from the equator. There is more cloud cover and less sunlight away from the equator than near it. Sunlight on the skin of humans results in the synthesis of vitamin D, a vitamin that assists in the necessary absorption of calcium into the body.[70] Because the digestion of lactose by lactase also assists with the absorption of calcium, consumption of lactose accompanied by lactase manufacture may have assisted the survival of human adults living away from the equator. Consistent with this hypothesis, most groups of people who possess large amounts of lactase tend to keep cattle, to drink milk from those cattle, and to live far from the equator.[71]

Implications

Clearly the ability to digest milk is determined by the genes. Infants and groups of adults who can digest milk drink it, and groups of adults who cannot digest it do not drink it. But does this mean that a preference for drinking milk is genetically determined? It may be possible to say that for a large proportion of all people, genetic input influences whether that group does or does not drink milk. Further, as will be discussed in more detail in Chapter 14, the genetic tendency of a group of people to manufacture or not to manufacture large amounts of lactase may be reflected in the traditional practices of food preparation and consumption within the group.

However, if someone in that group differs from the rest of the group in the ability to produce lactase, that person may learn to consume different amounts of lactose than are regularly consumed by the rest of the group. For example, in the United States the majority of adults are lactose tolerant, and milk is widely touted as a healthy food. But if an intolerant adult American consumes substantial amounts of milk as prescribed by the American culture and suffers the adverse consequences, he or she may learn to avoid further consumption of milk. Nevertheless, this decreased consumption may not reflect a change in his or her liking for milk, in the same way that avoidance of sugar by people who are fructose intolerant does not necessarily indicate a dislike for sugar.[72]

Although the preference for milk and milk products clearly has a genetic basis, it also illustrates how environment as well as genes may influence which foods an animal consumes.[73]

GENERAL EVIDENCE FOR GENETIC CONTRIBUTIONS

Because no trait is entirely determined by heredity or by the environment, investigations of the heritability of traits must often look where the weight of the evidence falls. In the cases of the preferences for sweet foods, salty foods, and milk, there is strong evidence for genetic determination, although the environment clearly also plays a role. The next sections consider more general evidence for the genetic contributions to food preferences.

Physiological Need

The preferences for sugar and salt are not the only preferences that change automatically following deprivation. Jeanne Pager[74] has shown that neural responses to the odors of some foods change when rats are deprived of food. There are more positive neural responses and fewer negative neural responses to these foods following deprivation.

Pager's data are consistent with those of George D. Mower, Robert G. Mair, and Trygg Engen,[75] who found that adult humans tended to rate the odors and tastes of food as more pleasant the more they were deprived of food. Nevertheless, the subjects' judgments of the intensity of the stimuli did not change as a function of their deprivation state. The subjects tasted various concentrations of sucrose and smelled various concentrations of orange, chocolate, and maple odors. Mower and his colleagues noted that all of the changes in pleasantness reported by their subjects were changes that, if reflected in changes in actual food consumption, would have helped to restore the homeostasis disrupted by the subjects' food deprivation.

Similarly, Judith J. Wurtman and Richard J. Wurtman have collected data consistent with the hypothesis that ingestion of certain types of foods can affect preference for other types of foods. Wurtman and Wurtman believe that this is because food intake modifies chemical transmission between neurons in the brain. This modification, they feel, then changes the probability of what will subsequently be eaten. For example, if breakfast has consisted mostly of carbohydrates, people tend to eat more proteins at lunch, and vice versa.[76] However, the degree to which Wurtman and Wurtman's results apply to daily eating situations outside the laboratory is controversial.[77]

Nevertheless, regardless of the precise mechanism, it appears that one of the strategies the body sometimes uses to restore homeostasis in cases of deprivation of certain substances is to automatically increase preference for those substances.

Facial Expression

In addition to the facial expression that accompanies sweet tastes, newborn humans also make characteristic facial expressions when they experience sour and bitter tastes (see Figure 5.2). The expression shown in response to a bitter taste has been described as follows:

Stimulation with the bitter fluid leads to a typical arch form opening of the mouth with the upper lip elevated, the mouth angles depressed, and the tongue protruded in a flat position. This expression involves primarily the mouth region of the face and . . . was typically followed by spitting or even by the preparatory movements of vomiting.[78]

The expression in response to a sour stimulus has been described as follows:

The sour stimulus leads to a lip-pursing, in a fashion known as the "Darwin's pursing of the lips," [that] may be either continuous or repetative [sic]. This is often accompanied or followed by a wrinkling of the nose and blinking of the eyes.[79]

The response to bitter was described as a rejection response by adults who watched videotapes of infants making that response.[80] It resembles the rejection response that rats make when they are given an aversive substance to taste.[81]

These data, together with the data on the characteristic facial response to sweet, suggest that there are two distinct inborn taste response systems: an acceptance system and a rejection system. These two systems are present in humans, rats, and perhaps other species, and they appear to be genetically linked to certain taste stimuli. The acceptance system appears to be genetically linked to sweet stimuli, and the rejection system to bitter stimuli. These two response systems increase the probability that newborns without taste experience, or animals experiencing new taste stimuli, will ingest substances that provide calories but will not ingest bitter substances that could be poisonous.[82]

Age Differences

Taste sensitivity apparently declines with age, as a result of physiological changes that are largely independent of environmental effects.

If taste sensitivity declines with age, perhaps food preferences also change with age. Declining taste sensitivity should be accompanied by increasing acceptability of a variety of foods, particularly strong-tasting foods. Several studies seem to confirm this hypothesis.

Henry C. Lindgren and his colleagues have found that older subjects dislike fewer foods than do younger subjects.[83] Similarly, E. V. Glanville and A. R. Kaplan[84] found that the taste sensitivity to 6-n-propylthiouracil (PROP), a bitter substance, declines with age, and that taste sensitivity to this substance correlates well with the subjects' stated preferences for bitter foods. Logue and Smith[85] found that older subjects tended to report lower preferences for sweet foods and higher preferences for spicy foods (e.g., chili pepper) than did younger subjects.

All of these data are consistent with the hypothesis that the decline in taste sensitivity with age affects food preferences. Other factors, however, such as increased familiarity with a variety of foods, could also be responsible for the findings reported here. These factors will be discussed in the next chapter.

Sensation Seeking

According to Marvin Zuckerman,[86] *sensation seeking* is the tendency to seek out new or unusual experiences. Zuckerman measures sensation seeking using a questionnaire. For each question, subjects are asked to indicate which of two alternatives best represents their feelings. For example, in one question subjects must choose between "I like 'wild' uninhibited parties" and "I prefer quiet parties with good conversation."

Several studies using Zuckerman's questionnaire have shown significant correlations of levels of sensation seeking with certain food preferences. For example, George B. Kish and Gregory V. Donnenwerth[87] found that subjects who scored high on sensation seeking also tended to report preferences for spicy, sour, crunchy foods, compared with bland, sweet, soft foods. Logue and Smith[88] found similar results, with subjects who scored high on sensation seeking tending to report a greater preference for spicy foods, and subjects who scored low on sensation seeking tending to report a greater preference for bland and sweet foods. Logue and Smith also noted that subjects who scored high on sensation seeking tended to prefer items such as alcohol and shellfish, foods that are often reputed to cause illness; but subjects who scored low on sensation seeking tended to prefer items such as bread and corn, foods that are rarely reputed to cause illness.

Because there appear to be many relationships between sensation seeking and food preferences, there may be a common basis for some aspects of sensation seeking and some food preferences. Based on studies comparing sensation-seeking correlations between identical and fraternal twins, Zuckerman[89] has argued that there is a genetic component to sensation seeking, that sensation seeking is heritable. To the extent that Zuckerman's data are reliable, his findings raise the possibility that some food preferences may also have a genetic component.

CONCLUSION

There appear to be substantial genetic contributions to many food preferences. Among these are the preferences for sweet foods, salty foods, and milk. The genes also appear responsible, at least to some extent, for the acceptance response system for sweet substances, the rejection response system for bitter substances, the tendency of certain food preferences to be correlated with levels of sensation seeking, and the increased preference for different and strong tasting foods with advancing age.

The changes in food preferences as a function of age may simply be due to the decrease in taste sensitivity that occurs with age, or they could be due to changes in nutritional requirements that also occur with age. Both mechanisms are largely independent of the environment.

Preferences for sweet foods, salty foods, and milk (away from the equator) as well as aversions to bitter-tasting foods, are traits that would usually have been advantageous to our evolving ancestors. Therefore it would not be surprising if humans have evolved possessing genes that contribute to these traits. Behaviors with a strong genetic component tend to be those whose performance is almost always followed by the same consequences, be they positive or negative. An organism is more likely to survive if it performs those behaviors correctly the first time, without a learning period.[90] Perhaps seeking out new experiences and sensations is also advantageous in certain situations, be it the experience of parachuting from a plane or of eating a new food, and perhaps this tendency has resulted in a genetic influence on sensation seeking.

But even though genes do affect our food preferences in some respects, the environment plays a strong role, as described in the present as well as in the next chapter.

CHAPTER
6
❦

Environmental Contributions to Food Preferences

The previous chapter discussed food preferences that tend to show little individual variation and that appear to be substantially genetically determined. The present chapter will be concerned with food preferences and aversions that are present only in some people and that are largely due to the effects of the environment.

That the environment plays a significant role in the determination of food preferences is immediately obvious. Across different cultures, or even across different socioeconomic classes within a single culture, food preferences vary widely. Yet when someone becomes part of a different culture or socioecomonic class, that person's food preferences change so as to be more similar to the new surrounding group of people.[1] For example, in the United

States, although most people's families did not originally come from cultures in which hamburgers were part of the cuisine, hamburgers are standard American fare, highly preferred by many people (Chapter 14 discusses the origins of cuisine in more detail).

The environment, therefore, must have considerable influence on food preferences. A good way to explore the influence of the environment on food preferences is to study the ways in which the environment can *change* food preferences. This chapter focuses on changes that result from an organism's direct experience with food and changes that result from an organism's interactions with other organisms. An understanding of the ways in which, and the degree to which, the environment affects food preferences will improve our ability to modify undesirable food preferences.

EXPERIENCE WITH FOOD

Four kinds of direct experience with food can change an organism's food preferences: mere exposure, consumption followed by changes in nutrition, consumption followed by illness, and consumption followed by other characteristic events.

Mere Exposure

Both humans and nonhumans exhibit *neophobia*, a fear of new things.[2] Neophobia applies not only to new objects and new situations but also to new foods. How many Americans would be willing to try fried grasshoppers, a traditional Chinese delicacy? In general, people and animals prefer foods and situations that are familiar.[3] Many kinds of research support this conclusion about food preferences. For example, small mammals (mice and voles) restricted to a diet consisting only of oats or wheat subsequently show a greater preference for this familiar diet.[4]

As early as 1966, Gordon M. Burghardt and Eckhard H. Hess explored whether effects like these might occur in newly hatched snapping turtles.[5] Burghardt and Hess gave their subjects either meat, fish, or worms for 12 days. At this point each turtle preferred the type of diet to which it had become accustomed. For the next 12 days, Burghardt and Hess fed each turtle a different diet from that it had been fed during the first 12 days. However, at the end of the 24 days, the turtles still preferred the diets to which they had originally been exposed. These results imply that some types of early exposure to food can result in increased preference for that food.

In humans, mere exposure to some foods also seems to increase preference for those foods. Two studies illustrate these points. Patricia

Pliner's[6] experiment used male undergraduates. The subjects were given 0 to 20 tastes of individual novel fruit juices. They were then asked to taste each juice and rate it in terms of how much they liked it. Juices that had been tasted more frequently in the first part of the experiment received the higher ratings.

Leann L. Birch and her colleagues used 2- to 5-year-old children in their experiments with novel fruits.[7] The children were exposed to each of the novel fruits between 0 and 15 times. For each child, exposure to some of the fruits consisted of simply looking at them. For the rest of the fruits, exposure consisted of tasting (and looking at) the fruits. Each child then rated the fruits, separately according to each fruit's appearance and according to each fruit's taste (and appearance). Preference for a fruit's appearance was greater the more times that a child had seen or tasted (and seen) that fruit. On the other hand, preference for a fruit's taste was increased only if a child had had previous exposure to that fruit's taste. Birch and her colleagues concluded that in order for experience with a food to increase preference for the taste of that food, experience with the actual taste of the food is necessary.

Note that all of the above studies, in which exposure increased preference for the taste of a food, included ingestion of the foods; the consequences of ingesting the foods could have been at least partly responsible for the subsequent increases in preference for the foods. Mere exposure may not have been the only factor involved, if exposure is defined simply as seeing and perhaps tasting a food. Situations in which the effects of food ingestion have been explicitly studied will be described in the next three sections.

In addition, it should be pointed out that humans and nonhumans do not invariably seek familiar foods. Although familiar foods and situations are generally preferred over unfamiliar ones, the preference for a food or situation is reduced immediately following exposure to it, a finding known as *sensory specific satiety*. In other words, exposure appears to result in a long-term increase in preference but a temporary decrease in preference.[8]

David J. Stang's experiment,[9] using adult female subjects and repeated tastings of different types of spices, supports these statements. The subjects' preference ratings for the spices decreased with repeated tastings but recovered after a week without tastings. In another experiment, Barbara J. Rolls, Edmund T. Rolls, and Edward A. Rowe showed that subjects would consume more sandwiches if the fillings in the sandwiches were repeatedly changed.[10] Because sensory specific satiety can develop so quickly (within 2 minutes) and then remains constant until it starts to decrease, it is thought to result from the sensations of food as it is ingested, not from the effects of the food after it has been ingested.[11]

Thus the findings demonstrating that people have preferences for familiar foods are not necessarily inconsistent with the findings demonstrating that some people tend to seek out new foods (described in Chapter 5). Apparently the tendency of organisms to prefer familiar foods, whether due to mere exposure or the consequences of food ingestion, coexists with a tendency to avoid recently consumed foods. For omnivores such as humans and rats, this combination of strategies is useful. It ensures that a variety of foods and thus a variety of nutrients are consumed.[12] For food preferences, familiarity does appear to breed (some) contempt, while absence makes the heart grow (somewhat) fonder.

Food Consumption Followed by Changes in Nutritive State

Changes in nutritive state following food consumption can also affect food preferences. In fact, this mechanism is believed to be responsible for much of the appropriate selection of foods by omnivores. Because they eat a great variety of foods, omnivores are relatively likely to encounter many new and different foods. An inborn preference or aversion for every possible food is impossible. Instead, omnivores learn which foods are beneficial and which are not by sampling them. When the consequences of consuming a food are nutritionally advantageous, omnivores increase their consumption of that food. When the consequences are harmful, they decrease their consumption.

Three kinds of studies illustrate these points: experiments in which organisms have been deprived of individual nutrients and then allowed to select from foods containing those nutrients, experiments in which organisms have been allowed to select from foods that together contain all needed nutrients, and experiments in which food consumption is followed by a specific change in nutritive state. The experimental results discussed in following sections differ from those on physiological need in Chapter 5 in that a deprived organism does not show an immediate change in preference; experience with the food and the consequences of its ingestion are necessary.

SELECTION OF AN INDIVIDUAL NUTRIENT.   Paul Rozin conducted a number of experiments in which he fed rats food containing all but one essential nutrient and then allowed the rats to select between two foods: the original food and the same food with the addition of the previously missing essential nutrient. When this was done using the essential nutrient *thiamine* (vitamin B_1), the rats consumed large amounts of the new food and almost none of the original, deficient food. Further, the rats were observed to overturn the feeding dish that contained the old food, treating this food the same way they treated a bitter, aversive food containing quinine. Even when recovered from the thiamine deficiency, the rats preferred to eat nothing when they were food deprived if the only choice was the old, deficient food.

The preference for the new food containing the missing nutrient is known as a specific hunger,[13] and it does not appear to be dependent on any distinctive tastes or smells of the various foods.[14] The most likely explanation for how specific hungers arise is that the rats acquire an aversion to the food associated with the deficiency. However, research with rats has also shown what appears to be a learned preference for a taste associated with recovery from thiamine deficiency.[15]

A possible example of specific hungers in humans comes from the clinical literature on pica. *Pica* is defined as the "repeated eating of a nonnutritive substance for at least one month."[16] It is usually found in children and in pregnant women, with some of the most commonly consumed items being paint, dry laundry starch, clay, and earth.[17] Because pica is most likely to appear in people with high nutritional demands, it has been proposed that it is the result of specific hungers for minerals, such as iron.[18] Herbivores, such as deer and sheep in Scotland, may be showing similar behavior when they consume an occasional seabird chick—such behavior is one of the only ways that these herbivores can obtain calcium.[19]

In summary, many species, under at least some conditions, appear responsive to the consequences of their diets and appear good at selecting nutritious foods. Two cautions must be entered here, however. First, experiments have shown that rats do not acquire aversions to all diets deficient in individual nutrients. For example, specific hungers in response to diets deficient in vitamins A and D have been difficult to demonstrate.[20] Second, rats in specific-hunger experiments are fed only the deficient diet in the first part of the experiment and are given a limited choice of diets in the second part. In more complex situations rats, humans, and other species might show less nutritional wisdom based on their past experience with various foods. The next section describes some data relevant to these questions.

SELECTION OF ALL NUTRIENTS.   Studies have been conducted in which rats and humans were deprived of a wide variety of nutrients and/or were given choices among many different foods. Curt P. Richter[21] reported a number of experiments in which rats were allowed to choose between a great variety of nutrients, and the rats' intake of each nutrient was measured. Experiments of this kind are known as cafeteria experiments. In general, Richter found that rats in a cafeteria paradigm did quite well at selecting nutrients consistent with their nutritional needs.

Clara M. Davis conducted a well-known and intriguing cafeteria study in the 1920s and 1930s using human infants.[22] She used 15 infants who at the start of the experiment ranged between 6 and 11 months of age. All of the infants had been weaned just before the experiment. Prior to weaning they had very limited experience with foods other than milk. All of the infants lived in a hospital for the 6 months to 4.5 years that they participated in the experiment. During the experiment, a nurse presented each child at meal times with a tray containing a variety of foods. The nurse would give the child any item to which the child pointed. The children sometimes went on binges during which they consumed large amounts of particular foods for long periods of time, but these binges were self-terminating. Over long periods of time the subjects ate a fairly well-balanced diet and grew well.

It would be easy to interpret these data as indicating, first, that infants and young children, and possibly older humans as well, would do perfectly well at selecting their own food if left to their own devices; and second, that extreme food preferences and food aversions need not be of any parental concern because in the long term children will eat what they need. However, it is possible that the nurses who were giving the foods to the infants unconsciously (or perhaps even consciously) affected the infants' choices, although the nurses were given instructions to avoid influencing the children. Effects of this kind are discussed in the subsequent section on food consumption followed by other consequences.

In addition, the sweetest choices available to the subjects were milk and fruit, and not surprisingly, those items were also the ones selected most often. These infants appear to have been demonstrating the genetic preference for sweet discussed in the previous chapter. Luckily the sweetest choices available to them, milk and fruit, were also quite nutritious. It seems unlikely that the children would have selected an equally nutritious diet if chocolate candy and other sugary foods with little nutritional value had been available. Surveys have shown that college students most prefer foods that are sweet, and that the food preferences reported by college students are inconsistent with a well-balanced diet.[23] Davis's study was valuable, however, because it yielded much suggestive, if not conclusive, results.

FOOD FOLLOWED BY A SPECIFIC CHANGE IN NUTRITIVE STATE.   In some experiments subjects are given something to eat, taste, or smell, and that experience is then followed by a specific change in nutritive state. Depending on the nature of this nutritional change, the subject's preference for the sample food may increase or decrease. For example, Robert C. Bolles, Linda Hayward, and Christian Crandall[24] conducted an experiment in which rats ate both a high-calorie food that contained one distinctive flavor, A, and a low-calorie food that contained another distinctive flavor, B. When the rats were given a choice between two foods differing only in flavor—one tasting of A and one tasting of B—they preferred the food flavored with A, the flavor previously associated with the high-calorie food. Many other experiments have also shown that nonhuman subjects can learn to prefer a food (or the taste or smell of a food) that is followed by caloric input,[25] even if that caloric input is delayed.

Fat is much denser in calories than are protein or carbohydrate (fat contains 9 calories per gram, but protein and carbohydrate each contain 4 calories per gram). Perhaps humans learn to like relatively high-calorie foods, including foods that are high in fat, because of their caloric consequences. Data from experiments using human subjects suggest this is true. D. A. Booth, who has done several experiments on this topic, has been able to show that adult humans can learn to eat smaller meals when those meals contain a disguised high-calorie starch load associated with a distinctive taste. Further, preference for this kind of meal increases as the subjects gain experience with these meals, particularly if the subjects consume them when food deprived. But if the subjects consume these meals when satiated, the opposite occurs; the subjects' preference for these meals decreases as the subjects gain experience with them.[26] Leann L. Birch and Mary Deysher have extended Booth's findings to preschool children.[27] These researchers demonstrated that preschool subjects learn to eat smaller meals following a taste that has been previously associated with a high-calorie snack, and larger meals following a taste that has been previously associated with a low-calorie snack.

It is not surprising that humans and other animals are able to learn which foods are dense in calories and that they prefer those foods. Such behavior would be adaptive for species such as ours that evolved in food-scarce environments. Unfortunately, now that food is no longer scarce for most people in the United States, our preferences for high-calorie food make it difficult to keep fat consumption low, as recommended by the Surgeon General (see also Chapter 10).[28]

CONCLUSION. Caloric consequences can help humans as well as other species regulate the size of their meals and select among different foods. Nevertheless, although animals appear fairly good at selecting foods that provide most of the essential nutrients,[29] humans given a wide selection tend to consume too much salt and calories and not enough of other essential nutrients (see Chapter 5). In these respects, human behavior does not appear to be governed by the direct nutritional consequences of the foods consumed. However, one consequence can greatly affect the food preferences of both humans and nonhumans, and that consequence is illness.

Chapter 6

Food Consumption Followed by Illness

BASIC CHARACTERISTICS.   A likely explanation for specific hungers, as stated previously, is that an aversion is acquired to the deficient diet. In more detail, this explanation postulates that an organism fed a deficient diet will feel ill, and that consumption of that diet is thus associated with illness and that the diet is therefore avoided.[30]

This statement is supported by a now-extensive literature[31] reporting a decrease in preference for a particular food when consumption of that food has been followed by illness. Such decreases in food preference were first observed by farmers trying to get rid of rats. The farmers would lace some bait with a strong poison, but they found it was difficult to kill rats in this way. The rats would take only small samples of any new food, and if they then became ill, they would subsequently avoid the bait. This behavior was labeled *bait shyness*.[32]

The first laboratory investigations of this phenomenon began in the 1950s when John Garcia and his colleagues were examining the effects of irradiation on rats' behavior. Garcia noticed that the rats ate less after being irradiated. He was able to show that the rats appeared to develop an aversion to eating any food paired with irradiation. Apparently the irradiation made the animals gastrointestinally ill, and they associated the illness with the food.[33] Subsequent experiments used injections of *lithium chloride (LiCl)* as the illness-inducing agent instead of irradiation because LiCl is easier to administer and control.[34]

Garcia described this learning as a type of *classical conditioning*. In classical conditioning, a particular *unconditioned stimulus (US)*, such as food, elicits a particular reflexive response, such as salivation. The *conditioned stimulus (CS)* is a previously neutral stimulus that, after being paired with the US, also elicits the reflexive response. According to Garcia, when rats avoid food after the food has been paired with illness, the illness functions as a US and the taste and smell of the food as a CS.[35]

In 1966 John Garcia and Robert A. Koelling published a paper whose findings were to rock the foundations of research on learning. Garcia and Koelling allowed thirsty rats to lick at a spout that delivered flavored water (see Figure 6.1 for the complete design of this experiment). In addition, each lick resulted in a flash of light and a click. Half of the rats were shocked whenever they licked. The other half, while licking, were made ill using either irradiation or LiCl. Several days later, after all the rats had recovered, they were again all water deprived and allowed to drink from a spout. But this time, for half of the rats, although the water was flavored, there were no light flashes or clicks. The other half of the rats received light flashes and

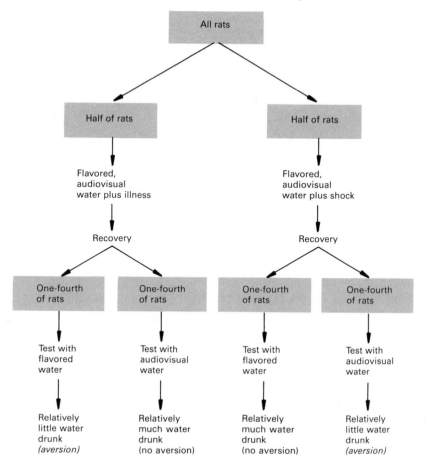

FIGURE 6.1   *Garcia and Koelling's procedure showing the tendency of rats to associate taste with illness and audiovisual stimuli with shock.* (After J. Garcia and R. A. Koelling, "Relation of Cue to Consequence in Avoidance Learning," *Psychonomic Science* 4[1966]:123–124.)

clicks following each lick, but the water was unflavored. The results showed that the rats that had been shocked drank very little of the water that was accompanied by light flashes and clicks, while the rats that had been made ill drank very little of the water that was flavored. Garcia and Koelling concluded that it was easier for rats to associate taste with illness and audiovisual stimuli with shock than vice versa.[36] Because of these results, bait shyness is now usually called *taste aversion learning.* (Keep in mind, however, that in most experiments a substance with a distinctive taste will also have a distinctive odor. Therefore it may be odors, or combinations of odors and tastes, that associate easily with illness.)

The fact that illness appeared to be associated more easily with tastes than with audiovisual stimuli at first seemed to violate one of the assumptions of traditional learning theory: that any event could be associated equally well with any other event.[37] This was not the only assumption of traditional learning theory that appeared to be violated by taste aversion learning. Psychologists quickly discovered that taste aversions could be acquired in a single trial with delays of up to 24 hours between consumption of the food and illness. According to traditional learning theory, learning would not occur if there were delays of more than a few seconds between two events.[38]

A third apparent difference between traditional and taste aversion learning concerned properties of the CSs involved in each case. In traditional learning, such as with shock (see Garcia and Koelling's experiment described above), the CS (lights and clicks) appears to function as a signal for the shock. The CS is avoided in those situations in which the shock has previously occurred, such as the experimental chamber, but not in other situations, such as the home cage. Preference for, but not liking of, the CS has changed. However, when illness is the US, the CS (the taste of a food) is avoided wherever it is encountered.[39] The taste therefore appears to change in hedonic value as a result of being paired with illness; the taste actually comes to taste *bad*, rather than simply signaling to the subject that illness is due shortly. Liking of the CS has changed.[40]

All of these unusual properties are useful in avoiding poisons. The presence of poison is more likely to be indicated by a particular taste than by a particular appearance or sound, it may take many hours before a poison will result in illness, and a poison is a poison no matter where it is encountered or how many times it is encountered. Therefore the peculiar characteristics of taste aversion learning seem well designed to assist organisms in avoiding illness-causing agents in foods. For example, large grazing mammals apparently easily learn to avoid grasses with the bitter taste of an alkaloid-producing fungus that makes the animals feel ill.[41] Psychologists therefore postulated that the rules governing this type of learning had been shaped by evolution.[42]

Research has pointed out, however, that even if one grants that evolution has shaped learning principles, this does not necessarily mean that different principles of learning apply in different situations. Although the principles of taste aversion learning do appear somewhat different from the principles of traditional learning, these differences tend to be differences in amount (for example, differences in the maximum CS–US interval), rather than differences in kind (for example, differences in whether or not the CS–US interval influences learning).[43]

Garcia's discoveries about the unusual characteristics of taste aversion learning should not be downplayed, however. His findings helped open a new area of research that awakened many learning theorists to the effects of evolution on behavioral change. Taste aversion learning is now being used to help understand and treat many eating and drinking disorders (see Chapters 9, 10, and 11).

EFFECTS ON DIFFERENT SPECIES. If evolution affects learning, then it is reasonable to think that different species may acquire taste aversions in different ways. An experiment reported by Hardy C. Wilcoxon, William B. Dragoin, and Paul A. Kral in 1971 supported this hypothesis.[44] Wilcoxon and his colleagues used both rats and quail in their experiment. The subjects all drank water that was both distinctively flavored and distinctively colored. They were then made ill and, after recovery, were tested for their consumption of water that was either only distinctively flavored or only distinctively colored. The rats tended to drink less of the distinctively flavored water, while the quail tended to drink less of the distinctively colored water.

Perhaps rats have difficulty acquiring aversions to visual stimuli because of their poor visual ability. Norman S. Braveman explored this interpretation in his experiments with guinea pigs, whose visual system is similar to that of rats. The guinea pigs easily acquired aversions to visual stimuli.[45] Because both quail and guinea pigs search for their food in the day, while rats search for their food at night, Braveman postulated that an animal tends to form aversions to stimuli that are perceived by the same sensory modes that the animal relies on when searching for food.

Nevertheless, research has shown that even in species that depend primarily on vision, taste appears basic to the formation of illness-induced food aversions. In all species, either illness-induced aversions are formed most easily on the basis of taste, or the concurrent presence of a taste will increase an aversion that is based on an odor or a visual stimulus associated with illness.[46]

Taste aversion learning has also been investigated in humans. For ethical reasons there have been relatively few experiments, using a fairly small number of subjects. These experiments have used rotating chairs[47] and dizzying visual illusions,[48] among other means, to induce illness (radiation therapy and chemotherapy for cancer have also been used; see Chapter 9). Most of the data obtained with humans have come from retrospective questionnaire studies, in which human subjects are asked to describe any taste aversions that they have acquired naturally. Although these data are not as conclusive as data obtained from experiments, they do offer some information regarding how humans acquire taste aversions.[49]

These questionnaire data show that humans apparently acquire taste aversions in much the same way that other species acquire them.[50] Humans acquire illness-induced food aversions most easily on the basis of taste; they can acquire these aversions with long delays between the consumption of the food and the illness; the aversive food is aversive no matter where it is encountered; and aversions appear to be more easily acquired when food consumption precedes rather than follows illness.

In many other ways as well, human taste aversion learning is similar to taste aversion learning in other species, as well as to the learning of other tasks. For example, aversions appear to be more easily acquired to novel, less preferred foods, and aversions tend to generalize to foods that resemble the food actually paired with illness. Sometimes an aversion is acquired to a food even though the subject is sure that the food did not cause the illness. In the introduction to his book on taste aversion learning, Martin E. P. Seligman described such an incident from his own experience. Seligman ate sauce béarnaise on steak and subsequently became ill with what was definitely flu. Yet Seligman acquired an aversion to the sauce béarnaise.[51] *Superstitious conditioning,* in which a response is acquired following an accidental pairing of the response and reinforcement, occurs frequently in all types of learning, even when subjects profess knowledge that there is no contingency between the response and reinforcement.

Humans appear to acquire taste aversions quite frequently. For example, in a study published by A. W. Logue, Iris Ophir, and Kerry E. Strauss in 1981, 517 college students reported a total of 415 taste aversions, a mean of almost one per person.[52] This is especially remarkable in view of the fact that the subjects were college students: they had not yet lived a complete lifetime and they might have had to remember taste aversions that they had acquired as many as 15 years previously. In general the aversions were strong and had persisted a long time, with 62 percent of the aversive foods having never been eaten again, even though those aversions had been acquired an average of about 5 years previously. Many of Logue and her colleagues' subjects were emphatic about their feelings toward the aversive food and wrote explicit comments in the margins of the questionnaire.

Because taste aversions appear to be acquired frequently in humans and to be strong and long-lasting, it is possible that taste aversion learning is responsible for some of the many food aversions of unknown origin that humans have. Young children frequently eat foods that are novel, and young children also frequently become ill; therefore it seems possible that people could acquire many aversions at young ages and later not be able to recall the origins of their aversions. Further, adults might acquire a taste aversion, possibly after only a mild illness, and never be aware of what caused the aversion, or forget the cause after only a short time.

INTER- AND INTRASPECIES RELATIONSHIPS.   The taste aversion paradigm has been used to investigate a variety of intra- and interspecies relationships.[53] This section discusses two of these relationships, species recognition and predator–prey interactions.

The taste aversion paradigm has been used to show that individual starlings can recognize other individual starlings. In the first part of this experiment, one starling was allowed to feed in the presence of another starling. Then the first starling was made ill while the other starling was present. In subsequent tests, the first starling was more likely to be aggressive toward, and less likely to associate with, the particular starling that had been paired with illness. The first starling also ate less in the presence of the particular starling paired with illness.[54]

Extensive research by Lincoln P. Brower, also using birds, has suggested that the aversion bluejays show toward monarch butterflies operates according to a taste aversion paradigm. Monarch butterflies contain cardiac glycosides, a toxic substance. Blue jays that eat monarch butterflies containing the cardiac glycosides become ill, as evidenced by their vomiting. Brower believes that the blue jays develop an aversion to the visual appearance of the monarch butterflies. He hypothesizes that it is for this reason that there are so many butterflies similar in appearance to the monarch: Mimicry of the monarch appearance is adaptive for butterflies because it prevents their being eaten.[55]

Other researchers have used taste aversion paradigms to influence natural predator–prey relationships. The most extensively reported efforts of this kind have been the attempts of Carl R. Gustavson and his colleagues to prevent coyotes from attacking sheep on western sheep ranches. The ranchers had been simply killing coyotes to prevent the attacks. Coyotes are a valuable part of the ecosystem, however, primarily because they keep the rodent population under control. Gustavson and his colleagues reasoned that if they could condition the coyotes to avoid only sheep, this would disrupt the ecosystem much less than would killing the coyotes. Gustavson and his colleagues placed lamb bait laced with lithium chloride on the range in areas frequented by wild coyotes. In addition, under more controlled conditions they attempted to induce captive coyotes to develop aversions to sheep.

Both wild and captive coyotes appeared to acquire an aversion to eating or to even approaching sheep. Not only did the coyotes develop an aversion to eating sheep, but they behaved submissively toward the sheep, running the other way when a sheep approached.[56] Consistent with these results,

William Timberlake and Ted Melcer have found that, under some conditions, rats will decrease their contact with, as well as their ingestion of, a prey food item following pairing of illness and the prey food item.[57]

Gustavson and his colleagues' work has been extremely controversial. There has been heated published discussion among some members of the U. S. Fish and Wildlife Service, Gustavson and his colleagues, and other researchers about the accuracy of these data.[58] At the very least Gustavson and his colleagues' work has great potential. As other research described above has shown, taste aversions are acquired easily and are usually quite strong. All of these findings encourage an approach like the one that Gustavson and his colleagues have used.

Food Consumption Followed by Other Events

Many events other than illness and changes in nutrition will modify food preferences when these events follow consumption of food or the taste or smell of food. For example, when two tastes are first paired and then one is made aversive by following it with illness, the other taste also becomes aversive.[59]

Conversely, if a taste is paired with a different, positive taste such as sweet, the preference for the first taste increases.[60] It has been hypothesized that this type of learning is responsible for the acquisition of preferences for initially aversive substances such as tea and coffee.[61] A new coffee or tea drinker usually adds more palatable substances such as sugar and milk to that beverage. Gradually, as the actual taste of the coffee or tea becomes associated with the taste of the sugar or the milk, the coffee or tea can be drunk with less, and finally no, sugar or milk. Debra A. Zellner and her colleagues were able to demonstrate such an effect experimentally by exposing humans different numbers of times to sweetened or unsweetened teas.[62]

The effects of following food consumption with pleasurable activities have been elegantly investigated by Birch, who works with preschool children in her experiments. She has shown that making participation in a pleasurable activity contingent on consuming a particular food results in a *decrease* in preference for that food.[63] She has also shown that if food is used as a reward for performance of some activity, there is a resulting *increase* in preference for that food.[64] A phenomenon that appears similar to this has been observed in rats. Rats consume smaller amounts of a less preferred solution if that solution has been regularly followed by a more preferred solution. In the literature on animal learning, this effect is known as *incentive contrast*.[65]

Accordingly, parents who want children to eat their spinach and not to eat so much candy may be working against themselves if they tell the children that they can only have candy if they eat their spinach. Nevertheless, it seems doubtful that telling the children that they can eat spinach if they first eat their ice cream (an experiment that has not yet been conducted) would result in the consumption of more spinach and less ice cream. The genetic preference for sweet is strong. But parents may want to keep Birch's findings and the incentive-contrast effect in mind when setting guidelines for their children's eating behavior.

EXPERIENCE WITH OTHER ORGANISMS

A number of studies have shown similarities between the food preferences of family members, but no greater similarities between identical than fraternal twins.[66] This pattern of results suggests that contact with other organisms is one of the ways in which the environment influences food preferences. Several influences of this kind, often without any food present, involving direct and indirect contact with other organisms, have been studied with both nonhuman and human subjects.

Direct Contact with Another Organism

NONHUMAN SUBJECTS. Bennett G. Galef[67] has performed some ingenious experiments with rats to identify the mechanisms that are necessary and/or sufficient for the transmission of food preferences between rats. A *necessary mechanism* is one without which food preferences cannot be transmitted; a *sufficient mechanism* is one that, if it alone is present, enables food preferences to be transmitted. Galef's research, which has provided detailed descriptions of the mechanisms by which rats transmit food preferences among themselves, has proven relevant as well to the transmission of food preferences among humans.

Galef's experimental design was basically the following. Two adult male rats and four adult female rats with their litters lived in a cage measuring approximately 3 feet by 6 feet. The cage contained several nesting boxes and food bowls. The rats had free access to water and were fed for 3 hours each day, during which time their behavior was monitored and videotaped. Usually two foods were presented, food A and the ordinarily preferred food B. Then some of the adult rats were made ill by sublethal amounts of poison added to food B. These rats then preferred food A to food B, making it possible to examine the transmission of that food preference.

Galef observed that the rat pups learned to choose the adults' preferred food A. He was able to isolate four ways in which this preference was transmitted. These were: chemical cues at the feeding site, such as are contained in feces, which attract pups to the site; pieces of food in the adults' fur, which, when the young come into contact with the adults in the nest, increase the young's preference for that food; the presence of adult rats at the feeding site, which, independent of the other cues, attracts pups to the site; and a chemical cue, specific to the mother rat's preferred food, which is present in a mother rat's milk and which increases the preference for that food in her nursing pups.

Apparently, then, there are at least four sufficient mechanisms for the transmission of food preferences from adult rats to pups. If one of these mechanisms is prevented from operating, for example, by removal of chemical cues present at the feeding site, food preferences can still be transmitted, because none of these mechanisms is *necessary*. In other words, if rats do not learn appropriate food preferences one way, they will learn them another way. It is clearly safer for omnivorous rat pups to learn food preferences by these multiple, sufficient mechanisms of social transmission than by their own trial and error.

The social transmission of food preferences has been demonstrated in the young of many other species as well. Chicks, kittens, and young monkeys learn to eat what the adults of their species eat, and their food preferences apparently can be acquired simply by observation of the adults.[68]

Galef and his colleagues have shown that food preferences can also be transmitted between adult rats. Preference for a particular food is increased in an "observer" rat following interaction of the observer with a "demonstrator" rat, a rat that has previously eaten that food.[69] This interaction need last only 2 minutes, but during that time period mouth-to-mouth contact between the observer and the demonstrator must occur. The resulting increase in the observer's preference for the food appears to be dependent on food stimuli (tastes and/or odors) present on the fur or emerging from the digestive tract of the demonstrator rat.[70] In addition, accompanying the food stimuli with *carbon disulfide,* a chemical compound present in rat breath, enhances rats' subsequent preference for the food.[71]

Adult rats are also more likely to follow other rats that have recently consumed nonpoisonous food than to follow rats that have recently consumed poisonous food.[72] Further, rats will more quickly learn to prefer the most nutritious of several foods if other rats that have been previously trained to prefer the nutritious food are present.[73] Apparently, many nonhuman animals are very good at acquiring food preferences from *conspecifics* (members of their own species), thus increasing the probability of consuming safe, nutritious food.

Food aversions, as well as food preferences, can be socially transmitted in animals. Another series of experiments with rats, this one by W. J. Carr, has illustrated how transmission of one such aversion, the aversion for consumption of conspecifics, might occur.[74]

Like humans, rats rarely eat members of their own species. Although a hungry adult rat will eat an unattended, live rat neonate of the same species without hesitation, the older the rat pup is, the lower is the probability that an adult rat of the same species will eat the pup. Further, adult rats are more likely to feed on dead adult rats of another species, or on dead adult mice, than on dead adult rats of their own species. The likelihood that an adult rat will feed on a member of its own species increases when the consumer rat has been made hungry or anosmic, when the carcass has been covered with the urine of another species, or when the carcass has been skinned. Finally, an adult rat's readiness to feed on a member of its own species can be increased by having that rat observe another adult rat performing this behavior. *Observational learning* appears to be important here as well as in the transmission of other food preferences.

Yet a question remains. How does a rat know that another organism is or is not a member of its own species? Carr's work on consumption of conspecifics offers an opportunity to investigate how animals identify conspecifics. The results of the experiments described above all seem to point to a chemical cue present in the fur of the animal.

To examine this hypothesis further, Carr experimented with Norway rats, rearing each rat in a cage adjacent to a cage containing another Norway rat or a cage containing a mouse. Rats raised beside a mouse were as unlikely to eat mice of that species as to eat members of their own species. However, all of the rats were unlikely to consume rats of their own species. This means either that adult rats are genetically programmed to avoid consuming members of their own species, or, what appears more likely, that experience with their own bodies is sufficient to engender an aversion to consumption of conspecifics. In any case, being raised beside a member of another species is also sufficient to prevent a rat from consuming members of that species.[75]

It is not known whether similar mechanisms are responsible for the tendency of humans to avoid eating other humans, but Carr's data certainly offer many suggestions about how consumption of conspecifics is governed.

Social influence on taste aversion learning has also been demonstrated in rats. Interaction with another rat that does not have a taste aversion to a particular food, but not simple exposure to that food, will decrease a rat's taste aversion to the food.[76] In addition, a rat can acquire a taste aversion if it eats a food and is then exposed to a sick rat.[77] Finally, lactating and nonlactating adult female rats that have given birth (but not adult female rats that have never given birth, nor adult male rats) can learn an aversion to a novel flavor when their consumption of that flavor is followed by exposure to a sick rat pup. Presumably this learning behavior is adaptive for mother rats, but not other rats, because it helps the mother rats to avoid foods that make their pups ill. As with so many other social effects on food preferences in rats (but not in humans, see below), an olfactory cue—in this case transmitted from the sick rat to the observer rat—seems to be the mechanism by which rats acquire food aversions after being exposed to sick rats.[78]

HUMAN SUBJECTS. Sibylle K. Escalona[79] was one of the first to record the social transmission of food preferences and aversions in humans. Working as a psychologist in the Massachusetts Reformatory for Women during the 1940s, Escalona was able to observe the inmates and some of their children. At this time, women who were incarcerated in this institution were often permitted to keep their children under 3 years of age in the prison nursery. The children lived in the nursery, and their mothers could frequently visit and care for them. Other inmates as well as reformatory employees also cared for the children. The nursery housed 50 to 60 infants. Approximately 70 percent of the children were infants under 1 year of age.

On many occasions Escalona observed what she believed were instances of subconscious influence on the children's food preferences by the caretakers. One of the more detailed descriptions of such a case is reported here:

> It came to attention accidentally that many of the babies under four months of age showed a consistent dislike for either orange or tomato juice. (These juices were offered on alternate days with equal frequency.) The number preferring each kind of juice was about equal. Furthermore, such preferences seemed to change and a baby who had refused orange juice for about three weeks occasionally would reverse his preference within two or three days, accepting orange juice and refusing tomato henceforth. A checkup revealed that where there was a sudden change in preference the baby's feedings had been re-assigned from one person to another. Next we determined the preference of the students who took care of these babies in such a way that they could not know why the question had been asked, in fact, were not aware of its having been asked. In the fifteen cases we were able to investigate in this manner, the student in charge of a baby showing a decided preference had the same preference, or rather the same dislike, as the baby. That is, babies who refused tomato juice were found to be fed by adults who also expressed a dislike for tomato juice. In three cases we were able to establish the fact that a baby reversing a preference had been changed to a student who possessed the dislike acquired by the baby subsequent to the change in personnel.[80]

These are sobering observations. Perhaps parents can influence their children's food preferences without any awareness whatever that they are doing so.

But by what mechanism does this influence occur? One possibility relates to the acceptance and rejection responses (reflexes) shown by many species, including humans (see Chapter 5). These responses are present at birth.[81] In addition, human infants as young as 36 hours of age are apparently able to imitate the facial expressions of adults.[82] Perhaps adults who are feeding young children consciously or unconsciously compose their faces in expressions of acceptance or rejection, depending on their own preferences for the food being fed, and the children then imitate the expression and consume more or less food accordingly. This may explain why people who feed children have eternally intoned "open the hangar" while simultaneously opening their own mouths and directing a spoonful of baby food at the child's mouth. Such a mechanism would be automatic, not requiring that the child have experience with the food; all that would be required is that the child come into contact with someone who has had experience with the food.

Birch has shown that if an adult repeatedly gives a child a food while being very friendly to the child, the child's preference for the food will increase. Note that the adult does not provide specific praise for eating the food; the adult just provides a general positive social context. Simply making the child more familiar with the food is not as effective at increasing preference for that food.[83]

In another experiment,[84] Birch arranged for certain preschool children (the target children) to repeatedly eat lunch with other children. All of the children ranged in age between 3 and 5 years. During lunch they sat in groups of four that remained constant throughout the experiment. One of the four children in each group was a target child. Adults came by with serving plates, asking the children to choose between a vegetable shown by pretests to be preferred only by the target child at a given table, and a vegetable shown by pretests to be preferred only by the other three children at the same table. The same pair of vegetables was served to each table for the four days of the experiment. On the first day the target child chose first, but on days 2, 3, and 4 the other children chose first. Not only did the target children increase their choices of their nonpreferred vegetables during the latter days of the experiment, but their reported preferences for those vegetables also increased. These effects were stronger for the younger children.

Lawrence V. Harper and Karen M. Sanders[85] showed that young children, 14 to 20 and 42 to 48 months old, were more likely to taste an unfamiliar food if an adult who was present tasted the food. This effect was stronger if the adult was the mother of the child rather than a friendly visitor. The effect also tended to be stronger for the younger children.

The above examples are all concerned with the social transmission of food preferences in humans. There is some evidence that humans can also transmit food aversions through observational learning. In Logue and her colleagues' study of taste aversions in college students,[86] several subjects reported acquiring taste aversions to specific foods after they saw someone else eat the food and then appear ill. For example, one subject who saw his baby brother eat baby food and then spit it out developed an aversion to baby food.

Indirect Contact with Another Organism

As discussed above, there is strong evidence that direct contact with another organism can result in modification of an organism's food preferences, in both humans and nonhumans. *Indirect* contact with another organism can also modify food preferences. In instances of this kind, preferences are modified by written and spoken descriptions of food and eating, such as the descriptions in television advertising. All of the data presented here involve human subjects, because humans are the only organisms that rely on printed and recorded information. However, similar influences may operate in other species as well, in instances in which an organism changes the environment in some way that later modifies the food preferences of other organisms.

TELEVISION ADVERTISING.   One of the clearest examples of the indirect influence of one organism on the food preferences of another is television advertising. Most of the research in this area has been concerned with the effects of television advertising on children. Many studies have shown that children in the United States spend more time watching television than they do in engaging in any other activity.[87] American children view an average of some 22,000 commercials per year, and more than 50 percent of these advertise foods that are poor in nutrition.[88] Good nutrition is critical to good health; if these commercials do affect the eating behavior of children, they could seriously harm children's health.

Several experiments have shown that when children are exposed to commercials for foods poor in nutrition, their reported preference for those foods as well as their tendency to buy or eat those foods increases.[89] On the other hand, there are reports that when children are exposed to commercials that present nutritional information, their preference for nutritive foods is not affected. To some extent these differential results may be due to the greater amount of effort and money that is put into producing commercials for foods poor in nutrition, compared with commercials carrying nutritional information.[90] The implications of this research are alarming. Most of the commercials that are seen by children appear to be teaching the children to prefer foods that are poor in nutrition.

OTHER CULTURAL INFLUENCES.   There is a great deal of evidence for the influence of "cultural" factors on food preferences, but much of this evidence is largely nonexperimental. Nevertheless, some of the points made by this literature will be mentioned here.

Culture can affect the types of substances that are considered appropriate to eat (see also Chapter 14). For example, Chapter 5 pointed out that people prefer salty foods when the foods are ones that they expect to be salty. Similarly, people learn through their culture at what temperature and at what time of day a food is usually served, as well as what its usual fat content is. They then prefer foods with these characteristics.[91] Mechanisms previously described in this chapter, such as mere exposure and observational learning, can help to explain in more detail precisely how such preferences are transferred within a culture.

Information transmitted verbally or in written form regarding the health benefits of various foods also appears to influence which foods are eaten. For example, American consumption of eggs and other high-cholesterol foods has decreased since the health problems associated with a high-cholesterol diet began receiving publicity.[92] But a change in the amount consumed for reasons of health does not necessarily indicate a change in food liking. A person may cut down on steak in order to cut down on cholesterol; but should a new study prove that cholesterol in the diet has nothing to do with cholesterol in the body, he or she might readily increase consumption of steak.

Cultural effects include any effects of social class on food preference. Reputedly, people tend to eat those foods that are eaten by members of the social group to which they wish to belong.[93] Perhaps a better way of describing this effect, a way that is more consistent with the previous evidence presented in this chapter, is to say that someone tends to eat those foods that are eaten by people who have control over many of that person's reinforcers. Thus children tend to eat those foods eaten by their parents and other adults, and people of lower income may tend to eat those foods eaten by people of higher income. This principle may help to explain the appeal of white bread; although less nutritious than whole wheat, until recently white bread was more expensive to make and therefore more available to people with relatively large incomes.

Many religions have rules regarding what may or may not be eaten, and these rules may be consistent with the food preferences of the members of

117

that religion. For example, many Jews do not enjoy the taste of pork when they happen to eat it.[94] Nevertheless, it is not accurate to state that Judaism causes an aversion to pork. Although those people raised as Jews may have a lower preference for pork than those raised as Christians, this difference in preference is probably due to other members of the religion exerting the types of indirect and direct influence described above. Chapter 14 describes in detail how the food-consumption tenets of a religion might evolve for reasons of survival.

CLASSIFICATION OF HUMAN FOOD AVERSIONS

Illness-induced food aversions are very common, but humans exhibit many other types of food aversions as well.[95] Much of the work on food preferences and aversions, as well as on the categorization of substances into foods or nonfoods, is summarized by Paul Rozin and April E. Fallon's classification of the four different types of food aversions shown by humans: foods that are rejected because they are distasteful, disgusting, inappropriate, or dangerous (see Table 6.1).[96] Some of these aversions seem to be determined by direct and/or indirect contact with humans, and other aversions are due to consequences from direct contact with the food.

Distasteful foods are those that most people would not mind eating if the taste of the food were covered up by sugar or if they only discovered what they had been eating after they had finished. *Disgusting foods* are those that most people would never want in their meal or stomach no matter how the foods were disguised and no matter how small the amount. *Inappropriate foods* are those items that are not considered food, and *dangerous foods* are those that could cause physical harm if eaten. Examples of common distasteful, disgusting, inappropriate, and dangerous foods are warm milk, urine, tree bark, and poisonous mushrooms, respectively. Foods may be considered distasteful or inappropriate because of genetically based reactions to the tastes of those items. Foods may qualify as distasteful, inappropriate, or dangerous because of direct experience with them. But foods are disgusting in large part because of direct and indirect contact with the reactions to these foods by other humans. Thus as children age and acquire increased experience with adults' reactions to certain potential foods, such as insects, that adults tend to treat as disgusting, the children themselves come increasingly to treat those potential foods as disgusting.[97] Foods may also be classified as disgusting because they have come into contact with something disgusting, or because their appearance is similar to that of

TABLE 6.1

Classification of Human Food Aversions

Type of Aversive Food	Description	Example	Possible Origins
Distasteful	Not aversive if cannot be tasted	Warm milk	Genetically based aversive taste, or consumption of the food has been followed by gastrointestinal illness
Disgusting	Aversive even if cannot be tasted or if in very small quantities; substances paired with a disgusting food also become disgusting (i.e., contamination occurs)	Urine	Direct or indirect contact with other humans who consider the food disgusting, or contact with another disgusting food, or similarity to another disgusting food
Inappropriate	Not considered to be food	Tree bark	Genetically based aversive taste, or direct experience with food or information from other humans indicates that food cannot be consumed and/or digested
Dangerous	Could cause physical harm if eaten	Poisonous mushrooms	Consumption of the food has ben followed by, or is reputed to be followed by, a nongastrointestinal illness

something disgusting. For example, a milkshake that once had (but no longer has) a cockroach floating in it is disgusting, as is fudge shaped to look like dog feces. These two ways in which food can become disgusting may be examples of the *principles of contiguity* and *similarity* from traditional *association theory*, clearly explicated over 200 years ago. According to these principles, we tend to associate stimuli that have been paired together or that are similar to each other.[98]

Marcia L. Pelchat and Paul Rozin[99] have further pointed out that taste aversion learning, in which the taste of a food is paired with gastrointestinal illness (principally nausea), usually results in a distaste for the food. Pairing consumption of food with another type of illness, such as respiratory distress (as with an allergic response), will result in considering the food dangerous, but not distasteful. When food consumption is followed by gastrointestinal illness, the subject does not want to eat the food again under any circumstances. But when food consumption is followed by another type of illness, the subject would be glad to eat the food again if a magic pill would just prevent the illness. Pelchat and Rozin's findings support the statements made earlier that taste aversion learning results in an actual change in the hedonic value (the liking) of the food, and that a change in consumption of a food for health reasons is not necessarily accompanied by a change in the hedonic value of that food.

CONCLUSION

Food preferences can be modified by experience, both nutritional experience and the social consequences of food consumption. Modeling, in which organisms imitate other organisms, also influences food preferences. The food preferences of the young of humans and other species seem especially sensitive to social interactions.

Explanations for the food-preference problems posed at the beginning of the previous chapter can now be attempted. Some of these problems, notably the decreased preference for milk with age and the extreme preferences for sweet and for salty foods, probably have a strong genetic component. In most adults milk becomes largely indigestible after the age of 3, and humans show a genetic preference for sweet and for salty foods. However, the degree to which an organism prefers to eat sweet foods, salty foods, and milk can be modified by experience. The acquired aversion to hot dogs after hot dog consumption had been followed by illness probably has a large environmental component. Organisms associate food consumption with subsequent nausea, resulting in a decreased consumption of that food. Finally, the child's aversion to eating vegetables (and President Bush's aversion to eating broccoli) may result from a number of different factors. Some people may find some vegetables bitter tasting because of a genetically based taste sensitivity to certain chemicals. In addition, vegetables, when eaten by themselves, are low in salt and sugar, both of which are innately preferred, and low in fat, which we learn to prefer due to its high concentration of calories. Finally, as Birch's research has shown, children can learn to prefer certain vegetables by observing others.

Therefore it would probably be easier to change, for example, the hot dog aversion than the milk aversion and the sweet preference. In the case of the hot dog, research indicates that preference is likely to be changed by repeated consumption of the food in a palatable sauce, under pleasant circumstances, and in the company of others who apparently enjoy hot dogs. Gradually, the sauce can be eliminated.

To a large degree, the ways in which our food preferences and aversions arise and change reflect our evolutionary heritage. We evolved in an environment in which calories and salt were scarce, and nutritious, nonpoisonous food sources had to be identified. That environment no longer exists, but our preferences for salty, caloric food and our aversions for foods associated with illness continue. This legacy of our past can cause serious problems, as will be discussed in Chapter 10.

The present chapter and the one preceding it were concerned with food preferences that organisms show when they may choose among equally available foods. The effects of availability on choice are the subject of the next chapter, which culminates the presentation of material regarding the normal behavior of choosing which food or drink to consume.

CHAPTER
7
❦
Choice

The preceding two chapters sought explanations for the preferences and aversions that animals and humans show when they can choose from a variety of readily available foods. But foods are not always easily and equally available. Sometimes it may be harder to obtain a particular food because of the amount of money or the amount of work necessary to obtain it. Choice among foods is affected not only by preference for qualities inherent in the foods but also by the cost and availability of those foods.[1]

These two aspects of food choice, preference based on qualities in foods that are easily available and preference influenced by cost and availability, are comparable to the distinction that psychologists make between learning and motivation. Learning concerns the acquisition of knowledge about the world, and motivation concerns whether or not that knowledge is acted upon.[2] Performance of a response to obtain a food item depends on how tired the organism is, how much effort is required to make the response, what other activities are available, and so on. Someone may readily consume M&Ms when they are available free of charge or effort. But if delivery of each M&M requires pushing a button 10,000 times, the person might very well ignore the button. If there were only one M&M left in the world, and it was on top of Mount Everest, the influence of that location on the choice to obtain the M&M would be a motivational effect.

EVOLUTION AND CHOICE

The preferences for salt and sweet, as well as the tendency to develop aversions to tastes (as opposed to visual stimuli) that have been followed by gastrointestinal illness, illustrate some of the ways in which genes are thought to play a role in the origins of food preferences and aversions (see Chapters 5 and 6). If evolution can affect an organism's inherent desire for certain foods, as well as the ways in which the organism's food preferences change, perhaps it can also influence the ways in which food preferences are expressed, that is, the ways in which an organism allocates its behavior to obtain food. Ideally, organisms should distribute their activities in ways that maximize their inclusive fitness.[3] Most researchers believe that evolution has provided animals with strategies for choosing between sources of food such that the animals obtain the optimal amount of food,[4] but three questions remain unanswered. What strategies do organisms actually use to optimize their acquisition of food, to what extent do these strategies actually maximize acquisition, and to what extent do organisms follow these strategies?

The two models of food choice that have gained widest acceptance, Herrnstein's matching law and optimal foraging theory, have each attempted to answer these questions, but from different perspectives. Both models are designed to make specific, quantitative predictions about how food choices will be made given several alternative choices. Each model includes mathematical formulas for this purpose. To introduce the sophistication of these two models, some simple versions of their formulas are presented below.

THE MATCHING LAW

Herrnstein's matching law starts with the premise that organisms are faced with some complex food-choice situations.

Choice Situation 1 Suppose a backwoods hunter has waited until the day before Thanksgiving to shoot the 10 wild turkeys needed for her family's Thanksgiving dinner. (It is a large family with large appetites.) Suppose further that the hunter knows that a turkey visits her apple orchard once an hour on the average, and that a turkey visits her adjoining field twice an hour on the average. Finally, suppose that once a turkey has arrived at the apple orchard or the field, it will stay there if undisturbed, and no other turkeys will join it because of the territorial conflicts between turkeys.

The question is how should the hunter distribute her time between the apple orchard and the field if she is to maximize the rate at which she obtains turkeys? At the start of her day of hunting, the hunter should go to the field, because turkeys come there more frequently. However, if she has spent an hour in the field obtaining any available turkeys, she should then go to the orchard, because a turkey is likely to be there. If she then spends half an hour in the orchard, obtaining any turkeys available there, she should return to the field, where another turkey has likely arrived.

There are many different choice situations, involving many variables. According to Richard J. Herrnstein, organisms are not able to maximize perfectly in every possible choice situation. Instead, Herrnstein has postulated, many species follow a strategy that frequently, but not always, maximizes their success in obtaining food. This strategy is called *Herrnstein's matching law.*[5]

This law states that on the average, organisms distribute their choices of foods in proportion to the distribution of the foods available. They "match" their choices with the distribution of those foods (that is, the rewards, the *reinforcers*). Thus, according to the matching law, the hunter should spend twice as much time in the field as in the apple orchard, because turkeys arrive twice as frequently in the field. For this combination of circumstances, the behavior predicted by the matching law is identical to a maximization strategy.

Researchers test the matching law by varying the distribution of reinforcers and observing whether the subjects' choice distributions match (are the same as) the reinforcer distributions. These experiments have been conducted using a great variety of species, including rats, pigeons, and humans, and using many different kinds of food reinforcement, including laboratory rat chow, grain, and snack foods. Researchers have found that the behavior of the subjects generally conforms well to the matching law in a variety of food-choice situations.[6] The matching law has even described well the food-choice behavior of a flock of wild pigeons.[7]

Self-Control

Another type of choice situation, involving choices between reinforcers of varying sizes and delays, has been examined using the matching law.
Consider the following example:

Choice Situation 2A Suppose a child's mother tells him on a Tuesday evening that if he eats all of his vegetables at dinner that night he can have three cookies for dessert. He eats his vegetables, but then the mother discovers that there is only one cookie in the cookie jar. (The father secretly eats the cookies in the cookie jar, always leaving one cookie because he thinks that way no one will notice what he has been doing.) Because she believes that it is important to keep promises to children, and because she feels badly that she does not have the cookies immediately available, she tells the child that he has two choices. He can either have the one cookie in the next hour or he can wait until tomorrow, Wednesday, and when she goes to the store she will get him three cookies for dessert after tomorrow night's dinner. But he cannot have both.

The matching law predicts the following.[8] If the child is given this choice many times, the ratio of the number of his choices of the three cookies divided by the number of his choices of the one cookie should be equal to the ratio of the numbers of cookies in the two choices (3 cookies/1 cookie), multiplied by the inverse ratio of the times to receive the three cookies or the one cookie (1 hour/24 hours), which is equal to $\frac{1}{8}$. Restated in equation form, the relations are as follows:

$$\frac{B_1}{B_2} = \frac{A_1}{A_2} \times \frac{D_2}{D_1} = \frac{3}{1} \times \frac{1}{24} = \frac{1}{8} . \tag{1}$$

The subscript 1 refers to choices of the three more delayed cookies, and the subscript 2 refers to choices of the one less delayed cookie. B_1 and B_2 are the numbers of choices of those two reinforcers, and A_1, A_2, D_1, and D_2 are the amounts (sizes) and delays of these two available reinforcers. As described by Equation 1, the child's choices are affected independently by the two different characteristics of the reinforcers, amount and delay. The bigger a reinforcer is, the more often it is chosen; but the more delayed a reinforcer is, the less often it is chosen. According to the matching law, the child should choose the one cookie available in 1 hour eight times as often as the three cookies available after tomorrow night's dinner.

If the child does choose the one less delayed cookie, this would be an example of *impulsiveness*, while a choice of the three more delayed cookies is an example of *self-control*. Many psychologists define choice of a larger, more delayed reinforcer over a smaller, less delayed reinforcer as self-control, and the opposite as impulsiveness.[9] In the present example with the cookies, the matching law predicts that impulsiveness is much more likely to occur than self-control. Note, however, that this prediction is not the same as maximization. To maximize total amount of received reinforcement, the child should choose the three delayed cookies.

CHOOSING EARLIER.   The matching law does suggest a way in which the probability of self-control can be increased. Figure 7.1a shows the matching law's description of the value of the two reinforcers, the one cookie available within 1 hour and the three cookies available in 24 hours, as a function of time. The solid vertical lines indicate the points in time at which the two reinforcers would be received. As one moves backwards in time, toward the left part of the graph, the values of the reinforcers decrease, as indicated by the decreasing curves. These decreases reflect the fact that if, for example, you are offered a candy bar that is available now, it would be worth a lot more to you than if you were offered a candy bar that would be available 10 years from now.

In Figure 7.1a, the X represents the point at which the child in our example is asked to make his choice. At this time, 6 p.m. Tuesday, the value of the one cookie is larger than the value of the three cookies. However, 15 hours earlier, at time Y, 3 a.m., assuming that the child could have been awakened, Equation 1 takes the following form:

$$\frac{B_1}{B_2} = \frac{A_1}{A_2} \times \frac{D_2}{D_1} = \frac{3}{1} \times \frac{(1+15)}{(24+15)} = \frac{48}{39} = \frac{1.2}{1} . \tag{2}$$

With 15 hours added to each reinforcer delay, the value of choosing the three cookies is greater than the value of choosing the one cookie. This is an example of what psychologists call *preference reversal*, and it is frequently seen in studies of self-control.[10]

Thus if the child can be induced to make his choice at time Y instead of at time X (in other words, if he can make his choice when both reinforcers are somewhat distant in time), he would be more likely to choose the three more-delayed cookies. As shown by Figure 7.1a, even earlier choices, say at dinnertime the previous night (time Z), will also result in self-control.

Choice Situation 2B Suppose it is late Monday night. The mother wants a snack and goes to the cookie jar, only to discover that her husband has once again eaten all but one cookie. The mother cannot go to the store the next day as she has to go out of town on business. She knows her child is going to have to get the one- versus three-cookie choice Tuesday after dinner, and she wants her child to show self-control. So she wakes her child up to give him the choice now; tomorrow morning would be too late. Everything goes as planned, and he chooses the three more delayed cookies, but there is still a problem. A babysitter is coming to give the child his Tuesday dinner as the

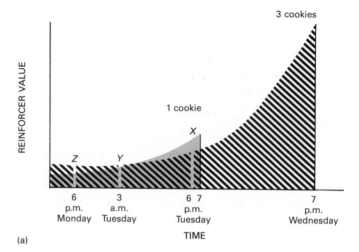

3 cookies

1 cookie

Z   Y   X

| 6 | 3 | 6 7 | 7 |

6
p.m.
Monday

3
a.m.
Tuesday

6 7
p.m.
Tuesday

7
p.m.
Wednesday

REINFORCER VALUE

TIME

(a)

REINFORCER VALUE

TIME

(b)

REINFORCER VALUE

TIME

(c)

mother will not yet be back from her business trip and the father will be at his weight-loss support group. The babysitter will give the child the cookie choice, and at that point the child will choose the one less delayed cookie. The child himself realizes this when he is awakened by his mother to make his choice, and he reminds his mother to leave a note for the babysitter that he has already made his choice and that the babysitter is not to give in to his pleas for the one cookie, no matter what.

A behavior of this kind, one that prevents an organism from making a future impulsive choice, is known as a *precommitment* device.[11] In most laboratory experiments, nonhuman animals have been unable to demonstrate self-control except with the use of precommitment devices. For example, pigeons are much more likely to wait for the larger, more delayed reinforcer if they have the opportunity, prior to their usual choice, to limit that choice to one between the larger, more delayed reinforcer and nothing. Many pigeons take advantage of such a precommitment opportunity.[12]

EVENTS DURING REINFORCER DELAYS.   There is another way to increase self-control in animals. This procedure is shown in Figure 7.2. It involves first giving subjects choices between equally delayed small and large reinforcers, and then very slowly decreasing the delay for the small reinforcer. James E. Mazur and A. W. Logue used this procedure with pigeons.[13] At the end of the experiment, Mazur and Logue's pigeons continued to choose the larger, more delayed reinforcer most of the time. Pigeons that had not been exposed to this fading procedure were consistently impulsive, choosing the smaller, less delayed reinforcer. Impulsive children exposed to a similar fading procedure also demonstrate increased self-control.[14]

Logue and Mazur[15] showed further that the increase in self-control demonstrated by the pigeons exposed to the fading procedure was stable over time, and was dependent on the presence of colored lights during the delay periods. In the experimental chamber, if a pigeon pecked the green

FIGURE 7.1   *The hypothetical values of two reinforcers as a function of time.* The two reinforcers are actually received at the times indicated by the solid vertical lines. The points X, Y, and Z indicate three times at which choices are made between the two reinforcers. In panel (b), reinforcer value as a function of delay declines relatively more slowly than in panel (a). In panel (c), reinforcer value as a function of delay declines relatively more quickly than in panel (a). (Adapted from A. W. Logue, M. L. Rodriguez, T. E. Pena-Correal, and B. C. Mauro, "Choice in a Self-Control Paradigm: Quantification of Experience-Based Differences," *Journal of the Experimental Analysis of Behavior* 41[1984]:53–67.)

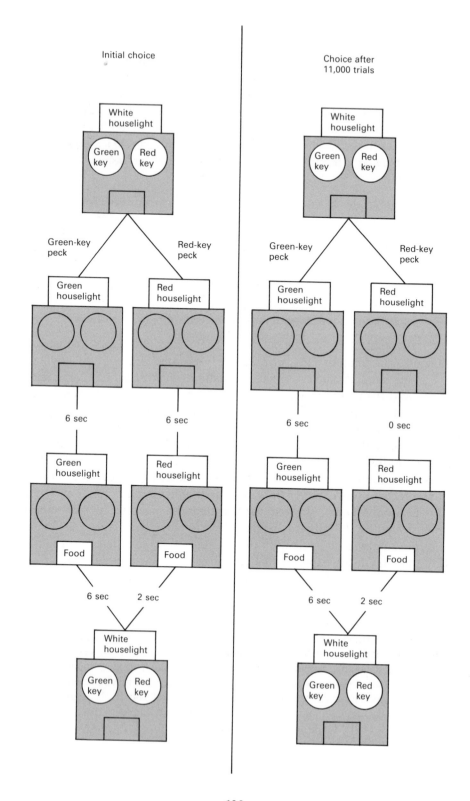

button that delivered the larger, more delayed reinforcer, a green light il-luminated the chamber; if it pecked the red button that delivered the smaller, less delayed reinforcer, a red light illuminated the chamber. Without these green and red chamber lights, the pigeons ceased to show the self-con-trol that they had acquired through the fading procedure.

These chamber-illumination lights may have functioned as reminders, linking the pigeons' choices with the reinforcers. Many experiments by Wal-ter Mischel and his colleagues have shown that the kinds of events that are present during the delays are crucial to a demonstration of self-control in children. These researchers have postulated that any events that result in the children's thinking about the motivating qualities of these reinforcers, such as how good those cookies would taste, decrease self-control; but thinking about other characteristics of the reinforcers, such as the round shape of the cookies and the little specks in them, increases self-control. These types of thoughts can be termed hot and cold thoughts, respectively. Further, playing games during the delay period, or even falling asleep, both of which presumably decrease hot thoughts, increase self-control in children.[16] The performance of alternative behaviors during the delay to the larger reinfor-cer may also help to increase self-control in pigeons.[17]

All of these findings, ways of decreasing and increasing self-control through manipulation of environmental events, are inconsistent with the matching law as expressed in Equations 1 and 2. These equations only ad-dress the quantitative values of the reinforcers. Therefore any subject ex-posed to the same reinforcers should make the same choices as any other subject exposed to those reinforcers, no matter what occurs during the rein-forcer delays and no matter what previous experiences the subject has had.

A modified version of the matching law described by A. W. Logue and her colleagues[18] dealt with these problems. This modification suggested that

FIGURE 7.2   *Fading procedure used to increase self-control in pigeons.* The pigeons are initially given a choice between 6 seconds of food delayed 6 seconds and 2 seconds of food delayed 6 seconds. They consistently choose the 6-second reinforcer. Then, over a year's time and approximately 11,000 trials, the delay to the 2-second reinforc-er is slowly decreased until the pigeons are choosing between 6 seconds of food delayed 6 seconds and 2 seconds of food that is available immediately. The pigeons continue to choose the 6-second reinforcer in most instances. (After A. W. Logue, M. L. Rodriguez, T. E. Pena-Correal, and B. C. Mauro, "Choice in a Self-Control Paradigm: Quantification of Experience-Based Differences," *Journal of the Experimen-tal Analysis of Behavior* 41[1984]:53–67; J. E. Mazur and A. W. Logue, "Choice in a 'Self-Control' Paradigm: Effects of a Fading Procedure," *Journal of the Experimental Analysis of Behavior* 30[1978]:11–17.)

sensitivity, that is, degree of reaction, to changes in reinforcer delay could differ across subjects and situations. When sensitivity to changes in reinforcer delay is small, the actual physical values of the delays could be described as seeming shorter for the subjects; the passage of time has little effect and time seems to go faster. This should increase self-control, because when time seems to go faster the subjects should be more likely to wait for the larger, more delayed reinforcer. This relation is borne out in Figure 7.1. Figure 7.1b shows how a decrease in the size of sensitivity to changes in reinforcer delay affects the curves shown in Figure 7.1a. The curves become less shallow and the crossover point, the point at which preference reverses, shifts to the right. There is now less time over which impulsiveness will be shown, less time over which the value of the smaller reinforcer is greater than that of the larger reinforcer, and so self-control is likely to increase. At the limit, where there is no sensitivity to variation in reinforcer delay, changes in delays have no effect, and the curves in Figure 7.1 would be horizontal straight lines, with the value of the larger, more delayed reinforcer always being greater than the value of the smaller, less delayed reinforcer, and with self-control always being shown. On the other hand, if sensitivity is increased, as shown in Figure 7.1c, the curves become much steeper and the crossover point shifts to the left, decreasing self-control. This modified version of the matching law can still describe changes in self-control resulting from changes in experience or from changes in the environment.

Different Types of Reinforcers

All of the choices described to this point have involved choices between two different frequencies, amounts, or delays of the same type of reinforcer. But in real life, humans and nonhumans often choose between two different types of reinforcers. For example, someone may have to choose between eating a hamburger or a piece of chicken, or between eating cookies now and dinner later. Can the matching law describe these types of situations?

In some cases it can. For example, H. L. Miller[19] conducted an experiment in which pigeons chose between different kinds of grain. He was able to describe choice between the different grains by simply expressing the amount of one kind of grain in terms applicable to the other type of grain. In other words, if a pea mixture were preferred to a hemp mixture, 1 second of eating the peas might be worth 1.5 seconds of eating the hemp. Once two grains had been expressed in common units, they could be used in the matching law as usual.

George R. King and A. W. Logue applied Miller's techniques to increase self-control in pigeons.[20] When the larger, more delayed reinforcer was also a more preferred grain, the pigeons were more likely to show self-control.

This finding suggests that it may be easier for people to wait for, say, a bag of M&Ms than for 6 ounces of broccoli, when the alternative is 2 ounces of broccoli that can be eaten immediately.

Conclusion

The matching law appears to provide a good, quantitative description of choice between different frequencies, amounts, and delays of reinforcement, and to describe self-control and impulsiveness as well. In some instances it can describe choice between different types of reinforcers. These results have been obtained using many different species. Often the choices made according to the matching law do maximize the total reinforcement obtained, but optimal foraging theory does have advantages over the matching law under some conditions, as will be described next.

OPTIMAL FORAGING THEORY

Definitions

To *forage* means to "wander or rove in search of food or other provisions."[21] Most organisms must forage repeatedly to survive. One version of *optimal foraging theory* builds on the assumption that evolution has shaped the behavior of organisms so that they forage in ways that maximize energy intake while minimizing energy output per unit of time spent foraging.[22] Thus optimal foraging theory is sometimes simply referred to as *optimization* or *maximization*.[23] It is important to keep in mind that two factors are involved—maximization of energy intake with concurrent minimization of energy output. Although the matching law sometimes makes predictions consistent with maximization, and sometimes does not, maximization is at the heart of optimal foraging theory.

Optimal foraging theory is closely tied to the field of ecology. Because optimal foraging theory proposes that in the course of evolution organisms have acquired behaviors that maximize their income while minimizing their costs, the natural habitat of each species is critical to understanding an organism's behavior. A particular foraging strategy may be optimal for a forest-floor habitat in Maine but not for a tree-dwelling existence in India. Without a knowledge of a species' habitat, it is impossible to determine whether or not that species forages optimally.

Most optimal foraging models contain three elements.[24] First, a model must concern itself with a particular aspect of food choice behavior, for example, choice between particular prey or choice between particular food patches. The particular food choice behavior with which a model is concerned may differ depending on the species studied. Some organisms eat only one kind of food. For example, the Koala bear eats only eucalyptus leaves. The Koala bear, a specialist, therefore has basically only one problem: to maintain its energy balance by regulating the amount of eucalyptus leaves that it finds and eats. Omnivores, on the other hand, are generalists, and they have a much more complex problem. Not only must they maintain an energy balance, as must the Koala bear, they must also regulate the amount of vitamins and other nutrients that they consume.[25]

Second, there must be a way of comparing the choices on a common scale. Most optimal foraging models use energy as their unit of analysis. These models involve mathematical equations, often extremely complex, that include energy obtained by foraging and energy used by moving and metabolic functions. These models are analogous to the earning and spending of money. Obtained food can be thought of as income, and energy expended in order to obtain that food can be thought of as cost. Therefore many researchers have proposed that optimal foraging research employ the terminology and the theoretical framework of economics.[26] Nevertheless, a common currency does not necessarily solve all problems of examining choice behavior between different types of reinforcers. For example, consider the intake of food and water. Most organisms need both of these. What is more, as discussed in Chapter 3, most organisms require food and water in specific packages—specific combinations of so much food and so much water. Any type of food is worth little to a hungry and thirsty organism unless water is also available, even though the availability of water changes neither the energy expended to obtain the food nor the energy received by consuming it.

Although the matching law has no way of expressing this distinction using its current equations, optimal foraging theory has been able to do so. The theoretical framework often used in the mathematical descriptions of optimal foraging comes from the work in economics on *substitutability*.[27] Food and water are essentially not substitutable; if an animal is thirsty but not hungry, it will not consume food as a substitute for unavailable water. Food and water are complements; food is worth more to a hungry and thirsty organism if it is accompanied by water. Thus, in choice situations of this kind, optimal foraging theory provides a better description of behavior than does the matching law.

The third element contained by most optimal foraging models is assumptions about the limits (that is, the *constraints*) on organisms' ability to forage optimally. For example, models may assume that organisms' ability to forage optimally is or is not limited by the degree to which they can obtain information about the environment. All organisms' foraging behavior is constrained to at least some degree.[28]

Economics and anthropology are primarily concerned with the behavior of large groups of people. Because experimental ecologists and animal learning researchers work mainly with individual animals, studies on optimal foraging theory using individual organisms have tended to be done by scientists whose background is in ecology or animal learning. In contrast, studies on optimal foraging theory using large groups have tended to be done by researchers whose background is in economics or anthropology. Nonetheless, principles of economics and ecology can be applied in optimal foraging studies, and studies of optimal foraging frequently use information from both economics and ecology.

Most studies of optimal foraging theory have examined choice situations for which it was possible to reasonably consider simple intake and output of energy. The sections that follow discuss two kinds of studies based on simple intake and output of energy—studies of the choice behavior of individual organisms and studies of the choice behavior of groups of organisms.

Micro Approach

GENERAL DESCRIPTION.   Many researchers have sought to use the principles of optimal foraging theory to describe the choice behavior of single animals. Several of these scientists have seen optimal foraging theory as a replacement for more traditional operant-conditioning models, such as the matching law, considering it a better description of the way laboratory subjects perform on various schedules of reinforcement, including schedules that involve choice.[29] Employing terminology from economics, these investigations can be termed *micro-approach studies*. The object is to describe and predict the behavior of individual animals.[30]

For example, many researchers have described what has been called the classical optimal foraging model for situations involving a choice between two types of prey.[31] According to this model, each of the two prey types can be described using three parameters: for a particular prey type i, λ_i (the frequency with which food is encountered while the forager is searching for food), h_i (the time taken to prepare the prey for consumption, i.e., handling time), and e_i (the gross energy gained by consuming the prey minus the energetic costs of obtaining the prey). The profitability of a particular prey type is then defined as e_i/h_i. If prey type 1 is more profitable than prey type 2, this model predicts that type 1 will always be chosen over type 2 unless:

$$\frac{1}{\lambda_1} > \frac{e_1}{e_2} h_2 - h_1 \ .$$

In other words, prey type 1 will always be chosen over prey type 2 unless the time between encounters of type 1 prey is large with respect to the differences in gross energy gained and handling time required for type 1 as compared to type 2 prey. More recent models have considered such issues as whether foraging behavior is random or systematic and whether encounters with prey are sequential or simultaneous.[32]

The variety of species whose food choice behavior has been investigated using this general type of approach is huge, including bees,[33] blue jays,[34] pigeons,[35] rats,[36] cats,[37] and monkeys.[38] One species whose food choice behavior has not been carefully studied from the perspective of optimal foraging theory for individuals is humans. For both ethical and practical reasons, it would be very difficult to manipulate and control the food intake as well as the energy consumption of humans.

Of the studies done with nonhumans, many have been conducted in the laboratory. Some have been conducted under natural and seminatural conditions. Some detailed examples from the work of Graham H. Pyke help illustrate how such foraging studies are conducted.

One series of Pyke's experiments compared the foraging of two species of birds: hummingbirds and honeyeaters.[39] Both of these species feed on the nectar of flowers, but to do this, hummingbirds hover and honeyeaters perch. For these experiments, Pyke used three methodologies. For the field studies he observed the birds' behavior under natural conditions, measuring as many of the relevant variables as he could, for example, the distance traveled between flowers, the time spent at each flower, and body weight. For the aviary experiments he constructed artificial "flowers" consisting of surgical needles filled with a solution of sucrose. He was therefore able to control the exact amount and spacing of food available. For the computer simulation studies, Pyke used estimates of the birds' optimal foraging behavior, employing a computer program that used several assumptions as well as actual observations concerning the birds' foraging behavior.

Through these methods, Pyke was able to show that the actual foraging behavior of the two kinds of birds—hovering for the hummingbird and perching for the honeyeater, the pattern of movement between the flowers, and the amount of time spent at each flower—was approximately optimal. Hovering allows a bird to move more quickly and easily between flowers, but more energy is required to sustain hovering than perching. Thus hovering is more suited to a smaller bird that requires less energy to hover, such as the hummingbird, than to a larger bird that requires more energy to hover, such as the honeyeater. Pyke noted, however, that the actual pattern of movement of the hummingbirds was only optimal if it were assumed that the hummingbirds were unable to use two types of information: the direction of likely flowers relative to the bird's previous direction of travel, and the sizes and distances of likely flowers.

Another example comes from the work of William A. Roberts and Tamara J. Ilersich.[40] These researchers examined the foraging behavior of rats in a four-arm radial maze (that is, a maze shaped like a simple plus sign). Each arm contained four possible locations in which there could be food. Roberts and Ilersich varied whether or not individual arms in the maze were open or closed, whether or not specific locations within an arm contained food, and whether that food was covered or exposed. Sometimes the food locations remained fixed, and sometimes they varied. One of the many findings of this study was that, when food locations changed randomly, the rats tended to visit, in order, all potential food locations in an arm before leaving the arm. Roberts and Ilersich performed a computer simulation of their rats' behavior to determine optimal performance in their experiment. In general, the real rats' behavior was similar to the optimal behavior simulated by the computer.

CONSTRAINTS. Many studies of optimal foraging in individual organisms have been forced to confront the issue of the subject's ability to forage optimally. If optimal is described simply as the maximum possible energy gain over a unit of time, independent of the characteristics of the subject, some ludicrous predictions would be made.

Choice Situation 3 Consider a deer foraging in a forest during the winter. Suppose the deer has stripped the bushes and trees of all remaining leaves and berries as high as it can reach. There are more leaves and berries at higher levels, but is the deer a nonoptimal forager because it does not eat them?

Choice Situation 4 Suppose it is early March and a 6-year-old deer must choose one of two mountains on which to forage for the next 6 months because in late March the melting snows will create a river between the two mountains that is too deep for the deer to cross until the river dries up in late September. Five years ago the deer chose mountain A, where there was an abundance of summer fruit and leaves. Four years ago the deer chose mountain B, where there was little to eat. For the past three summers the deer has been penned in a field during the summer and fed from a trough as part of a wildlife control program. Is the deer a nonoptimal forager if it now chooses Mountain B?

An organism's ability to forage optimally may be constrained by its own characteristics, for example, its ability to reach food and its ability to remember previous food locations, what could be called its cognitive capacity. In addition, how much information the organism has or can obtain about available food also influences its success in foraging optimally.[41] Many of these constraints on optimal foraging have been demonstrated experimentally. In these experiments the task of obtaining food was made more complex and the foraging efficiency of the subjects then decreased. For example, David S. Olton, Gail E. Handelmann, and John A. Walker conducted an experiment with rats in which the researchers increased the number of locations where food might be available; the rats spent more time visiting locations that did not contain food, and their foraging efficiency decreased.[42]

Similar limitations are shown by experiments in which subjects are repeatedly exposed to a situation that requires them to take into account the future availability of food. For example, subjects may be given an opportunity to work for food, although free food will be given some time later. Rats and pigeons in this situation do not behave optimally; even though there is little advantage to working for food, they continue to do so. These results have been interpreted as indicating that organisms integrate events over a fairly brief time; their *time window* is relatively short.[43]

Experiments on self-control in which pigeons repeatedly choose the smaller, less delayed reinforcer also help to demonstrate the time window constraint. For example, Mazur and Logue's fading procedure increased the pigeons' self-control, but this could also be described as an increase in the pigeons' time windows, which are normally quite limited.[44] The behavior of pigeons exposed to the fading procedure was controlled more by the more distant, larger reinforcer than was the behavior of pigeons that had not been exposed to the fading procedure. Adult humans show greater self-control in the laboratory than do pigeons; they have a greater window than do pigeons. This is apparently due to the fact that adult humans can count and can time events, and this allows them to integrate events over entire laboratory sessions.[45]

Organisms are also limited in their ability to forage efficiently by the performance of other behaviors necessary for their survival. For example, salamanders forage optimally only in territories that they have marked with their own pheromones. In other territories they spend much of their time and energy on marking or engaging in submissive posturing.[46] Presumably this is still adaptive, because it decreases the chances that the salamander will later have to engage in territorial conflict.

RISK AVERSION AND RISK PREFERENCE. Optimal foraging theory predicts that under situations of extreme food deprivation, when only a large reinforcer would be sufficient to keep an organism from dying, an organism should be more likely to choose a "risky" alternative that sometimes delivers a large amount of food and sometimes delivers a little food, compared with "a sure thing," an alternative that always delivers a medium amount of food.[47] This prediction has been confirmed by Thomas Caraco and his colleagues with several species of birds.[48] However, similar findings were not obtained with rats.[49] Additional work is needed to determine under what conditions risk aversion and risk preference occur.

SELF-CONTROL AND IMPULSIVENESS. The optimal foraging analysis of risk aversion and risk preference makes it apparent that it can sometimes be adaptive for an organism to choose an alternative that could result in the organism's receiving a relatively small amount of food. Another example of how this can happen occurs with experiments on self-control. Optimal foraging researchers have pointed out that it can be adaptive for organisms to discount delayed events (similar to having a relatively short time window) because during a species' evolutionary history it is likely that delayed events have actually been less likely to occur than immediate events.[50] For example, suppose a bear chooses to wait for the berries on a large bush to ripen rather than going to the other side of the mountain where there is a small bush that has ripe berries now. During the delay period, the bear might be interrupted because it had to go find a mate, or because it was killed by a hunter, and thus may not end up being able to eat the ripe berries. During this same period the semiripened berries might be eaten by birds, or they might be destroyed in a big storm. Finally, the ripe berries might or might not appear at the end of the waiting period (the berries on some bushes do not ripen no matter how long you wait).

Therefore, particularly if an organism needs some food quickly in order to survive, it can be adaptive for that organism to choose a smaller, immediate reinforcer over a larger, delayed reinforcer. Further, species that have evolved in environments characterized by a great deal of change and unpredictability should be more likely to be impulsive than species that have evolved in fairly constant environments.[51]

INDIVIDUAL DIFFERENCES. Optimal foraging theory can also describe individual differences. Anteaters show large individual differences in the type of ant they prefer to consume and in the type of habitat in which they prefer to forage. An anteater whose food preferences are somewhat different from those of nearby anteaters is likely to find more food and therefore to have an increased chance of survival.[52] Individual differences can sometimes help to maximize food intake, and in those instances they are predicted by optimal foraging theory.

Optimal foraging theory does describe well the food-choice behavior of individual organisms of many species in a great variety of situations. The next section considers the food-choice behavior of groups of organisms in light of optimal foraging theory.

Macro Approach

Employing the terminology of economics, optimal foraging analyses applied to the food-choice behavior of large groups of organisms of the same species can be termed *macro-approach studies*. One argument that has been made in support of macro-approach studies is that group behavior is a consequence of the behavior of the individuals that make up the group. Therefore if economic principles apply to the behavior of individuals, they should apply to group behavior as well.[53] Further, when people shop for food they often purchase for an entire household, and the standards of desirability for foods are usually a function of the opinions of a group of people, not of a particular person.[54] Finally, sometimes the only data available are group data. This has been true for archeological attempts to study the food choices of extinct cultures.[55] For all of these reasons many group studies of optimal foraging theory have been performed, the majority using human subjects.

Some examples of the macro-economic effects on food-choice behavior have been described in Chapter 5. There, it was pointed out that when the price went down for sugar products and the availability went up, consumption of sugar products increased. This is a general phenomenon as countries industrialize.[56] Similar relationships have been demonstrated for the consumption of other nutrients as well.[57]

Optimal foraging theory has also been increasingly used in the field of anthropology. In particular, it has been applied to explaining three types of problems: territorial behavior in *hunter-gatherers* (people who obtain food by hunting, fishing, and gathering food items from the wild), group foraging strategies, and food sharing.[58] For example, it has been found that chimpanzees' group structure while foraging maximizes efficiency in obtaining fruit.[59] As another example, the Ache foragers in Paraguay and the Hiwi foragers in Venezuela only attempt to obtain a food when the net energy they expect to receive from it is greater than the energy they would have if they ignored that food, again consistent with optimal foraging theory.[60]

THE MATCHING LAW VERSUS OPTIMAL FORAGING THEORY

Many researchers have argued over whether the matching law or optimal foraging theory provides a better description of behavior, and many experiments have been conducted to test these views.[61] The matching law would seem to have an advantage in that it appears relatively easy for organisms to behave as it predicts; they need only distribute their responses as reinforcers are distributed. Both the matching law and the optimal foraging theorists agree that no organism can be expected to have perfect knowledge or perfect ability to determine and to carry out optimal food-choice behavior. However, the matching law has trouble describing choice between foods that are not substitutable, and it does not take effort into account. On the other hand, to adequately test optimal foraging theory it is usually necessary to measure energy expenditure and energy income, and that is often impossible. To some extent, when the subjects' food-choice behavior does not conform to the researchers' expectations, both the matching law and the optimal foraging theorists take refuge in explanations such as that the procedure was too complex for the subject or something must not have been measured properly. Perhaps the best resolution to this argument is provided by J. E. R. Staddon:

> Optimal behavior is always subject to *constraints* and in the limit these constraints define the *mechanism* that animals use to achieve something like reinforcement maximization under many, but never all, conditions. . . . Optimality theory remains useful because when it fails it points to limits on animals' ability to optimize, and thus to constraints and mechanisms. When it succeeds it is useful because it makes sense of behavior in many situations.[62]

In other words, optimality is a useful concept for developing ways to describe food-choice behavior. One of these ways could be the matching law. Organisms may not always be able to behave optimally because of various constraints. They may therefore behave according to simple principles that frequently coincide with optimal behavior, so-called rules of thumb,[63] such as the matching law.

Thus optimal foraging theory, identified most closely with the field of biology, and the matching law, from the field of psychology, are not necessarily competing, exclusive explanations. Instead they are complementary, with the matching law tending to focus on behavioral mechanisms and optimal foraging theory tending to focus on net energy gain and inclusive fitness (see Figure 7.3). Both approaches are concerned with the same behavior in the same environments, and both have much to contribute with regard to food-choice behavior.

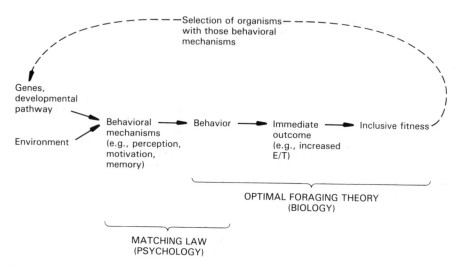

FIGURE 7.3   *Relationships between psychological and optimal foraging mechanisms in describing choice betweeen different food items.* (Adapted from S. J. Shettleworth, "Learning and Foraging in Pigeons: Effects of Handling Time and Changing Food Availability on Patch Choice," *Quantitative Analyses of Behavior* 6[1987]:115–132.)

The matching law and optimality theory are the two most frequently investigated quantitative models of choice, but there are many others: Edmund Fantino's delay reduction model,[64] John Gibbon's scalar expectancy theory,[65] and Peter R. Killeen's incentive theory,[66] to name a few. Through investigations of these models we may someday be able to describe and predict many of the effects of food availability on the choice behavior of all organisms.

CONCLUSION

This chapter concludes the section of the book on the determinants of normal eating and drinking behavior. The present chapter and the past two chapters have sought to explain how different foods are selected for consumption. A number of examples of largely genetic and largely environmental determinants of food preferences, as well as models describing choice as a function of food availability, were described. Explaining and predicting food selection is complex and difficult but not impossible, and progress is being made. The next section of the book turns to the effects of food on behavior.

Part III

EXPERIMENTS WITH NUTRITIVE AND NONNUTRITIVE SUBSTANCES

The chapter that follows takes a somewhat different perspective from the others in this book. Instead of examining what factors are responsible for our consumption of foods and drinks, Chapter 8 looks at how the nutritive and nonnutritive substances we consume affect our behavior, and how these behavioral effects are studied by experimental researchers. Because an evaluation of experimental findings rests on a thorough understanding of experimental methods, the chapter begins with a discussion of research methodology.

CHAPTER
8
❧
The Effects of
Food on Behavior

The bodies of all organisms, including humans, derive from the nutrients the organisms consume, whether through the umbilical cord in fetal mammals, through the egg yolk in fetal birds, or through the mouth in young and adult organisms. If we accept that all behavior, in every organism, is ultimately determined by the body, then behavior must be affected by what is eaten. In the extreme, if no food is eaten, there will be no behavior, because without food organisms die. But there are many other ways in which the consumption of food can affect behavior.

For example, daily fluctuations in the diet influence the function of neurons in the brain. Neurotransmitters are synthesized from specific chemical precursors, such as *choline*, the precursor for *acetylcholine*. Behavior is influenced by the levels of the neurotransmitters, which in turn are in-

145

fluenced by the levels of the precursors, which in turn are influenced by the daily diet.[1]

This chapter draws on research that has investigated these types of changes in behavior as a function of food consumed and emphasizes how the food an organism chooses can affect its behavior. Experiments demonstrate the necessity of normal food intake for normal behavior in two ways—by removing food, with resulting abnormal behavior, and by giving certain foods, with resulting abnormal behavior. The effects of food on abnormal behavior are described here by these two kinds of experiments, with the exception of the effects of consumption of alcohol, which will be described in Chapter 11.

Recent popular interest in the possible effects of food on behavior has been substantial. After all, if modern manufactured chemicals such as diazepam (Valium) and thorazine can affect our actions, why not the chemicals present in foods? Fortunately, the research establishment has also been showing an interest in this topic, and many carefully performed experiments have now been published.[2]

Before delving into the data, it will be helpful first to briefly review some of the basic methodological strategies and issues involved in evaluating the effects of any environmental manipulation.[3] Conducting a good experiment on the effects of a particular treatment is extremely difficult, and an understanding of what is required will provide a foundation for interpreting the experimental findings presented in this chapter and the ones that follow.

RESEARCH STRATEGIES AND ISSUES

Suppose you are a psychologist working for a large food-products manufacturer. This company has developed a new artificial food color, AAA, and the company wants to use AAA in its new product, Bright and Early Cereal. Your company's medical research department has already shown that AAA does not cause cancer, heart attacks, rashes, or any other medical problems. It is now your job to determine whether AAA causes any adverse behavioral reactions. How do you do this? It is not an easy job.

Designing the Experiment

CONTROLLING WHO KNOWS WHAT.   One strategy would be to give AAA to some people but not to others. You would have to make sure that the people getting the food color did not know when they were getting it. Otherwise your subjects might react the way they believed appropriate for having received AAA, thus failing to demonstrate their actual reaction to

AAA. Behavior of this kind is known as *demand characteristics*. Since you can hardly slip AAA into your subjects' morning coffee at home, you could give some of your subjects AAA but others a placebo. A true placebo looks, feels, smells, and tastes exactly the same as a real substance, in this case AAA, but is actually an inert substance that causes no reaction whatsoever.

But suppose it is your job both to prepare the AAA and the placebo for administration by forming them into pink pills and to give the pills to the subjects. Therefore you know who is receiving AAA and who is receiving placebo. But remember, it is possible for you to unintentionally communicate to individual subjects how you expect them to react to the particular substance that you are giving them (see Chapter 6). This is another example of demand characteristics. A better strategy would be for one of your assistants to prepare the pink pills and to note which is which, so that when you distribute the pills you have no idea who is getting AAA and who is getting placebo. When neither the experimenter nor the subjects are aware of which treatment a subject receives, the experiment has a *double-blind design*.

SELECTING THE SUBJECTS. You have decided to use a double-blind design. Now you need to choose your subject population. You could require all of the company's secretaries to participate as a condition for receiving their next paycheck, but that is not ethical. It would be better to ask for volunteers, perhaps using a monetary incentive. However, your company's human-subjects ethics committee warns you that, if you use human subjects, there must be adequately informed consent, which means that the subjects cannot consent to participate in the experiment until after you have told them the purpose of the experiment, explained that they might receive an experimental food color or placebo, and outlined any possible harmful consequences that may affect them.

Even faced with all these requirements to be satisfied, you still feel that it is better to use humans than rats. You know that the eating behavior of rats is very similar to that of humans and that your company has used rats in many previous experiments. But you realize that results obtained with rats may not be as applicable to the selling of your company's Bright and Early Cereal as would results obtained with humans. Further, the medical department has assured you that the chances of any adverse reactions to this drug are extremely small, and adequately informed consent is not a problem for your experiment if you use the double-blind design.

You post signs around your company's plant describing the experiment and offering $10 for participation; 100 people volunteer. According to your statistical estimates, you only need 50 subjects in order to see whether AAA has an effect: 25 to receive the placebo and 25 to receive the AAA. How do you choose which 50 people will be in the experiment? If you look through

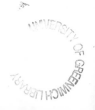

the list of volunteers and pick those people that seem about right, you may be using some unspecified, and therefore undesirable, selection criteria. You may be introducing some bias in the sample by choosing certain characteristics that may, unbeknownst to you, affect the subjects' reactions to AAA or placebo. Ideally the two groups should differ only in the substance each group receives, either AAA or placebo. Therefore you should probably pick the subjects randomly.

But random selection may cause another problem. At the end of the experiment you want to compare the reactions of the subjects who received the placebo with those who received the AAA. Suppose that, even though you randomly pick the subjects for each group, the placebo subjects are all older than the AAA subjects. Then it might be difficult to tell whether any differences between the two groups were due to AAA or to age. This problem can be solved by ensuring that the placebo and AAA subjects are picked randomly, but with the constraint that the average age of the two groups is similar. In fact, the two groups of subjects should be *matched* on any variable that you think could conceivably cause a difference in their reaction to AAA.

The subjects who are given the AAA will be called the *experimental group*, and the subjects who are given the placebo will be called the *control group*. This terminology is used to indicate that the experimental subjects receive the experimental manipulation, AAA, and the control subjects test whether or not any factors other than the consumption of AAA affect the subjects' behavior (the control subjects "control for" any effects other than that of AAA, for example, any effects due solely to the administration to the subjects of the pink pills).

In this case it is possible to match the two groups perfectly by giving each subject the AAA on one occasion and the placebo on the other occasion. Now the groups receiving AAA and the placebo are identical, and each subject serves as his or her own control. This type of design is known as a *within-subject design;* experiments in which different groups of subjects receive different treatments use what is known as a *between-subject design* (Figure 8.1). Generally the within-subject design is statistically more *powerful,* meaning that fewer subjects are needed to determine statistically whether a treatment has had any effect. The only situations in which a within-subject design is not advisable are those in which the effects of one or more of the treatments are lasting, so that they interfere with determining the effects of subsequent treatments.

ADMINISTERING THE TREATMENTS.   You are fairly sure that any effects of AAA do not last, so you can use a within-subject design. In using a within-subject design in this experiment, you will have to ensure that half of the subjects receive the AAA first and half receive the placebo first. This controls

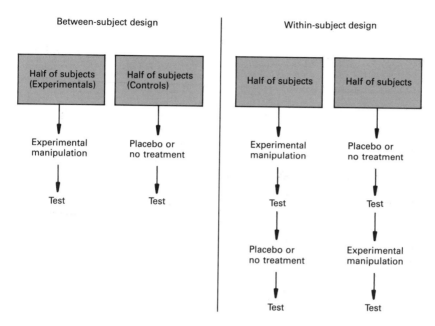

FIGURE 8.1   *Between-subject and within-subject experimental designs.* In a between-subject design, half of the subjects, the experimentals, receive the experimental treatment, and half, the controls, receive no treatment or a placebo. In a within-subject design each subject serves as its own control, receiving both the treatment and the placebo.

for (i.e., tests for the existence of) any effects that arise from the order in which treatment is administered. A subject might react differently simply because it is the second, rather than the first, time that he or she has received a substance.

Now you have to decide how much AAA to give and whether to give it along with any other foods. Since you work for a food-products manufacturer, it is important to you that your results be useful to your employer. Therefore you want whatever manipulations you make to be comparable to natural conditions. In other words, the amount of AAA that you give should be reasonably close to what a subject would normally receive. Further, since people would probably be getting AAA in cereal, you might want to deliver it or the placebo in cereal rather than in pink pills so that you could determine the actual effects of AAA when eaten with cereal.

Another strategy would be to give the subjects nothing to eat for 24 hours before and after AAA or placebo administration in order to isolate the effects of AAA. A procedure such as this one, in which only one substance is administered in order to assess that substance's acute effects, is known as a *challenge design*. However, while the challenge design might maximize the chances of seeing any effects of AAA, it is not comparable to natural conditions. Your goal is to determine the effects of AAA in actual eating situations; therefore you decide not to use a challenge design but to give the subjects the AAA or the placebo in cereal, using the approximate amounts that the manufacturer would use.

MEASURING THE EFFECTS.   You have only one other major design problem: how to measure the effects of the AAA versus the placebo on your subjects' behavior. Simply having people report how they feel is sometimes but not always indicative of the effects on behavior that actually occur. Therefore you decide both to ask the subjects structured questions about how they feel and to observe their behavior on various learning and social-cooperation tasks. You choose the particular questions and tasks based on their proven success, in previous studies, in detecting subtle behavioral changes following subjects' exposure to artificial food colors other than AAA.

Evaluating the Data

You conduct the experiment and obtain your data. Let us suppose, for the sake of simplification, that you are able to distill all of the collected measures into one number for each subject. These numbers range from 0 to 100, with a score of 0 being normal behavior and a score of 100 being extremely abnormal behavior. Your subjects obtain an average score of 15 when they are given the placebo but an average score of 25 when they are given the AAA. Your subject sample is large enough that, with the aid of various statistical computations, you can state that in 95 percent of similar experiments, results this different between the placebo and the AAA treatments would have been due to the AAA treatment, not to chance. Therefore you can state fairly confidently that AAA did cause behavioral changes in your experiment; the AAA resulted in a *statistically significant* change in behavior.

But was that change *clinically significant?* Is a difference of 10 in the scores a meaningful change in terms of behavior in the natural environment? Under normal conditions would anyone notice a difference between someone scoring 15 and someone scoring 25? The manufacturer might decide that statistical significance by itself is insufficient grounds for not putting AAA into the cereal.

Now suppose that the difference between these average scores, 15 and 25, is not statistically significant; the probability that these results could have occurred due to chance is greater than 5 percent. Does this mean that AAA has no effect? There is still some probability that the results are not due to chance. In addition, suppose there are one or two subjects who show huge increases in their behavioral scores when they are given AAA, but the remainder of the subjects show no change or a change in the opposite direction. What if AAA causes behavioral problems in some subjects but not in others? Most statistical tests are not designed to determine whether there is a small minority of subjects who show a reaction.[4] It is difficult to determine whether these few subjects actually are more sensitive to AAA or whether this is just a chance occurrence. By chance alone you would expect a few of the subjects to show increases in their scores after having been given AAA. A solution might be to conduct the experiment again, but only with the subjects who had shown a strong reaction to AAA, to see whether they again showed the effect. If so, you would try to determine what was different between these subjects and those who had not shown the effect, so as to be able to predict who might show the effect in the future.

Conclusion

These are only a sample of the methodological and ethical problems that complicate experiments on the effects of various treatments or manipulations, including the effects of removing or consuming foods and food additives. In many instances there is no clear indication of which method to follow; the researcher must simply pick the one that seems best, given the goals of the particular experiment.

EFFECTS OF REMOVING NUTRITIVE SUBSTANCES

Some nutritional deficiencies affect virtually everyone, while other deficiencies cause behavioral problems only in some people. The sections that follow present data illustrating each of these types of effects.

Effects in the General Population

ALL NUTRIENTS. Depriving an organism of many nutritious substances over a relatively long period of time can be psychologically damaging. During infancy and early childhood malnutrition can hinder language development and result in lower IQ scores, and these effects may persist even after the malnutrition has been reversed.[5] A single missed breakfast can cause children to perform worse on IQ tests and on other cognitive tasks given later in the day.[6] These findings may be related to the fact that persistent malnutrition in infants, malnutrition over weeks and months, decreases the rate at which cells divide in the developing brain. Results from many different species suggest that this effect is permanent, resulting in a smaller brain even after the child is no longer malnourished.[7] Researchers have had difficulty showing that specific abilities, and not just overall energy level, are affected by malnutrition. Consequently they have been developing increasingly sophisticated tests for determining precisely what is affected by early malnutrition. One possible technique involves studying the effect of malnutrition on an organism's ability to learn food preferences through observation of its fellow organisms (observational learning), based on Galef's research on the social transmission of food preferences (see Chapter 6).[8] The advantage of using this type of task is that the animal can learn without making any overt movements.

SPECIFIC NUTRIENTS. The behavioral effects of depriving subjects of specific nutrients have also been investigated. For ethical reasons many of these studies have used animals, although some field studies with humans have also been performed.

Several experiments have been done in which animals were specifically deprived of protein. In general these experiments appear to show that current protein deprivation results in poorer learning in rats and monkeys.[9]

A deficiency in iron intake is the world's most common nutritional disorder, and unfortunately this disorder most frequently occurs between the ages of 6 and 24 months, when the brain is ending its growth spurt.[10] Rudolph L. Leibel, Ernesto Pollitt, and Daryl B. Greenfield[11] investigated the effects of iron deficiency on learning in 3- to 6-year-old children. They showed that these iron-deficient children learned discrimination tasks and performed other tasks requiring attention less well than did the nondeficient matched control subjects. When the iron deficiency was removed, however, the previously deprived children performed as well as the controls. Unfortunately this experiment does not rule out the possibility that the iron deficiency affected overall energy level or some other general factor, rather than specific aspects of cognitive functioning. In addition, other studies have found that iron deficient infants' developmental impairments persisted even after the iron deficiencies were removed.[12]

Effects in Some Members of the Population

Some researchers have hypothesized that for physiological reasons some people are deficient in one or more nutritive substances even though they receive what are normally adequate diets. These researchers reason that such deficiencies can cause these people to behave abnormally, and that the abnormal behavior can be treated or prevented by removing the deficiencies. Linus Pauling has called this approach *orthomolecular psychiatry.*[13]

One example of this sort of deficiency is seen in people with an irreversible memory disorder, *Korsakoff's syndrome*. People who suffer from this disease have difficulty remembering recent events.[14] Korsakoff's syndrome is caused by two factors. One is a genetic aberration in the activity of a particular enzyme, *transketolase*, necessary for the metabolism of glucose and the production of *RNA* (ribonucleic acid). The other is a diet deficient in thiamine. When both of these factors are present the syndrome will develop. Korsakoff's syndrome tends to be seen in alcoholics because they are frequently malnourished (see Chapter 11 for more discussion), but it can also occur in nonalcoholics if they have the genetic abnormality and a thiamine deficiency.[15]

But Pauling expanded the sphere of orthomolecular psychiatry far beyond diseases such as Korsakoff's syndrome. According to Pauling, many people are suffering from nutrient deficiencies that can be cured by changes in diet. For example, Pauling has contended that schizophrenics suffer from a deficiency of vitamin C and that schizophrenia can be successfully treated by giving large doses of vitamin C.[16] Such contentions have caused a great deal of controversy and some research.[17]

Thomas A. Ban and his colleagues have performed several experiments designed to determine whether large doses of vitamins will improve schizophrenia.[18] The experiments have all used placebos as well as double-blind designs. Many different types of schizophrenics have been used in these studies, as well as varying amounts of, and durations of exposure to, different vitamins. The vitamins used have included niacin, C, niacin plus C, niacin plus pyridoxine (B_6), and niacin plus pyridoxine plus C. There were no consistent improvements in the schizophrenics using any of these vitamins. Additional research has confirmed that niacin is ineffective in treating schizophrenia.[19] The possibility remains, however, that some of the treatments helped a few of the schizophrenics.

There have been suggestions in the research literature that consumption of certain amino acids and their derived products—notably tryptophan, tyrosine, and choline—can relieve such behavioral problems as depression, reactions to uncontrollable stress, and memory deficits.[20] However, definitive demonstrations of such effects have not been performed with human subjects.

Although there are some indications for the use of some nutrients in the treatment of some abnormal psychological behaviors, the public should nonetheless beware of unsubstantiated claims. False hope created by useless treatments can bring much harm to those who believe in them. False hope can mean money lost, time wasted, severe disappointment, avoidance of other more useful treatments, direct physical harm (for example, there may be direct physical harm to a patient who is given large doses of some nutrients, such as vitamins A, D, niacin, and pyridoxine), and possible physical harm to a patient who is supposed cured and is therefore subsequently poorly monitored.[21]

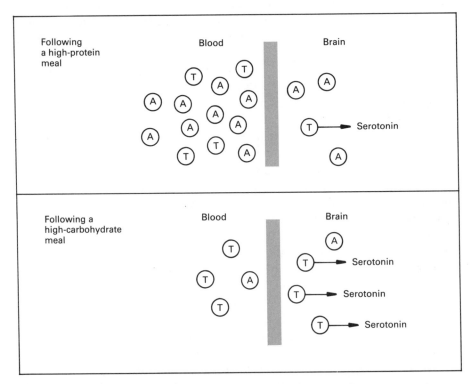

FIGURE 8.2   *Conceptual diagram of how tryptophan affects sleep behavior.* Tryptophan (T) in the blood competes with other amino acids (A) for access through the blood–brain barrier to the brain. After a high-protein meal is eaten, many amino acids enter the bloodstream; few of these are tryptophan. Therefore, because of competition, relatively little tryptophan enters the brain, and therefore tryptophan does not affect sleep. However, after a high-carbohydrate meal, very few amino acids enter the bloodstream. In addition, insulin is released. Insulin transports most of the amino acids, but not tryptophan, to the skeletal muscles. Therefore, because there is little competition, a relatively great amount of tryptophan enters the brain. In the brain tryptophan increases serotonin, and thereby sleep. (After H. R. Lieberman, S. Corkin, B. J. Spring, J. H. Growdon, and R. J. Wurtman, "Mood, Performance, and Pain Sensitivity: Changes Induced by Food Constituents," *Journal of Psychiatric Research* 17[1982/83]:135–145.)

EFFECTS OF GIVING NUTRITIVE SUBSTANCES

Effects in the General Population

NEUROTRANSMITTER PRECURSORS.   A large number of experiments have demonstrated that consumption of a meal can affect activity level, performance, and/or perceived time duration—sometimes increasing these measures of behavior and sometimes decreasing them, depending on the time of day that the meal is consumed and what it contains.[22] Specific effects of meals on the availability of neurotransmitter precursors, and thus on neurotransmitters in the brain and on behavior, have been consistently shown with *tryptophan* (a precursor) and serotonin (its neurotransmitter). Tryptophan is an amino acid. Serotonin is a neurotransmitter that is important in the regulation of sleep. Many studies have shown that direct administration of tryptophan improves sleep in adult and newborn humans.[23]

Normal variations in diet also affect tryptophan and thereby sleep, although not, perhaps, in the way that one might expect (Figure 8.2). The plasma concentration of tryptophan is increased by a high-carbohydrate (not a high-protein) meal. This seeming paradox occurs because protein foods contain very little tryptophan, although they do contain a great deal of other amino acids. After a high-protein meal the other amino acids in the blood compete with the small amount of tryptophan for access across the *blood–brain barrier,* allowing little tryptophan to enter the brain. (The blood–brain barrier is the functional barrier between the blood and the brain; some substances have more difficulty than others diffusing from the blood to the brain.[24]) The *insulin* secreted to digest whatever carbohydrate has also been ingested transports some of these other amino acids (but no tryptophan) to the skeletal muscles; however, the amount thus transported is insufficient to remove tryptophan's disadvantage in crossing the blood–brain barrier. On the other hand, after a high-carbohydrate meal, the insulin transports most of these other amino acids to the skeletal muscles. After a high-carbohydrate meal, therefore, tryptophan in the plasma has little competition for crossing the blood–brain barrier, and this allows more tryptophan to enter the brain.[25] Consequently a high-carbohydrate meal, not a high-protein meal, should improve sleep.

Bonnie Spring and her colleagues were able to partially confirm this hypothesis.[26] In their study, female subjects reported fatigue only following a single high-carbohydrate meal, but not following a single high-protein or a single carbohydrate and protein meal. Spring and her colleagues were able to demonstrate that the fatigue following the high-carbohydrate meal was not related to blood sugar level. However, the onset of fatigue coincided with the elevation of tryptophan in the blood.

Spring and her colleagues have also shown that subjects tend to perform worse on a task requiring sustained attention following a high-carbohydrate meal than following a high-protein meal.[27] Combined with the data described above regarding decreased cognitive performance of children after missing breakfast, Spring and her colleagues' results seem to suggest that regular meals containing some protein may assist in the performance of cognitive tasks.

Given Spring and her colleagues' results, it is not surprising that in a double-blind, placebo experiment by Judith L. Rapoport, children given a single dose of sugar showed lowered activity levels.[28] This was found despite the fact that subjects were recruited by newspaper advertisements soliciting children who were more active after having consumed sugar. The mothers of the children in the study claimed that their children showed immediate behavioral changes after consuming smaller doses of sugar than were given in the study. No such reactions were found. In fact, the children were less active after having consumed sugar. Additional well-controlled experiments have found either no change or a decrease in activity level following sugar consumption.[29] All of these data are consistent with the hypothesis that carbohydrates, including sugar, increase sleepiness.

Several other precursor–neurotransmitter relationships are well known. Examples are the precursor amino acid *tyrosine*, present in high-protein foods, and its neurotransmitters norepinephrine and *epinephrine*; and the precursor vitamin choline, present in foods containing the fat *lecithin*, and its neurotransmitter acetylcholine. In both of these cases, variations in diet have been shown to affect the availability of neurotransmitters in the brain.[30] However, the changes in human behavior seen following alterations in tyrosine and lecithin consumption have not been established to the extent that they have for serotonin.[31] Perhaps future experiments will find consistent behavioral effects for dietary lecithin and tyrosine. In any case the results with serotonin have clearly demonstrated that it is possible for diet to affect the brain and thereby behavior.

MSG.   *Monosodium glutamate (MSG)* is the sodium salt of an amino acid that is frequently added to foods as a flavor enhancer. Nevertheless, taste researchers have known for many years that MSG does not enhance flavors already present in food; instead it adds its own taste.[32] As is well known, the consumption of MSG gives many adults what is known as the *Chinese restaurant syndrome*, or, to be more accurate, *Kwok's disease*. This is an acute reaction frequently characterized by a tightening of the muscles of the face and neck, headache, nausea, giddiness, and sweating.[33] In the brain, MSG acts as an excitatory neurotransmitter. When it is present in excessive amounts, it becomes an *excitotoxin;* it can actually stimulate neurons to the point of death.[34] It has been shown that MSG given in high doses to rat pups can cause brain lesions and later difficulties in learning, even when the MSG is part of a normal diet. The effects of lower doses are not known.[35] Because of these findings, MSG has been removed from baby food, and there is continuing controversy about whether or not the Food and Drug Administration should ban it from all food.[36] A statement by M. E. Rubini provides a summary commentary on the use of MSG, particularly in baby food:

> More knowledge is needed for a rational understanding of what monosodium glutamate offers, both as advantage and as risk. Although it can be argued that the removal of glutamate from baby foods was premature and not based on sound scientific evidence, perhaps one should also ask why it was added in the first place. There seems to be reasonable evidence that changes in the taste of food (according to an adult taster) do influence infant behavioral response, but whether this is taste in the same sense that an older child experiences taste is uncertain. If the baby can taste, its taste must be atrocious. Was the taste or flavor of a slurry of pureed apricots and minced veal—or a gruel of powdered bone cereal and sieved liver—really improved by the addition of monosodium glutamate? For the infant? For its mother? Ugh.[37]

Effects in Some Members of the Population

Some scientists have hypothesized that for physiological reasons some people are sensitive to particular nutritive substances present in normal diets. These researchers believe that sensitivities of this kind can result in abnormal behavior after the food is consumed. The study of these food sensitivities is included in the discipline known as *clinical ecology,* the study and treatment of organisms' reactions to environmental stimuli. Although clinical ecologists often refer to food sensitivities as food allergies, they are not implying that the ordinary medical requirements for an allergy (an immunologic antigen–antibody relationship) are satisfied. For clinical ecologists a food allergy is demonstrated when consumption of a food alters someone's reactivity to the environment.[38]

A well-documented food sensitivity that results in psychological symptoms is shown by children with *PKU* (*phenylketonuria*). Approximately 1 in every 20,000 children born in the United States has this disease. These children are born missing the gene for a particular enzyme. People who lack this enzyme cannot metabolize *phenylalanine,* an amino acid. It therefore accumulates in the body, resulting in profound and permanent retardation. Luckily it is possible to test newborns for PKU. If an infant with PKU is put on a low-phenylalanine diet immediately after birth, he or she will usually develop normally.[39]

Experimental research is scanty concerning more subtle psychological effects of normal diet. One study was conducted by David S. King,[40] who performed a double-blind study with 30 subjects. First he determined which substances the subjects might be allergic to. He did this by asking the subjects how frequently they ate various substances and how much they craved those substances, as well as by examining their reports of psychological reactions following consumption of those substances. The substances that he used most frequently in the experiment were extracts of wheat, beef, milk, cane sugar, and tobacco smoke.

King placed these extracts under the subjects' tongues. A placebo of distilled water was also used. King took extra precautions in this experiment to make sure that demand characteristics were not a factor. He did not tell the subjects that there would be any placebos until the experiment was over. In addition to conducting the experiment in a double-blind manner, immediately after giving an extract King asked each subject to guess what the substance was; and he recorded any trials in which he thought that he himself had guessed the identity of the substance. Data from the trials in which the subject correctly guessed that no substance had been given, and from trials in which King thought that he had known what substance he was delivering, were excluded from the analyses.

King's subjects reported significantly more cognitive-emotional symptoms (such as depression and irritability) following administration of extracts than following administration of placebo. However, they did not report significantly more somatic symptoms (such as nasal congestion and flushing) following the extracts. Therefore King's data do appear to provide some support for the hypothesis that some food substances can cause psychological reactions in some people. It is not yet clear to what extent these reactions are indeed characteristic of only some people, rather than the general population. In addition, keep in mind that King used food extracts, not natural foods, and so his results might not apply to natural eating conditions.

NONNUTRITIVE SUBSTANCES IN FOODS AND HYPERACTIVITY

Some substances are nonnutritive, but for various reasons they are present in foods. These substances include artificial colors, flavorings, and preservatives, as well as unintended contaminants and toxins. Food ingestion frequently results in concurrent consumption of these types of substances. Therefore, to the extent that their consumption results in any psychological symptoms, these substances are of concern here. Nonnutritive substances that tend to cause psychological reactions in everyone who consumes them will be considered first, followed by the possible role of food additives in making some children hyperactive.

Effects in the General Population

CAFFEINE.   Caffeine is widely prevalent in the diet. It is contained in significant amounts not only in coffee and tea but also in soft drinks and chocolate. People consume a great deal of caffeine. For example, in Sweden, one of the leading coffee-consuming nations, caffeine consumption is approximately 425 milligrams of caffeine per person per day. In the United States, per capita consumption of caffeine is approximately 211 milligrams per day.[41] In Sweden this is equivalent to every man, woman, and child drinking about four cups of brewed coffee per day, and in the United States about two cups of brewed coffee per day. Add to this the fact that many soft drinks contain at least as much caffeine as a half cup of brewed coffee[42] and it is clear that the effects of caffeine consumption need thorough investigation.

The effects of relatively small amounts of caffeine on the behavior of children and adult humans have been well documented. Caffeine consumption increases subjective reports of wakefulness and energy, as well as increasing measures of attention and speech rate.[43] Judith L. Rapoport[44] found that adults report more mood changes following caffeine consumption than do children, while children show more changes in objective behavioral measures than do adults. She correctly observes that it is difficult to determine whether children subjectively experience fewer mood changes following caffeine ingestion than do adults, or whether children are just poor at reporting such changes.

A double-blind study by Roland R. Griffiths, George E. Bigelow, and Ira A. Liebson[45] carefully examined the ability of caffeine to serve as a reinforcer. The subjects were residents in a behavioral pharmacology research ward, and all had a history of consuming large amounts of coffee and caffeine. In one experiment, each subject chose between a caffeine capsule or a placebo capsule. In another experiment, on different days subjects could work to obtain caffeinated coffee, decaffeinated coffee, caffeine capsules, or placebo capsules. In both experiments, whether or not subjects had been abstaining from caffeine, and independent of whether they consumed coffee or capsules, the subjects preferred to consume caffeine. In other words, these subjects demonstrated a preference for caffeine that was not a result of caffeine tolerance, caffeine dependence, or a preference for coffee liquid. In and of itself, caffeine is a reinforcer for some people.

Long-term consumption of caffeine can result in physiological dependence. In addition, in some people consumption of as little as two cups of coffee can result in a disorder called *caffeinism* or *caffeine intoxication,* which is marked by "restlessness, nervousness, excitement, insomnia, flushed face, diuresis, and gastrointestinal complaints."[46] Given that caffeine is a reinforcer for and can harm the behavior of at least some people, it appears advisable for everyone to be cautious in their consumption of caffeine.

ERGOT.   *Ergot* are the *sclerotia* (food-storage forms) of a fungus that grows on grains, particularly rye. Consumption of ergot results in a type of food poisoning, known as *ergotism.* The symptoms of ergotism include temporary deafness or blindness, sensations of pinching or of ants crawling under the skin, and convulsions. Several researchers have postulated that undiagnosed ergotism has been responsible for historical events such as the 1692 Salem witch trials. In 1692 ergotism was unknown. The majority of the "bewitched" accusers of the Salem witch trials complained of symptoms identical to the most common symptoms of ergotism. In addition, most of the bewitched were teenage girls, and ergotism is more likely to affect people, such as teenagers, who are consuming a great deal of food relative to their body mass. Finally, the geography, weather, and growing patterns of Salem in 1692 all make it likely that a great deal of rye contaminated with ergot was eaten at that time. Therefore, researchers believe, ergotism caused some people to feel that they were bewitched, resulting in accusations and executions.[47] Food contaminants can change the course of history.[48]

OTHER TOXINS.   There are many other nonnutritive substances present in food that can cause psychological as well as physiological damage. Such toxins need not be accidental contaminants; they may be put into foods and consumed on purpose, although perhaps without any knowledge of the toxin's effect. In the late nineteenth and early twentieth centuries absinthe was a popular drink in France. *Absinthe,* a pale green liqueur, contains oil of wormwood, alcohol, and extracts from plants such as anise. It was usually drunk diluted with sugar and water due to the bitterness of the wormwood. People said they liked to drink absinthe because it made them experience things in unique and unusual ways. However, the wormwood in the absinthe contains a toxin, thujone, which actually causes hallucinations, mental impairment, and, eventually, irreversible brain damage. Van Gogh is said to have been addicted to absinthe, and the drink to have contributed to his psychosis and suicide. As people became aware of the harm caused by absinthe, its popularity slowly waned.[49]

Another toxin whose effects on behavior have been investigated is lead. Rhesus monkeys reared on a diet including lead show poorer learning than do control monkeys.[50] Large doses of dietary lead also hinder children's learning, even causing retardation. What is not clear is how much lead must be present in a child's diet before there will be subtle decreases in the child's ability to learn. Some researchers believe that even relatively low doses of lead can harm IQ scores.[51] Although lead has been banned as an ingredient for indoor paint, old peeling paint that contains lead is still present in some houses, and young children are consuming it. Therefore, lead consumption with resulting psychological damage may still be a problem for some children.[52]

Lead poisoning has even been responsible for the deaths of large numbers of adults. In 1845 the 134-member Franklin expedition left England for the Arctic with the assigned task of mapping the Northwest Passage. During the course of the expedition, many of the expedition's members began to behave strangely, and all of them died before they could complete their task. Recent examinations of the bodies of the members of this expedition have indicated that the cause of the deaths was lead in the expedition's food supply. The recovered bodies contained high amounts of lead, and the cans that contained the expedition's food supply were probably made with large amounts of lead.[53]

Toxins can cause mental retardation if a fetus consumes them through the food intake of its mother. This has occurred with the toxic chemical *methylmercury*. Adults who consume methylmercury also suffer neurological symptoms, such as visual and motor disturbances and headaches. Methylmercury can pass into bodies of water, and thus to fish, from industrial sources. Humans are then exposed to methylmercury when they eat the contaminated fish.[54]

Hyperactivity

Some nonnutritive substances present in food cause psychological abnormalities in most people. However, it has also been claimed that some people are especially sensitive to some food additives. The most thoroughly investigated and controversial claim of this nature concerns *attention-deficit hyperactivity disorder*.[55]

Hyperactivity is most often seen in children, and more often in boys than girls.[56] One study found that each of the following descriptive statements was used by at least two-thirds of mothers describing their hyperactive children, but by less than one-third of other mothers: "overactive," "doesn't finish projects," "fidgets," "can't sit still at meals," "doesn't stay with games," "wears out toys, furniture, etc.," "talks too much."[57] But not all hyperactive children show the same symptoms; the hyperactive population is not homogeneous.[58]

For many years drugs called *amphetamines* have been used to treat hyperactive children. Although amphetamines appear to speed up adults' behavior, they appear to slow down the behavior of children, including hyperactive children. The reason seems to be that, for both adults and children, amphetamines increase attention to cognitive tasks. Because sustaining attention on a cognitive task is particularly a problem for children, and because activity and attention are incompatible, hyperactive children administered amphetamines are less active.[59] However, amphetamines are powerful drugs with many side effects. For example, children given amphetamines for long periods of time may not grow as tall as children not given amphetamines.[60] In addition, amphetamines result in only short-term improvements in behavior. Teaching hyperactive children new behavior patterns may be a more effective long-term treatment.[61]

Approximately 20 years ago Ben F. Feingold proposed that hyperactivity is due to the increased tendency of some children to react to some food additives in their diets. Feingold asserted that the offending substances are artificial flavors, artificial colors, the preservatives *BHT* and *BHA,* and *salicylates,* substances related to salicylic acid that occur naturally in foods such as almonds, apples, and tomatoes. Feingold reasoned that if these substances were removed from the diet, the hyperactive behavior should significantly decrease. Thus was born the *Feingold diet* for hyperactive children.[62] Many parents of hyperactive children swear by this diet,[63] but the research literature is not so clear-cut.

SUPPORT FOR THE FEINGOLD DIET.   Several studies have used nonhuman subjects to investigate the effects of food dyes on behavior. For example, George J. Augustine and Herbert Levitan[64] applied a food dye to a *neuromuscular synapse* (a synapse between a neuron and a muscle) in the frog. When a certain dose of food dye, or a larger dose, was applied, an increased amount of neurotransmitter was released at the synapse. These results indicate that food dyes could possibly increase motor behavior. James R. Goldenring and his colleagues[65] used rat pups for their experiment. Goldenring and his colleagues infused food dyes into the pups' gastrointestinal tracts. On the average, the rat pups' activity level subsequently increased, while their ability to avoid shock subsequently decreased. Bennett A. Shaywitz, James R. Goldenring, and Robert S. Wool[66] also used rat pups. Shaywitz and his colleagues gave food dyes orally to their subjects. The pups were more hyperactive and had problems learning after they had been given the food dyes.

James M. Swanson and Marcel Kinsbourne's experiment using 40 children has also provided some support for the Feingold diet.[67] For half of these children a diagnosis of hyperactivity had been confirmed and for half that diagnosis had been rejected. All of the children were put on the Feingold diet for five days. In a challenge design, each child was given a capsule containing a blend of food dyes and a capsule containing a placebo, one on day 4 of the Feingold diet and one on day 5 of the Feingold diet. On both of these days all of the children were given a learning task. On the average, performance on the learning task was worse for the hyperactive children on the day that they received the food dyes, compared with the day that they received the placebo. The nonhyperactive children, however, showed no difference in their learning behavior on the two days.

Not directly supporting, but also not directly refuting, the use of the Feingold diet are results from a study conducted by Bonnie J. Kaplan and her colleagues.[68] In this ambitious study 24 hyperactive preschool-aged boys and their families consumed a diet free of artificial colors and flavors, as well as of various other substances, for 4 weeks. In addition, for 3 weeks the subjects and their families consumed a control diet that was similar to that which they normally consumed. A double-blind procedure was used such that neither the subjects, their families, nor any of the study's personnel who came into contact with the subjects or their families knew when the experimental diet was being administered or when the control diet was being administered. Each day, parents observed their children's behavior and physical symptoms (if any). The results showed that 10 of the 24 children demonstrated approximately a 50 percent improvement in their behavior when consuming the experimental diet, and another 4 children demonstrated approximately a 12 percent improvement. In addition, when the children were consuming the experimental diet they also tended to sleep better. Note however, that the experimental diet used here was substantially broader in its exclusions than the typical Feingold diet. In addition to the usual restrictions of the Feingold diet, the present experimental diet also eliminated MSG, caffeine, and most simple sugars. To allow for children with a possible history of problems with cow's milk, all dairy products were removed as well. Other substances were removed in individual cases if a child seemed to have had problems with that substance in the past. Due to all of these varied dietary exclusions, it is possible to conclude from this study only that a substantial proportion of hyperactive children can demonstrate improved behavior through dietary intervention. It is not possible to identify definitively which substances, including those specified by the Feingold diet, are most likely to improve behavior if they are removed from the diet.

CRITICISMS OF THE FEINGOLD DIET.   The above results seem to suggest strongly that the Feingold diet could help hyperactive children. However, many criticisms have been made of the previous studies and of the Feingold diet approach to treating hyperactivity. To begin with, according to one study,[69] parent ratings of their children's hyperactivity are often inconsistent with experimenter laboratory observations. Therefore parental testimonials about the benefits of the Feingold diet must be regarded with extreme caution.

Second, studies that have used nonhumans may be criticized for just that. Hyperactivity in nonhumans may not be comparable to hyperactivity in humans, particularly when dyes are administered by infusing them into the gastrointestinal tract or by applying them to a neuromuscular junction. Third, in many of the studies the dosages of dye used were far in excess of what is usually encountered in normal diets, particularly considering that in the animal studies these doses were given internally. In Swanson and Kinsbourne's study with human subjects the children received doses equivalent to what is consumed by the 10 percent of the children in the normal population who are consuming the most. Fourth, the challenge design has been deemed inappropriate if the purpose of the experiment is to determine whether food dyes affect children on normal diets. Findings obtained from experiments using a challenge design may lack clinical significance.[70] Fifth, Swanson and Kinsbourne's experiment did not state whether or not the experiment was conducted double blind. If it was not, the experimenters' expectations might have influenced the children's behavior.

Another study with human subjects casts further doubt on the usefulness of the Feingold diet. Bernard Weiss and his colleagues[71] investigated the behavior of 22 children with a diagnosis of hyperactivity, all of whom had been on the Feingold diet for months. On some days of Weiss and his colleagues' experiment a subject received a drink containing artificial colors, and on some days a drink containing no artificial colors. The placebo and dye-containing drinks were concocted so that there was no way to tell the difference between them based on appearance, taste, or smell. The dosage of food dyes used was comparable to the mean dose of food dyes ordinarily consumed by children. Weiss and his colleagues' study was performed double blind. Mothers' reports of their children's behavior were used to assess the effects of the food dyes.

Weiss and his colleagues found that only 2 of the 22 children seemed to show ill effects from the food dyes. For 1 child the effect was dramatic. This child was given the food dyes on eight separate days, and on five of these days the mother was immediately able to detect a difference in the behavior of her child. On only one day did the mother incorrectly think that her child had been given the dyes. Nevertheless, the fact remains that for at least 20 of the 22 children, the food dyes had no discernible effect, despite the fact that a challenge design was used, and that the subjects were children who had been previously reported as having their behavior improved by the Feingold diet.

Several other studies using human subjects have had difficulty obtaining support for the Feingold diet in all but a small fraction of the subjects tested.[72] As a result, both the Nutrition Foundation and an expert panel convened by the National Institutes of Health have recently recommended extreme caution in the use of the Feingold diet. Neither could find any consistent scientific evidence showing the worth of this diet for treating hyperactivity except for perhaps a very few children. On the other hand, neither panel thought that use of the diet would cause physical harm to children, so that the diet could be used if parents wished. As stated before, however, physical harm is not the only harm that may ensue from a useless treatment. Loss of money, wasted effort, disappointment, and the possible avoidance of other more effective treatments can all result from pursuing a useless treatment.

CONCLUSION

Psychologists and other research scientists have made some dramatic discoveries in the past few decades about the effects of food consumption on our behavior. Although diet may not influence hyperactivity in children to any great degree, it may influence how sleepy we are, how well we learn, how depressed we are, and whether or not we feel as if ants are crawling under our skin. The future will undoubtedly bring additional speculations and research testing statements such as the following by Galileo who, in this interpretation by Bertolt Brecht, is a dedicated scientist who believes that plentiful supplies of food and drink are essential to his research:

> How can I work, with the tax collector on the doorstep? And my poor daughter will never acquire a husband unless she has a dowry, she's not too bright. And I like to buy books—all kinds of books. Why not? And what about my appetite? I don't think well unless I eat well. Can I help it if I get my best ideas over a good meal and a bottle of wine? They don't pay me as much as they pay the butcher's boy. If only I could have five years to do nothing but research! Come on. I am going to show you something else.[73]

Part IV

EATING AND DRINKING DISORDERS

Part IV concerns eating and drinking behavior that is not characteristic of a species in
its natural environment, that is, abnormal behavior. By definition, most organisms eat and
behave normally most of the time, but when
they do not, the consequences can be devastating. The three chapters in this part explore the
consumption of abnormal amounts of food
and the consumption of alcohol. Coverage of
these topics revolves around two focuses: possible origins of abnormal behavior and possible treatments of abnormal behavior. Origins
and treatment are not independent; having a
thorough understanding of the factors responsible for a particular behavior can make
changing that behavior considerably easier.
Similarly, successful treatments may provide
clues about how the abnormal behavior arose.
Wherever possible in the next three chapters,
discussions of both origins and treatment are
related to the concepts concerning normal behavior and its origins that have been set out in
the preceding parts of this book.

Chapter
9

❦

Anorexia and Bulimia

There are instances when individual animals and humans consume inappropriate amounts of food. If inadequate amounts are consumed even though sufficient food is available, these individuals are said to exhibit *anorexia*, literally, lack of appetite. Anorexia may occur for many different reasons. Some animals consume little food when behaviors other than eating have a great value, for instance, during hibernation or incubation (see Chapter 2). Other causes of anorexia include the effects of cancer and of drugs; anorexia may also occur as part of various psychological disorders such as depression, mania, anxiety, and anorexia nervosa. Anorexia may also occur as part of bulimia nervosa, a disorder characterized by intermittent periods of excess consumption. Each of these variations of anorexia, including bulimia, will be discussed in the present chapter. Cases in which individuals consistently consume too much food will be discussed in the following chapter, "Overeating and Obesity." The focus of the present and the next chapter is on how much is eaten, as in Chapter 2. But in these two chapters the concern is with cases in which too little or too much is eaten with deleterious results, rather than with simply the reasons why individuals eat or do not eat.

Recent studies with nonhumans indicate that there are some health advantages (and also disadvantages) of long-term low-calorie diets.[1] Nevertheless, studies with humans have yet to be performed and during the past 15 years there has been increasing medical concern over people who are thin. Physicians now believe that the medical dangers to humans of being thin are greater than they first realized.[2] The weights for specific heights that by definition constitute "thin" have even been revised upward. For many years the standards were provided by height and weight tables issued in 1959 by the Metropolitan Life Insurance Company. These tables were compiled using information about mortality rates as a function of people's reported weights. It appears, however, that some of the people whose data were used to compile the 1959 tables may have underreported their weights. In any case it has been recognized that the weights recommended by the 1959 tables were too low in some instances.[3]

The Metropolitan Life Insurance Company therefore corrected this problem and published a new set of tables (Tables 9.1a and 9.1b). In many instances recommended healthy weights were revised upward. In addition, the new set of tables includes an easy, objective way of estimating body frame size using a standardized measure of the distance between two bones in the elbow (Table 9.2; for other methods of estimating thinness and obesity, including adjusting standards according to peoples' ages, see Chapter 10).

The revised tables do not mean that problems associated with obesity have disappeared; many people are still too heavy according to the new tables. However, the dangers of being too thin were emphasized. Some of the causes of being too thin are the focus of the next sections.

CANCER ANOREXIA

Cancer is responsible for 22 percent of all deaths in the United States. Anorexia and weight loss frequently accompany and often contribute to death from cancer.[4] Explanations of the anorexia and weight loss accompanying cancer have cited changes in cancer patients' taste sensitivities, food preferences, metabolic rates, endocrinology, and biochemistry. These changes may result from the cancer treatment or from the cancer itself.[5]

The taste aversion paradigm has proven particularly useful in understanding and treating cancer anorexia (see Chapter 6 for discussion of the

TABLE 9.1a

Comparison of 1959 and 1983 Metropolitan Height and Weight Tables: Men*

Weight in pounds (without clothing)

Height (without shoes) in feet and inches	Small frame				Medium frame				Large Frame			
	1959	1983	Change since 1959	Percent change	1959	1983	Change since 1959	Percent change	1959	1983	Change since 1959	Percent change
5 1	105–113	123–129	18 16	17 14	111–122	126–136	15 14	14 11	119–134	133–145	14 11	12 8
5 2	108–116	125–131	17 15	16 13	114–126	128–138	14 12	12 10	122–137	135–148	13 11	11 8
5 3	111–119	127–133	16 14	14 12	117–129	130–140	13 11	11 9	125–141	137–151	12 10	10 7
5 4	114–122	129–135	15 13	13 11	120–132	132–143	12 11	10 8	128–145	139–155	11 10	9 7
5 5	117–126	131–137	14 11	12 9	123–136	134–146	11 10	9 7	131–149	141–159	10 10	8 7
5 6	121–130	133–140	12 10	10 8	127–140	137–149	10 9	8 6	135–154	144–163	9 9	7 6
5 7	125–134	135–143	10 9	8 7	131–145	140–152	9 7	7 5	140–159	147–167	7 8	5 5
5 8	129–138	137–146	8 8	6 6	135–149	143–155	8 6	6 4	144–163	150–171	6 8	4 5
5 9	133–143	139–149	6 6	5 4	139–153	146–158	7 5	5 3	148–167	153–175	5 8	3 5
5 10	137–147	141–152	4 5	3 3	143–158	149–161	6 3	4 2	152–172	156–179	4 7	3 4
5 11	141–151	144–155	3 4	2 3	147–163	152–165	5 2	3 1	157–177	159–183	2 6	1 3
6 0	145–155	147–159	2 4	1 3	151–168	155–169	4 1	3 1	161–182	163–187	2 5	1 3
6 1	149–160	150–163	1 3	1 2	155–173	159–173	4 0	3 0	166–187	167–192	1 5	1 3
6 2	153–164	153–167	0 3	0 2	160–178	162–177	2 -1	1 -1	171–192	171–197	0 5	0 3
6 3	157–168	157–171	0 3	0 2	165–183	166–182	1 -1	1 -1	175–197	176–202	1 5	1 3

*Comparison of recommended weights for different heights and frame sizes for men aged 25–59 published in 1959 and 1983 by the Metropolitan Life Insurance Company based on data compiled by the Society of Actuaries and Association of Life Insurance Medical Directors of America. Method of estimating frame size is shown in Table 9.2. (Courtesy of the Metropolitan Life Insurance Company.)

TABLE 9.1b
Comparison of 1959 and 1983 Metropolitan Height and Weight Tables: Women*

Weight in pounds (without clothing)

Height (without shoes) in feet and inches	Small frame 1959	Small frame 1983	Change since 1959	Percent change	Medium frame 1959	Medium frame 1983	Change since 1959	Percent change	Large Frame 1959	Large Frame 1983	Change since 1959	Percent change
4 9	90– 97	99–108	9 11	10 11	94–106	106–118	12 12	13 11	102–118	115–128	13 10	13 8
4 10	92–100	100–110	8 10	9 10	97–109	108–120	11 11	11 10	105–121	117–131	12 10	11 8
4 11	95–103	101–112	6 9	6 9	100–112	110–123	10 11	10 10	108–124	119–134	11 10	10 8
5 0	98–106	103–115	5 9	5 8	103–115	112–126	9 11	9 10	111–127	122–137	11 10	10 8
5 1	101–109	105–118	4 9	4 8	106–118	115–129	9 11	8 9	114–130	125–140	11 10	10 8
5 2	104–112	108–121	4 9	4 8	109–122	118–132	9 10	8 8	117–134	128–144	11 10	9 7
5 3	107–115	111–124	4 9	4 8	112–126	121–135	9 9	8 7	121–138	131–148	10 10	8 7
5 4	110–119	114–127	4 8	4 7	116–131	124–138	8 7	7 5	125–142	134–152	9 10	7 7
5 5	114–123	117–130	3 7	3 6	120–135	127–141	7 6	6 4	129–146	137–156	8 10	6 7
5 6	118–127	120–133	2 6	2 5	124–139	130–144	6 5	5 4	133–150	140–160	7 10	5 7
5 7	122–131	123–136	1 5	1 4	128–143	133–147	5 4	4 3	137–154	143–164	6 10	4 6
5 8	126–136	126–139	0 3	0 2	132–147	136–150	4 3	3 2	141–159	146–167	5 8	4 5
5 9	130–140	129–142	–1 2	–1 1	136–151	139–153	3 2	2 1	145–164	149–170	4 6	3 4
5 10	134–144	132–145	–2 1	–1 1	140–155	142–156	2 1	1 1	149–169	152–173	3 4	2 2

*Comparison of recommended weights for different heights and frame sizes for women aged 25–59 published in 1959 and 1983 by the Metropolitan Life Insurance Company based on data compiled by the Society of Actuaries and Association of Life Insurance Medical Directors of America. Method of estimating frame size is shown in Table 9.2. (Courtesy of the Metropolitan Life Insurance Company.)

TABLE 9.2

To Make an Approximation of Your Frame Size

Men		Women	
Height without shoes	**Elbow breadth**	**Height without shoes**	**Elbow breadth**
5'1"–5'2"	2½"–2⅞"	4'9"–4'10"	2¼"–2½"
5'3"–5'6"	2⅝"–2⅞"	4'11"–5'2"	2¼"–2½"
5'7"–5'10"	2¾"–3"	5'3"–5'6"	2⅜"–2⅝"
5'11"–6'2"	2¾"–3⅛"	5'7"–5'10"	2⅜"–2⅝"
6'3"	2⅞"–3¼"	5'11"	2½"–2¾"

Extend your arm and bend the forearm upward at a 90-degree angle. Keep fingers straight and turn the inside of your wrist toward your body. If you have a caliper, use it to measure the space between the two prominent bones on either side of your elbow. Without a caliper, place thumb and index finger of your other hand on these two bones. Measure the space between your fingers against a ruler or tape measure. Compare it with these tables that list elbow measurements for medium-framed men and women. Measurements lower than those listed indicate you have a small frame. Higher measurements indicate a large frame.

*SOURCE: Metropolitan Life Insurance Company, 1983

taste aversion paradigm). Ilene L. Bernstein and her colleagues have conducted an imaginative and difficult series of experiments in which they have shown that children or adults given a novel-tasting ice cream prior to their chemotherapy acquired an aversion to the novel-tasting ice cream. Apparently the illness resulting from the chemotherapy was paired with the taste of the ice cream, and a taste aversion resulted. These researchers have also shown that patients can acquire aversions to familiar foods consumed near in time to chemotherapy. Bernstein and her colleagues have used experiments with nonhuman subjects to confirm and expand on their findings with human subjects.[6] Clearly any food that might be given to cancer patients prior to their chemotherapy or radiation treatments should be chosen with care. However, more research is needed to determine precisely which aspects of cancer therapy result in the formation of taste aversions.[7]

Some cancer patients, perhaps as many as 40 percent, report nausea and even vomiting in anticipation of chemotherapy.[8] In such instances, nausea has apparently been paired with the environmental stimuli associated with a chemotherapy treatment. As soon as those stimuli are encountered the subject begins to feel ill, even though chemotherapy has not yet been given.[9]

It should be pointed out here that, although it is easier to associate tastes than audiovisual stimuli with illness (see Chapter 6), it is nonetheless possible to associate audiovisual stimuli with illness. However, stronger illness and more pairings of the stimuli with the illness may be necessary for learning to occur.[10] After many treatments a chemotherapy patient might come to feel ill simply upon stepping into the room where the chemotherapy treatments are usually given.

A number of treatments have been tested to determine whether they would eliminate anticipatory nausea and vomiting. Various medications designed to reduce nausea and anxiety have not been particularly effective.[11] However, a particular type of treatment technique developed from learning theory has proved helpful in combating anticipatory nausea and vomiting. This technique is known as *systematic desensitization*. It involves systematically exposing a patient, while the patient is completely relaxed, to gradual approximations of the object or stimulus that is causing the aversive response in the patient. In the case of cancer drug nausea, patients are taught to relax while imagining the environmental stimuli that induce their nausea. This technique has been helpful in reducing patients' reports of nausea preceding chemotherapy.[12] To the extent that systematic desensitization can decrease the anticipatory nausea experienced by a cancer patient who is receiving chemotherapy, this technique should decrease the conditioned taste aversions that result in cancer anorexia.

Taste aversions resulting from treatment-induced illness are apparently not the sole cause of anorexia in cancer patients. Bernstein has also investigated the possible role of illness arising from a tumor itself. She concludes that some tumors, but not others, apparently cause an illness that can serve as the unconditioned stimulus in taste aversion learning. Food consumption is paired with this illness, and anorexia results.[13]

Although all of the threads are not yet tied together, great advances in understanding and treating the anorexia that accompanies cancer are being made through the work of Bernstein and others.

THE EFFECTS OF DRUGS ON ANOREXIA

Some drugs have been found to increase anorexia and some to decrease it. The number of anorexia-increasing drugs is much larger than the number of anorexia-decreasing ones.[14] In the former category are drugs that act centrally, either with or without stimulant properties, and drugs that act peripherally, including hormones.[15]

One of the most widely investigated drugs that increases anorexia is amphetamine. This is a centrally acting drug with stimulant properties. Although it is known that animals and people who take amphetamine generally decrease their food intake, the mechanism for this reduction is not completely clear. The increased and disrupted behavior resulting from the stimulant properties of amphetamine may be a factor.[16] Many hypotheses have suggested that amphetamines affect the neurotransmitters responsible for feeding.[17] Specific amphetamine receptor sites, primarily in the hypothalamus, that appear to be involved in the anorexic effect of amphetamines, have been identified.[18]

A complication in determining the mechanism responsible for amphetamine anorexia is that amphetamines do not always suppress food intake, particularly in animals.[19] The effects of many antidepressant drugs, which were traditionally thought to increase food intake (a notable exception being fluoxetine), are also variable. In some, but by no means all, cases, antidepressant drugs increase humans' preferences for sweet foods and/or result in humans' gaining weight.[20] But although these drugs apparently increase food consumption in humans, they appear to decrease food consumption in nonhumans.[21] John E. Blundell has hypothesized that such differences may be due not to species differences but to differences in the ways in which the drugs are administered to human and nonhuman subjects. Humans are usually mildly food deprived or satiated and are given repeated small doses of drugs while having free access to food. Nonhumans, on the other hand, are usually severely food deprived and are given a few large doses while having limited access to food.[22]

To test whether or not the manner of drug administration could account for the species differences that had been reported, Blundell conducted a series of experiments in which antidepressant drugs were administered to rats under conditions comparable to those that usually prevail when humans receive these drugs.[23] Instead of simply suppressing food consumption, the antidepressant drug *alaproclate* suppressed intake of palatable food but increased intake of laboratory chow. Other antidepressant drugs, such as *amitriptyline,* showed small effects on food consumption. Type of drug, as well as the conditions of testing the effects of the drug, can influence the degree to which food consumption is increased or decreased.

Blundell has taken these conclusions a step further, stating that feeding in general is dependent on many factors other than mere drug-induced internal chemical reactions. Drug and other effects on feeding are a function not only of the drugs that the subject has taken but also of the subject's environment.[24] A diagram of Blundell's model is shown in Figure 9.1. Blundell's statements concerning the effects of the environment are similar to those made by Hogan and others about the determinants of hunger (see Chapter 2) and by Toates about the determinants of thirst (see Chapter 3). Many theorists have become increasingly aware that the explanation and prediction of eating and drinking behavior is complex; many internal and external factors must be considered.

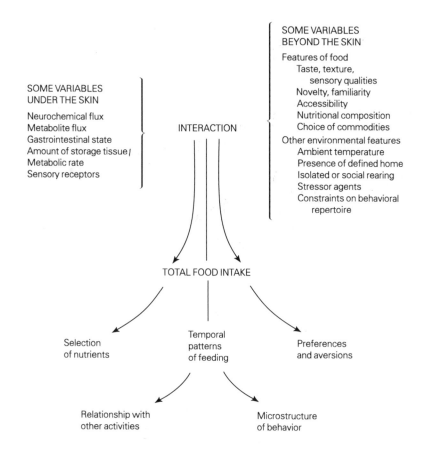

FIGURE 9.1 *Feeding as affected by both internal and external factors.* (After J. E. Blundell, "Systems and Interactions: An Approach to the Pharmacology of Eating and Hunger," in *Eating and Its Disorders*, eds. A. J. Stunkard and E. Stellar, New York: Raven Press, 1984.)

MOOD AND ANOREXIA

Mood has been shown to covary with anorexia. People who are depressed, as well as people who are manic, usually eat less than people of normal affect, although depressed people sometimes eat excessively.[25]

The majority of the research on mood and food consumption has concentrated on depression. Several researchers have investigated the type of eating disturbance associated with depression and have found that people who are normally restrained eaters, dieters, tend to increase the amount of food they consume when they become depressed. On the other hand, people who are normally unrestrained eaters, nondieters, tend to decrease the amount of food they consume when they become depressed.[26]

[Some instances of depression and suppression of food consumption are so closely linked that they may have a common cause.] As mentioned previously, many people who become depressed also consume less food. Further, the rate at which saliva is secreted decreases during a depressive illness.[27] Finally, as also mentioned previously, drugs that alleviate depression tend to increase food consumption in some people. Therefore researchers have proposed that the specific brain mechanisms responsible for some cases of depression may also be responsible for lowering food intake.[28]

Additional support for this hypothesis was provided by an experiment conducted by Elzbieta Fonberg.[29] Fonberg lesioned the lateral hypothalamus (LH) in dogs. Lesioning the LH results in a decrease in food intake (see Chapter 2). The dogs in Fonberg's experiment decreased their food intake and also showed symptoms of depression and apathy, including decreased movement, drooped ears and tail, indifference to many stimuli, lack of friendliness, and opposition or lack of response to commands. When the dogs were given antidepressant drugs, they showed fewer of these symptoms and tended to consume more food.

The mechanisms responsible for the decrease in food consumption seen with mania or anxiety have not been investigated as thoroughly as have the mechanisms that decrease food consumption with depression. For mania, it seems likely that less food is consumed because manic people, like people given amphetamines, are continually active, which may interfere with feeding behavior.[30] The manic behaviors themselves, not any neurochemical disturbance responsible for the mania, may be the cause of the decreased food consumption.

ANOREXIA NERVOSA

Characteristics and Prevalence

Anorexia nervosa is an eating disorder. Hilde Bruch, a well-known therapist who has specialized in treatment of eating disorders, defined this disorder as "the relentless pursuit of thinness through self-starvation, even unto death."[31] Many books have been written about anorexia nervosa, some of which are listed in the notes for this chapter.[32] It is a disorder that usually occurs in females ranging in age from their teens to their 30s. Only about 5 percent of anorexics are male. In addition, most people with anorexia nervosa are white and upper-middle or upper class. It is a very serious disorder, with mortality estimates ranging up to approximately 18 percent.[33]

There have been few adequate studies on the prevalence of anorexia nervosa. However, a study conducted in nine London schools by A. H. Crisp, R. L. Palmer, and R. S. Kalucy[34] provided good evidence that anorexia nervosa is quite common. Crisp and his colleagues counted only severe cases of anorexia nervosa and examined only specific age ranges. Despite these restrictions they found that in the schools that were the English equivalent of American private schools, approximately 1 out of every 100 girls over the age of 16 was suffering from anorexia nervosa. However, in the other two schools, 1 out of every 1000 girls was suffering from anorexia nervosa. Other studies have found that 1 in 800 girls suffers from anorexia nervosa.[35]

Many authors believe that the prevalence of anorexia nervosa is increasing. It is possible, however, that the tendency of anorexics to seek treatment or the tendency of psychiatrists to give a diagnosis of anorexia nervosa has changed over time. Nevertheless, most researchers believe that the actual prevalence of anorexia nervosa, not just the reported prevalence, has increased during the past 25 to 35 years.[36]

There are many characteristic symptoms of ongoing anorexia nervosa. A defining characteristic is the lack of food consumption. Contrary to what the name anorexia nervosa might imply, this lack of food consumption is not accompanied by a lack of appetite. Anorexics are completely obsessed with food and food consumption. They carefully calculate just how many calories they can and do consume. They think and dream about food constantly. Patients have made the following comments to Bruch: "Of course, I had breakfast; I ate my Cheerio." "I won't even lick a postage stamp—one never knows about calories."[37]

Not surprisingly, the result of the lack of food consumption is a significant loss of weight. By definition, someone cannot be diagnosed as anorexic unless that person weighs at least 15 percent less than his or her minimal normal weight.[38] For example, a 25-year-old women who is 5 feet 6 inches tall with a medium frame could be diagnosed as suffering from anorexia nervosa if she lost weight to the point at which she weighed only 110.5 pounds (15 percent less than 130 pounds, see Table 9.1b). Some anorexics weigh less than 50 percent of their ideal weight.[39]

Along with this loss of weight, females must stop menstruating to be classified as anorexic. Or, if they develop anorexia nervosa prior to reaching puberty, menarche must be delayed.[40] These hormonal disturbances have been attributed to the lowered fat content of the body. Studies have claimed that a certain percentage of fat is needed for the female body to maintain proper hormonal functioning.[41] Presumably this protects females in case of pregnancy's additional nutritional demands (see also Chapter 12).

Some patients diagnosed as having anorexia nervosa will occasionally go on feeding binges. Following a binge, to rid themselves of the calories consumed, they will either self-induce vomiting or use laxatives.[42] Feeding binges will be discussed in more detail in a subsequent section on bulimia nervosa. Here it should be pointed out that, in contrast to bulimics, only some anorexics binge, and then only occasionally.[43] However, it is possible for someone to be diagnosed as simultaneously suffering from both anorexia nervosa and bulimia nervosa.[44]

Another common symptom of anorexia nervosa is excessive exercise. Many patients exercise vigorously for many hours each day. Through all of this self-starvation and exercise they claim to feel perfectly fine: not tired and not hungry.[45]

Finally, anorexics by definition have a different perception of their body size, compared with the impression that other people have of them. Anorexics tend to see themselves as being heavier than they really are.[46] David M. Garner and his colleagues demonstrated this tendency using an unusual method called the *distorting photograph technique* (see Figure 9.2).[47] With this technique a subject can adjust someone's photograph to between

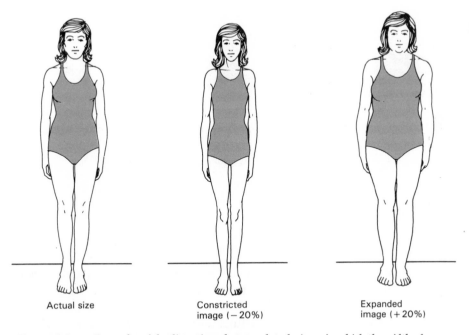

Actual size   Constricted image (−20%)   Expanded image (+20%)

FIGURE 9.2   *Examples of the distorting photograph technique, in which the width of a person's photograph can be adjusted* (After P. E. Garfinkel and D. M. Garner, *Anorexia Nervosa*, New York: Brunner/Mazel, 1982, p. 134.)

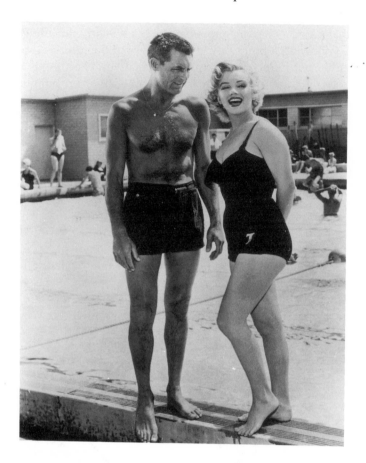

FIGURE 9.3a   *A "perfect" figure from the 1950s: Marilyn Monroe (with Cary Grant).*

+20 percent and –20 percent of the actual photograph's normal width. When Garner and his colleagues used this technique with anorexic and normal subjects, the anorexics showed a greater tendency to adjust pictures of themselves so that the adjusted pictures were larger than their actual size. However, this tendency was not shown when the anorexics adjusted pictures of people other than themselves. Apparently the anorexic's tendency to distort body image is limited to herself.

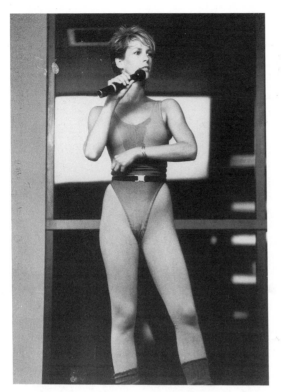

FIGURE 9.3b *A "perfect" figure from the 1980s: Jamie Lee Curtis.*

Possible Explanations and Causes

A great variety of explanations and causes have been proposed for anorexia nervosa, including societal, psychological, and physiological factors.[48] With regard to societal factors, many authors have argued that the present fashion image of thinness is a major contributing factor to the increased incidence of anorexia nervosa.[49] Figures 9.3a and 9.3b show two "perfect" figures from the 1950s and the 1980s: Marilyn Monroe and Jamie Lee Curtis. Monroe is clearly much heavier than Curtis. A quick perusal of the fashion magazines of then and now will demonstrate the same point. Fashionable women 35 years ago were heavier than are fashionable women now. Even *Playboy* centerfolds and Miss America Pageant winners have become thinner. Who can forget Twiggy, who made thinness the ultimate ideal in the 1960s?

Perhaps due to this current fashion image of thinness, it appears that the majority of today's girls and young women, but not the majority of today's

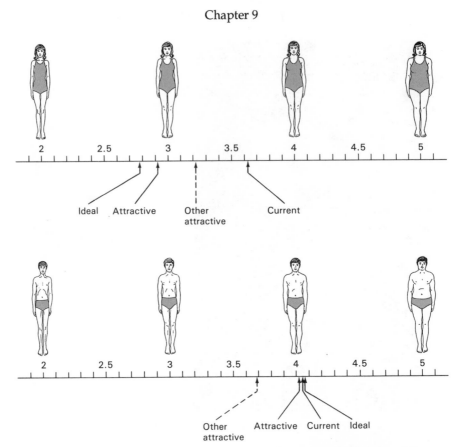

FIGURE 9.4   *Mean ratings of figures.* Mean ratings by women (top) and men (bottom) of current figure, ideal figure, and figure most attractive to the opposite gender; mean ratings by men of the female figure that they find most attractive (top, labeled *other attractive*) and equivalent mean ratings by women, on the bottom. (After A. E. Fallon and P. Rozin, "Sex Differences in Perceptions of Desirable Body Shape," *Journal of Abnormal Psychology* 94[1985]: 102–105.)

boys and young men, feel that they need to be thinner in order to be attractive.[50] For example, in a landmark study April E. Fallon and Paul Rozin had 475 male and female undergraduates use sets of male and female figure drawings ranging from very thin to very heavy to indicate: (a) the figure that looked most similar to their current shape, (b) the figure they most wanted to look like, (c) the figure they felt would be most attractive to the opposite sex, and (d) the figure of the opposite sex to which they felt they would be most attracted (see Figure 9.4). The men chose very similar figures as representing their ideal figure, their current figure, and the figure most attractive to women; the women, however, chose a heavier figure as representing their current figure and a thinner one as their ideal. In addition, although the male figure judged by men to be most attractive to women was actually heavier than what women preferred, the female figure judged by women to be most attractive to men was actually thinner than what men preferred. Thus most of the women in this study, but not most of the men, were dissatisfied with their current figure in such a way that could encourage them to diet and to become anorexic.[51]

Several other explanations of anorexia nervosa have focused on acquired behaviors of the individuals who develop the disorder. Anorexics are seen as using anorexia as a way of gaining attention, as an attempt at individuality, as a denial of sexuality (in addition to not menstruating, girls who are severely underweight lack secondary sexual characteristics), and as a resolution of various problems in interacting with overdemanding parents.[52] These explanations are generally put forward by clinicians who observe many patients but who do not conduct controlled studies of general anorexic populations.

Much of the recent theorizing regarding possible causes of anorexia nervosa has focused on physiological explanations. One of the critical findings that initiated physiological hypotheses was the observation that menstruation appears to stop in some anorexics before they lose the percentage of their body weight that is deemed necessary for menstruation to cease.[53] Therefore, it was reasoned, there may be some common physiological factor responsible for both the menstrual irregularities and the anorexia nervosa. The likely candidate would be a dysfunctional hypothalamus, since the hypothalamus is critically important both in feeding behavior and in hormonal functions. Hypothalamic functioning in anorexics is abnormal in many different ways.[54]

Still, the question remains whether this abnormal functioning is a cause or an effect of the lack of eating. Because most of the hypothalamic functions return to normal once eating is resumed and weight regained, including the functioning of the hormones that cause menstruation, these abnormalities are probably an effect, rather than a cause, of the anorexia nervosa. The cases in which menstruation ceases prior to a large weight loss have been attributed to emotional factors, coincidence, or possibly inaccurate reporting.[55]

It should be kept in mind that starvation and weight loss, which are what anorexics undergo, result in many profound physiological changes.[56] Dawdling over food, obsession with food, and hyperactivity, all symptoms of anorexia nervosa, have also been observed in humans and nonhumans who have been deprived of food either in the laboratory or under natural conditions.[57] Therefore some of the psychological, as well as some of the physiological, symptoms may be due to the effects of lack of food. It is hard to tease apart what is cause and what is effect in anorexia nervosa because experimental simulation of the disorder in humans is unlikely to be approved by human-subjects ethics committees. Results from clinical studies in which patient characteristics are simply observed with an eye toward elucidating etiology, or from documented cases of starvation in nature, are often the only data available, and conclusions from such studies must be treated with caution.

Case Histories

With many books and articles attempting to provide the definitive description of anorexia nervosa, it is important to remember that not all anorexics are alike. The way that the disorder begins, and the way that it progresses, may differ substantially between patients. A few case histories will help to illustrate the varied nature of anorexia nervosa:

> Hazel as a young teenager had enjoyed being popular and was quite flirtatious. She heard her father say, "Is she now going to be a teenager?" and this sounded to her as if he were disgusted and might reject her. Background for this anxiety was a much older half-sister who, according to the family saga, had been her father's declared darling but who had disappointed him. . . . [Hazel] wanted to deserve her father's love and admiration by excelling academically and in sports, and she restricted her food intake more and more. For her the issue became "mind over body," and she practiced it in the most literal sense. She expressed it: "When you are so unhappy and you don't know how to accomplish anything, then to have control over your body becomes a supreme accomplishment." You make out of your body your very own kingdom where you are the tyrant, the absolute dictator.[58]

> Sarah was the only child of rather elderly parents who were both somewhat obese. She had herself been plump from infancy and by the time she was sixteen she weighed [154 pounds]. She was used to being called "fatty" or "the lump" at school and was always embarrassed when she had to undress to change for games. She was a keen horsewoman and had some success in competition. Her occasional attempts at dieting became more determined after she came to the conclusion that her increasing weight was becoming a handicap to her riding. She dieted with the encouragement of her parents and set out to lose [30 pounds]. However, she passed this weight after less than three months, but continued to avoid fattening foods. After a further

three months she weighed less than [98 pounds] and was unequivocally in a state of anorexia nervosa.[59]

[Grace] was the youngest of three girls, and the two older sisters had begun to menstruate at eleven. The sister next to her was very heavy and was continuously criticized for not having the willpower to diet. Grace weighed one hundred and ten pounds when her eleventh birthday approached; she was taller than most of her classmates and knew of no others who menstruated. She became alarmed when she noticed the first bloodstains, knowing that this was a harbinger of menstruation, and she felt unable to cope with the responsibilities involved, was fearful of being teased or having an odor or spotting her clothes. She wanted to postpone this event until she was fourteen or fifteen. Her determination to do something about it became even greater when a film about sexual development was shown in school. She dropped twenty-seven pounds within six weeks, and the signs of approaching puberty disappeared; she did not begin to menstruate until two years later.[60]

These case histories illustrate many different possible precipitating events for anorexia nervosa: a desire not to be overweight, a need for love and attention from parents and friends, a desire to improve sports fitness, and a desire to prevent sexual development. The first three of these are not necessarily unhealthy goals; problems arose only when these goals were carried too far, to an unhealthy standard of thinness. The variation within these passages illustrates that anorexia nervosa may have different causes. Perhaps different treatments will succeed with different patients, depending on the cause of each patient's anorexia nervosa.

Treatments

Susan Swann Van Buskirk[61] has pointed out that it is helpful to divide potential treatments for anorexia nervosa into two groups. The first group consists of treatments designed primarily to induce an immediate weight gain in the patient, sometimes without her consent. These are treatments that focus on short-term effects. Common examples are nurturance, drug therapy, and behavior therapy. A second group consists of treatments designed primarily to maintain or prolong a weight gain. These are treatments that focus on long-term effects. Common examples are individual, group, and family psychotherapy, and self-help groups. Each of these types of treatment and their advantages and disadvantages will be briefly described.

Nurturance can consist of one or more different treatments that attempt to improve the patient's nutrition. In the simplest form, bed rest, the patient is simply confined to her bed so that her potential for exercise is diminished. A high-calorie diet is simultaneously offered. Other forms of nurturance entail various ways of directly administering nutritive substances. This may be done, for example, through a tube down the patient's throat or through a needle in one of her veins.[62] Force feeding of this sort can sometimes be followed by medical complications, although it is the most successful treatment in obtaining a quick weight gain.[63] Initial weight gain is important because, without it, it appears to be difficult for any long-term changes to occur in an anorexic's behavior due to the psychological changes wrought by starvation.[64]

"*Behavior modification* is a general term denoting behavior change resulting from the systematic application of behavioral principles. Behavior modification methods may be applied to any behavior in any setting, but when specifically applied to the alleviation of the behavior disorders, the term *behavior therapy* has generally been used."[65] It should be noted that, contrary to some definitions given in the popular media, psychosurgery and drug therapy are *not* classified as behavior therapy. Typically, when behavior therapy is used with anorexics, engaging in activities known to be pleasant for the anorexic is made contingent on eating.[66]

Behavior therapy is fairly successful in inducing an initial weight gain, although there seems to be some question about whether it is successful over the long term.[67] Given Birch's results described in Chapter 6, one wonders whether making engaging in pleasurable activities contingent on eating might, over time, decrease the value of eating. Perhaps such an effect hinders the long-term effectiveness of behavior therapy, particularly when the behavioral contingencies are no longer present. Gloria Rakita Leon[68] has suggested that the long-term efficacy of behavior therapy can be improved by using *cognitive-behavior therapy* instead. In this type of therapy learning principles are used to modify the patient's reported thoughts and images. Leon would use these techniques to change anorexics' beliefs about the value of the excessive self-control that they are demonstrating with regard to food consumption.

A great variety of drugs have been given to anorexics. Some of these drugs, such as insulin, increase appetite. Other drugs, such as *tricyclic antidepressants*, elevate mood. Drugs are usually given to anorexics in the initial stages of treatment to help induce an immediate weight gain.[69]

A review of the literature has suggested that drug therapy does not add any benefit when other types of therapy are used.[70] Other observations have suggested that drug therapy may be useful in inducing initial weight gains in some patients in severe cases.[71] Given the potential medical problems with using any drug, particularly over long periods of time, it seems that drug therapy should be approached with caution.

There are many different types of psychotherapy, including *individual, group,* and *family psychotherapy.* In individual psychotherapy the patient works with the therapist on a one-to-one basis. In group psychotherapy a group of patients discusses their problems together with the therapist. In family psychotherapy the therapist treats the whole family as a unit, rather than just treating the individual.[72] With each of these types of psychotherapy, the therapist may use a behavioral, a psychodynamic, or some other type of approach. Bruch has reported success with an approach focusing on active participation by the patient, which she feels helps the patient to be more independent.[73] Psychotherapy can also vary according to its length; each of the above types of psychotherapy can last for as little as a few weeks or for as long as several years.

Unfortunately there have been few controlled studies on the long-term effects of different treatments of anorexia nervosa.[74] This means that there is little information on the benefits of the various kinds of psychotherapy that are used to help treat this disorder. Psychotherapies are often used in conjunction with other types of therapy, so that it is difficult to isolate their effects from the effects of the other therapies. What is known is that the overall treatment package used for patients, usually consisting of some form of nurturance plus psychotherapy, seems to have fairly good results, although the success of this type of treatment does not appear to have improved over the past 50 years.[75]

More research is needed to determine what aspects of treatment are most helpful in the long-term maintenance of weight gain. It may be that, due to the multidetermined nature of anorexia nervosa, any one treatment in isolation is unlikely to be successful; the best treatment may be a treatment package.[76]

Hospitalization, when needed, may involve one or more of the above types of treatment. Which treatments are used depends on the nature of the treatment facility and the particular patient involved. One or more of the treatments described above, with the exception of force feeding, may also be given to anorexics being treated on an outpatient basis.[77]

One way in which nonhospitalized anorexics frequently find therapists, information, social support, and other types of assistance is through *self-help groups.* (A list of some such groups is offered at the end of this book.) Self-help groups are popular because they are relatively inexpensive and because they provide a number of services often not easily available through traditional mental health care institutions. More research is needed to determine the appropriate role of self-help groups in the treatment of anorexia nervosa.[78]

Prognosis

Although anorexia nervosa is a life-threatening eating disorder, most treated patients improve. There is some indication that treatment is more successful the younger the patient is when treatment begins,[79] perhaps because psychotherapy is more influential with a younger child, or because the patient is still living with her parents, which makes family therapy useful, or because cases of earlier onset may be less severe. We now turn to another, more recently recognized but related eating disorder, bulimia.

BULIMIA NERVOSA

Characteristics

Although anorexics may occasionally binge eat, repeated binge eating is called bulimia nervosa. The American Psychiatric Association describes the essential characteristics of bulimia nervosa as:

> recurrent episodes of binge eating (rapid consumption of a large amount of food in a discrete period of time); a feeling of lack of control over eating behavior during the eating binges; self-induced vomiting, use of laxatives or diuretics, strict dieting or fasting, or vigorous exercise in order to prevent weight gain; and persistent overconcern with body shape and weight.[80]

Craig L. Johnson and his colleagues surveyed 316 bulimic women and found that most of these women binged at least once per day, usually in the evening. The binges averaged 4,800 calories and ranged between 1,000 and 55,000 calories. The foods used for the binges were primarily sweet or salty carbohydrate foods. At the time of the study, most of the women were using various purging techniques to rid themselves of the calories they consumed during a binge; 81 percent relied on self-induced vomiting and 63 percent on laxatives. Johnson and his colleagues' data indicated that most of the subjects began to use purging techniques approximately 1 year after they began binging.[81]

Despite the frequent vomiting, bulimic women apparently do not develop taste aversions to the food they eat during binges (see Chapter 6 for discussion of taste aversion learning). This could be due to the fact that the vomiting is self-induced rather than externally imposed. In addition, bulimics sometimes report that they are extremely used to vomiting; it is not aversive to them.[82] Data obtained with rats indicate that a US is more successful at inducing a taste aversion if it is novel, and the average bulimic vomits many times.[83]

Most bulimics maintain a weight that is approximately within normal limits.[84] However, the repeated binging and purging can have devastating physiological effects. Some of the less serious effects include sore throat and swollen glands caused by repeated vomiting. The vomitus is acidic and it eats away at the enamel of the teeth, making bulimics prone to tooth decay. More serious is that both the vomiting and the use of laxatives can disrupt the balance of the electrolyte potassium in the body, with dehydration and cardiac arrhythmias as possible results. Urinary infections and renal failure can also occur, as well as epileptic seizures.[85] Bulimics have an additional problem in that they have significantly lower metabolic rates than do non-bulimics, thus making it easier for bulimics to gain weight. It is not yet known what is responsible for this low metabolic rate, but it may be due to binging and then purging (see Chapter 10 for more information on how food deprivation can decrease metabolic rate).[86]

Some researchers have found that insulin secretion in response to a specific test meal does not occur normally in bulimic women, but other researchers have found no such differences between women who are and are not bulimic.[87] However, whether or not bulimics' insulin responses to food are normal, bulimics do consume more food than women who are not bulimic, even in a laboratory setting.[88] Perhaps these two research areas can be combined so as to determine whether bulimics' insulin responses are abnormal when they binge, thus giving a more complete answer to the question of whether or not bulimics' insulin responses are abnormal when bulimics consume food under natural conditions. The answers to questions such as these can lead to hypotheses regarding specific physiological causes and effects of bulimia nervosa.

Prevalence

As with anorexia nervosa, most bulimics are apparently young adults. This information is based on the types of cases reported by clinicians.[89] However, if subjects of different ages vary in their tendency to seek help for bulimia nervosa, these data would be biased and would not represent the actual prevalence of bulimia nervosa among different age groups.

Again, as with anorexia nervosa, the majority of bulimics are women, although there is not yet sufficient data to specify precisely the female to male ratio.[90] Some information is provided by recent studies of the frequency of bulimia nervosa in college and university populations.[91] The percentage of students suffering from bulimia nervosa as identified by these studies has ranged from 1 percent to 19 percent of females, and from 0.1 percent to 5 percent of males; and the ratio of female-to-male students reporting bulimia nervosa has ranged from 3.8-to-1 to 19-to-1. That these results vary so widely is undoubtedly due, at least in part, to the varying methodologies that the studies used. Some of the studies included graduate student subjects, but others did not. Some had high response rates (e.g., 97 percent of those contacted), but others did not (e.g., 66 percent of those contacted). Some, but not all, used the American Psychiatric Association's most recent stringent diagnostic criteria for bulimia nervosa. Finally, some, but not all, collected their data at elite, private universities. Depending on which study is read, the current prevalence of bulimia nervosa may or may not seem alarmingly high.[92]

Despite the lack of agreement among the various studies, all of them found a high frequency of disordered eating among college populations, with these symptoms including instances of binging and/or purging. Only recently has there been much publicity about bulimia nervosa, and thus it is difficult to determine whether the frequency of binging and purging has always been this high or whether their prevalence has recently increased.[93] Perhaps the college population of our weight-conscious society has been discovering what at first glance appears to be the perfect solution to dealing with both the wide availability of palatable food in college and the desire to be physically attractive according to prevailing standards: binge and purge. As one patient said, "I thought I had the problem licked; I couldn't understand why everyone didn't eat and then vomit."[94] What bulimics often do not realize is that their disease can have serious medical complications.

Possible Explanations and Causes

Many of the possible explanations and causes that have been proposed for anorexia nervosa have also been proposed for bulimia nervosa. The weights reported as desirable by bulimics are far below healthy weights. Bulimics, like anorexics, seem to have a distorted view of their own weight.[95] The overeating has also been seen as fulfilling some emotional need, because it is influenced by such factors as exposure to certain social situations.[96] Further, bulimics, like anorexics, are obsessed with controlling their food intake. However, unlike anorexics, who are successful at this control, the bulimic will regularly slip and consume huge amounts of food. Once the binge starts, it seems uncontrollable. Then the bulimic attempts to purge herself of the food.[97]

For the bulimic, the continual struggle with binging and purging results in a preoccupation with food: how much to eat, when to eat, how to do it without the knowledge of others, and how to get enough food for a binge. It has been argued that bulimics' binging results from their dieting (i.e., from their being *restrained eaters*): the binges result from homeostatic mechanisms attempting to return food-deprived bodies to their respective set points. However, the opposite theory—that binging causes the dieting—has also been proposed.[98]

Bulimics' preoccupation with eating too much and too little has been linked by many authors to the depression that seems to be a common feature of bulimia.[99] However, bulimics' depression may not be a consequence of their bulimia. Bulimics tend to come from families with a history of affective disorders.[100] Further, many affective disorders appear to have a genetic component. It has therefore been suggested that a single, genetically based chemical disorder may be at least partly responsible for both depression and bulimia.[101]

The possibility that bulimia may have a biological basis related to the biological basis of depression is intriguing. It opens up new avenues for treatment, which will be discussed below. However, it is unlikely that a simple model, such as depression leading to bulimia or bulimia leading to depression, will explain all or even most cases of bulimia and depression. There has been no definitive proof of a causative link between bulimia and depression, in either direction. Further, there is too much heterogeneity among both bulimics and depressives with respect to their symptoms as well as with respect to the ways in which their illnesses develop and progress.[102]

Treatments

As with anorexia nervosa, various types of psychotherapy have been used with bulimia nervosa. For example, traditional behavior therapy, as well as cognitive-behavior therapy, has been used to treat bulimia nervosa.[103] One treatment technique derived from behavior therapy allows patients to eat large amounts of food until they feel the urge to vomit. However, they are prevented from vomiting and are encouraged to concentrate on the anxiety thus created. This is known as *exposure and response prevention*. The theory behind this treatment is that, because the patient is exposed to anxiety accompanying excessive food consumption but is not allowed to remove this anxiety through purging, the patient habituates to the anxiety and the cycle (binge, anxiety, and removal of anxiety through purging) is broken.[104] One experiment found that cognitive-behavior therapy combined with exposure and response prevention resulted in significantly greater decreases in bulimics' binging and vomiting than did cognitive-behavior therapy used alone. In fact, 1 year after treatment, patients treated with cognitive-behavior therapy plus exposure and response prevention were completely free from binging and purging.[105] Dietary advice and guidelines may also be helpful in treating binging.[106]

Consistent with the hypothesis that the causes of bulimia nervosa and depression are in some way physiologically related, several researchers have reported improvement in the eating behavior of bulimics after administration of antidepressants.[107] For example, Harrison G. Pope and his colleagues conducted a double-blind study with 22 bulimic women using an antidepressant and a placebo. These authors found that the drug tended to decrease the frequency of binge eating, but the placebo did not. In fact, 1 to 8 months after the original study 90 percent of the entire sample had significantly decreased their frequency of binging following treatment with an antidepressant.[108] However, some therapists have observed that antidepressants relieve only depression in bulimics, not binging or purging.[109] In addition, it may be necessary to use cognitive-behavior therapy to increase the (usually small) number of nonpurged calories consumed by bulimics and to achieve long-lasting maintenance of treatment effects.[110] Yet the majority of studies appear to indicate a role for antidepressants in the treatment of bulimia nervosa: Antidepressants are a relatively inexpensive treatment that frequently ameliorates the binging and purging of bulimia nervosa.[111]

CONCLUSION

There are a number of different situations in which food consumption can decrease to the point at which intake is inadequate. Drugs, disease, and mood disorders may all result in anorexia. Psychologists and physicians are making progress in alleviating these life-threatening conditions. Their efforts are even more essential considering the recent emphasis on the medical dangers of being too thin.

CHAPTER
10
❦
Overeating and Obesity

This chapter is concerned with food consumption so excessive that it is considered abnormal, and with obesity, a body weight significantly greater than average. One of this chapter's aims will be to show that, contrary to popular opinion, overeating and obesity do not necessarily depend on each other.

There is no single objective standard for specifying the weight that constitutes obesity for a given individual. Many different criteria have been used based on the different techniques for estimating body fat. For example, one way of estimating thinness or heaviness is to divide an individual's weight (in kilograms) by the square of that person's height (in meters), thus generating the *body mass index* or *(BMI)*. The higher this number, the more mass someone has per inch of height. Someone is defined as overweight if his or her BMI is 25–30 kg/m^2, and as obese if his or her BMI is greater than 30 kg/m^2. However, these values should probably be adjusted such that they rise as age increases beyond 24 years.[1] The problem with this measure is that it does not distinguish between lean body mass, such as muscle and bone, and stored fat. Another measure consists of determining the thickness of the skinfold at the upper back of the arm. The thicker the fold, the more subcutaneous fat has been stored. By still another method, a person's weight is measured in the usual way and then is measured under water. Because the specific gravity of fat is less than that of lean body tissue, it is possible to use this technique to estimate the percentage of the body that consists of stored fat.[2]

A common way of estimating obesity is simply to measure someone's height and weight and then compare those values to the ones given in the standard height–weight tables (see Tables 9.1a and 9.1b). Although this method, like the BMI, does not estimate how much of the body weight is lean tissue and how much is fat, it does at least take the person's frame size into account. It is also the easiest method to use.

The previous chapter on anorexia and bulimia pointed out that the weights in the height–weight tables have recently been increased. These changes in the tables were made because there is now greater knowledge of the dangers of being too thin. The changes in the tables should not be interpreted as diminishing the health hazards of being extremely overweight, however. Although ideal weights have been raised, a body weight significantly in excess of these weights can still entail some medical risk. Diseases associated with extreme obesity include hypertension, diabetes, cancer, and heart attack. It has been estimated that over 15 percent of the U.S. population between the ages of 30 and 62 has a BMI of 30 or more (i.e., is obese).[3] In addition, the incidence of extreme obesity in American children has been continually increasing.[4] Obesity has been and continues to be a health problem. However, if someone is simply described as *obese* in this chapter, without an indication of the degree of the obesity, this indicates only a greater than ideal weight and does not necessarily imply that the person has a health problem.

This chapter will first describe the demographic characteristics, eating behavior, and moods of people who are obese. The second section discusses the possible factors involved in the origins of obesity. The chapter closes with a discussion of the methods that have been used to decrease overeating and obesity.

CHARACTERISTICS OF THE OBESE

Relative Prevalence

The prevalence of obesity varies from one group of people to the next. More women than men are obese. Obesity increases with age up to the age of about 60 years, and thereafter it begins to decrease. However, this decrease appears more likely to occur in men.[5] In the United States, obesity is much more prevalent among women in lower than in higher socioeconomic groups. In developing countries, men, women, and children are all more likely to be obese the higher their socioeconomic status.[6] However, it should be emphasized that obesity occurs in all groups; it is simply more common in some groups than others.

Eating Behavior

The eating behaviors of obese people vary, although some general statements can be made. Lynn Spitzer and Judith Rodin conducted an extensive survey of the literature on the eating behavior of obese and normal-weight people.[7] They found that, in general, the obese are more likely to eat large amounts of palatable food than are people of normal weight. In addition, people who are obese are less likely to slow their rate of eating during the course of a meal than are normal-weight individuals. However, over entire meals there are no differences in the eating rates of obese and normal-weight people. Spitzer and Rodin were struck by the general lack of clear, consistent differences in the eating behaviors of normal-weight and obese people. Many of the studies that Spitzer and Rodin reviewed had found differences in the eating behavior of the obese and nonobese, but subsequent studies had not replicated these differences.

Two specific characteristic eating behaviors that have been investigated in the obese should be mentioned here. First is the question of whether obese people consume more calories than do nonobese people. One study found that women who were in the dynamic phase of obesity, that is, whose weight was increasing, tended to consume approximately 480 calories per day more than women who were in the static phase or who were of normal weight. However, there were no significant differences in the number of calories consumed by women of normal weight and by women who were in the static phase of obesity.[8] Other studies have found no differences in calories consumed even between subjects who are and are not gaining weight.[9] Second, approximately 25 percent of obese people demonstrate symptoms of severe binge eating.[10] But this also means that 75 percent of obese people do not demonstrate these symptoms.

Considered together, the data suggest that there are few consistent differences in the eating behavior of obese and normal-weight people.

Mood

Most people have heard at one time or another that fat people are jolly. Santa Claus and Captain Kangaroo are both legendary jovial characters who are quite overweight. But does a happy mood accompany overeating? How does mood vary as excess food consumption varies? There have been some investigations of these questions.

Robert Plutchik[11] gave thin, normal-weight, and obese people a questionnaire that contained questions about mood and eating behavior. The more overweight a subject was, the more likely that subject was to report eating when depressed or anxious. Similarly, Joyce Slochower and Sharon P. Kaplan[12] found that experimentally induced anxiety was likely to result in food consumption by obese subjects. However, in normal-weight subjects, experimentally induced anxiety was likely to result in diminished food consumption. Consistent with the results from both of the studies just described were the results from a study conducted by Joyce Slochower, Sharon P. Kaplan, and Lisa Mann.[13] They found that obese female college students ate more during exam periods when they reported anxiety, whereas normal-weight subjects ate less during exam periods when they reported anxiety. Note that the reported degree of anxiety by itself did not differ between the obese and nonobese subjects. All of these studies seem to suggest that obese people are more likely to eat when they are experiencing aversive moods.

However, a number of findings appear to indicate that *dieting* is a better predictor of eating during depression than is obesity.[14] Apparently neither Plutchik nor Slochower and her colleagues assessed whether or not their subjects were dieting. If more of the obese subjects in these three studies were dieting than were the leaner subjects, the results would be consistent with the hypothesis that dieters, but not nondieters, tend to eat more when depressed. Although the eating behavior of dieters and nondieters may differ, once again it appears that there are few consistent data indicating differences in the eating behavior of the obese and the nonobese.

There is one subgroup of obese people, however, who may indeed differ from leaner persons with respect to mood and eating behavior. These are people suffering from *seasonal affective disorder (SAD)*. SAD tends to occur among susceptible people during the winter months, when these people are exposed to less light. SAD is characterized by depression, a craving for carbohydrates, overeating, and weight gain. Only a small proportion of obese people suffer from SAD, however.[15]

If the obese do not, on average, differ in mood or eating behavior from the nonobese, are there other differences between obese and nonobese people that could cause obesity? The next section discusses some such possible causes.

CAUSES OF OVEREATING AND OBESITY

There has been a great deal of research on the possible causes of overeating and obesity. Naturally, most of this research has been conducted with an eye toward ways of preventing and decreasing obesity. In this section investigations of the genetic, physiological, and environmental bases for overeating and obesity will be presented.

Genetic Bases

There is no question that obese parents tend to have obese children. Only about 10 percent of children who have no obese parent become obese. Approximately 40 percent of children with one obese parent become obese; approximately 70 percent of children with two obese parents become obese.[16] How much of this concordance between obesity of parents and offspring is due to eating or exercise habits transmitted environmentally from parents to children, and how much is due to genes transmitted from parents to children?

Evidence supporting a genetic basis for obesity comes from studies with nonhuman subjects. It is possible to breed rats and mice that have a propensity to become obese.[17] This is done by repeatedly breeding the most obese animals.

Two types of studies have been used to examine genetic predisposition for obesity in humans. Twin studies compare the weights of identical and fraternal twins, and adoption studies compare the weights of biological parents and their offspring and of adoptive parents and their children. These studies generally find that weight tends to be more similar between identical twins than between fraternal twins, and more similar between biological parents and their offspring than between adoptive parents and their children. Although it is possible to find criticisms of most of these studies, the evidence leans toward the conclusion that there is a genetic component in the determination of obesity.[18]

Nevertheless, a genetic component is not the same as complete genetic determination. Significant correlations have been found between the weights of adoptive mothers and their children.[19] There is no question that the environment also plays a role in the determination of obesity. In addition, simply knowing that there is a genetic component does not tell us the mechanisms by which that genetic component exerts its effects. The following sections suggest some candidates for such mechanisms, as well as some candidates for more environmentally based mechanisms.

Adipose Cells

The amount of fat stored in the body is thought to be related to body-weight set point, the long-term weight maintained by the body (see Chapter 2). *Adipose cells* store fat. When the adipose cells are full, there is less hunger; when the adipose cells are not full, there is more hunger. Therefore someone whose body has stored a certain amount of fat in a particular number of adipose cells would generally feel hungrier than someone whose body has stored the same amount of fat but in fewer adipose cells.[20]

Heredity plays a role in the number and distribution, and therefore the appetite-generating ability, of adipose cells.[21] In addition, there is now evidence that although the number of adipose cells can increase when a person gains weight, that number can never decrease. The increase in number of adipose cells appears to occur most easily in childhood, a period of rapid growth, but can occur at other times of life as well.[22] Therefore people who have been overweight at some time in their lives, whether or not they are presently overweight, have a relatively large number of adipose cells; such people must continually struggle if they wish to eat amounts of food less than those needed to maintain their maximum attained weight.

Energy Expenditure

Someone gains weight when energy intake exceeds energy expenditure. Given that, as described above, much research has demonstrated no large differences in eating behavior between people who are and are not obese, recent work has focused on the other possible major factor responsible for weight gain: energy expenditure. An individual's total energy expenditure is composed of: (a) basal metabolic rate, (b) energy used as a result of physical activity, and (c) *thermogenesis* (the production of heat, mainly following food consumption).[23] A low value for any of these three types of energy expenditure could increase someone's tendency to gain weight and to become obese. This section considers each of these three types of energy expenditure as possible explanations for obesity.

Individuals having identical body weights may have different metabolic rates; the lower the metabolic rate, the greater the person's tendency to become obese.[24] Various factors can influence metabolic rate. For example, lean tissue (i.e., muscle and bone) supports a higher metabolic rate than does fat. Someone who is obese may actually have a higher basal metabolic rate than someone who is not obese, due to the increased muscle tissue that develops in order to support the excess adipose tissue.[25] A factor that can decrease metabolic rate is low levels of food consumption. The body conserves energy when food intake is low. This was adaptive when humans had limited access to food sources. Now, when low food intake in the United States is frequently by choice, this decrease in metabolic rate is counterproductive; it tends to counteract the effects of dieting.[26] The decrease in metabolic rate following sustained food deprivation may even continue for months after the food deprivation has ceased. For example, Diane Elliot and her colleagues[27] measured basal metabolic rate in seven obese women before and after weight loss from a protein-sparing modified fast (of approximately 300 calories per day). At the start of the fast, which lasted 10 to 23 weeks, basal metabolic rate decreased 22 percent. Four weeks after the diet was over, the subjects' basal metabolic rates were still about 22 percent below baseline values. There was some increase in basal metabolic rate 8 weeks after the diet was over, but only in some subjects. No subsequent data were reported for these subjects.

Metabolic rate can also be increased through exercise. This increase is not permanent, but it can last for more than 12 hours. It is not yet known what intensity and duration of exercise are needed to obtain the carryover effect, but it can occur following acute strenuous exercise such as playing football.[28] Not every study, however, has demonstrated an increase in metabolic rate as a function of exercise. For example, S. A. Bingham and his colleagues[29] observed no change in subjects' basal metabolic rates during a 9-week exercise training program. However, because the caloric intake of the subjects was held constant throughout the 9 weeks, while their amount of exercise was gradually increased, they were experiencing an energy deficit by the end of the experiment. Given that an energy deficit caused by dieting decreases metabolic rate, the fact that the metabolic rates of the subjects in this study did not decrease suggests that exercise did increase metabolic rate. Other research has demonstrated that subjects who exercise show a small decrease in metabolic rate when dieting.[30] Further, Jasper Brener has shown that environmental uncertainty, such as occurs when a novel task must be performed, results in greater energy expenditure than performance of a familiar task, even though both tasks require the same amount of physical work.[31] The exercise required by Bingham and his colleagues' experiment involved walking and/or jogging for the entire 9-week program. The familiarity of this exercise could have inhibited the subjects' total energy expenditure.

Many studies, although not all, have shown that on the average obese people are less active than are nonobese people. Perhaps this difference in activity has something to do with the origin or maintenance of the obesity. However, most of the studies that have looked at this question appear to have examined activity level, not number of calories used in exercise. Obese people may expend as many calories as lean people, even though the obese people are exercising less, simply because a greater number of calories are needed to move a greater weight.[32] Consistent with this hypothesis, research has shown that energy expenditure over a 24-hour period is identical for both lean and obese women.[33]

It is thought that decreased activity may, in part, explain the significant correlation between number of hours of television viewing with degree of obesity in children. Children who are watching television use less energy than those who are playing in the park. They are also inclined to snack while they watch and to prefer the salty and sweet foods and drinks that they see advertised on television (see Chapter 6). For all of these reasons, television viewing is thought to be a major contributor to obesity in children.[34]

Finally we turn to the effect of food consumption on thermogenesis in lean versus obese people. A number of experiments have suggested that so-called brown (as opposed to white) adipose tissue is responsible for thermogenesis; however, the evidence so far is limited to nonhuman subjects.[35] Whatever the responsible mechanism, food consumption increases thermogenesis. This effect is larger following a high-carbohydrate than a high-fat meal.[36] Further, if food consumption is greater than usual, thermogenesis is also greater. Similar to the decrease in metabolic rate that accompanies food deprivation, the increase in themogeneseis following increased food consumption helps organisms to stay at a constant weight. However, if rats' weights are increased by giving the rats continued free access to a high-fat diet, their adipose cells increase in number, and eventually the increased thermogenesis disappears; a new set point has been reached.[37] Some research has suggested that the thermogenesis response of obese subjects following food consumption is impaired, although this impairment may be seen only after high-carbohydrate meals.[38] The finding that the size of the thermogenesis response may have a genetic component[39] suggests the possibility that obese people become obese in part because of an impaired thermogenesis response—that the impaired thermogenesis response is a cause, not just a consequence, of obesity. Additional research will be needed to confirm this hypothesis.

Neurotransmitters

As was mentioned above, some people—for example, those suffering from SAD—become obese due to carbohydrate craving. It has been hypothesized that the carbohydrate craving seen in people with SAD, and in some other obese people, is due to a dysfunction in serotoninergic transmission in the brain, because serotonin is involved in the appetite for carbohydrates (see Chapters 5 and 8). More specifically, carbohydrate craving is hypothesized to arise from insufficient amounts of serotonin stimulating the brain.[40]

Type of Food Consumed

Our gustatory system, including taste preferences, evolved during times of food scarcity, before food manufacture became a common human occupation (see Chapters 5 and 6). Our genetic preferences for sweet and for salt, and our predisposition to learn to prefer highly caloric food, were useful when those substances were hard to obtain. Now, too many sweet, salty, and highly caloric substances are consumed in industrial societies because of our evolutionary history and because these substances are widely and cheaply available.

Generally the food that is available in industrialized societies is both abundant and geared to the preferences of the population. It is therefore not surprising that in countries such as the United States there is a great deal of overeating and obesity. Recall from the preceding discussion that the obese have a greater tendency to eat large amounts of palatable food than do the nonobese; thus their excess weight may be at least partly due to their residence in an industrialized society. Experiments with both rats and humans have shown that subjects will eat more of palatable than unpalatable foods and that when large amounts of highly palatable foods are available, subjects will overeat and become obese.[41] Amount of food consumed can also be increased by composing a meal of a variety of foods (thus removing the sensory specific satiety effect, discussed in Chapter 6).[42] Within-meal variety is another common characteristic of food consumption in industrialized countries such as the United States.

Many researchers have paid special attention to the role of the taste of sweet in inducing overeating and obesity. In order to separate the effects of the taste of sweet from the postingestive effects of sugar consumption, artificial sweeteners—which provide a sweet taste with no postingestive effects (i.e., no calories)—have been used in many of these investigations. Many, but not all, of these experiments appear to indicate that the taste of sweet can increase general appetite, sometimes to the point of obesity, and that this is true for artificial as well as caloric sweeteners.[43] This effect may be due in part to the cephalic phase insulin response (see Chapter 2) or to the liver's increasing hunger through lowering blood sugar and increasing storage of ingested fuel as fat.[44]

Chapter 10

Responsiveness to External Stimuli

In 1971 Stanley Schachter published a now-classic paper entitled "Some Extraordinary Facts about Obese Humans and Rats."[45] This paper synthesized Schachter's attempts to relate the behavior of obese humans and of rats with the ventromedial hypothalamus (VMH) syndrome to the behavior of nonobese humans and rats. Recall that if a lesion is made in a rat's brain near the VMH, the rat tends to consume huge amounts of food until it becomes extremely obese (see Chapter 2).

Schachter conducted a number of unusual and clever experiments to make his comparisons. For example, one comparison that he investigated involved the willingness of obese and nonobese humans to work for food. VMH-lesioned rats are much less willing to work for food than are nonlesioned rats. To obtain relevant data, Schachter and several of his colleagues visited many Chinese and Japanese restaurants. As each patron entered the restaurant, one of the researchers would classify that person as either obese or nonobese. Subsequent observations determined whether the person ate with chopsticks. The results showed that 22 percent of the nonobese, but only 5 percent of the obese, ate with chopsticks. Because it presumably takes more work to eat with chopsticks than with a fork, these data are consistent with those comparing VMH-lesioned and -nonlesioned rats.

Table 10.1 summarizes some of Schachter's comparisons. A preload of food decreased food consumption by the nonobese but not by the obese. Note that giving a preload involves manipulation of the subjects' internal

TABLE 10.1

Summary of Schachter's Comparisons between the Obese and the Nonobese

	Relative effects on eating	
Manipulation	Nonobese	Obese
Preload	Yes	No
Food visible	No	Yes
Taste	No	Yes
Work	No	Yes

Source: S. Schachter, "Some Extraordinary Facts about Obese Humans and Rats,"

state. In contrast, external manipulations, such as making the food very visible, very tasty, or very easy to get, increased the food consumption of the obese but not of the nonobese. Schachter therefore proposed that obese humans and VMH-lesioned rats are relatively sensitive to external stimuli and relatively insensitive to internal stimuli. Figure 10.1 is a pictorial representation of his model.

Because of the similarities that Schachter found between obese humans and VMH-lesioned rats, he went even further and proposed that obesity in humans and VMH-lesioned rats might both be related to the hypothalamus. This hypothesis is subject to the same criticisms made of the hunger and satiety centers theory of hunger in Chapter 2. In addition, Schachter's primary hypothesis, that the obese are relatively more responsive to external stimuli, has also come into question.

Judith Rodin found that there are many externally responsive people (people whose eating is affected by external cues) at every weight level, some of whom find ways of restraining their eating so that they do not be-

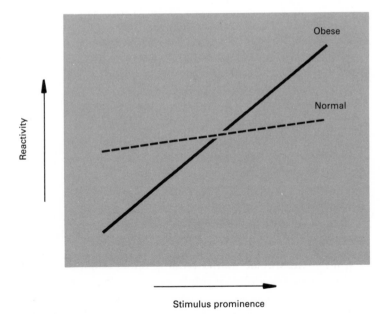

FIGURE 10.1   *Reactivity as a function of stimulus prominence for both obese and normal subjects.* (After S. Schachter, "Some Extraordinary Facts about Obese Humans and Rats," *American Psychologist* 26 [1971]: 129–144.)

come obese. Whether or not they restrain their eating, people who are externally responsive generally demonstrate particular physiological responses to the sight of food. According to Rodin, when externally responsive people see food, their insulin level increases. This, in turn, increases hunger and the likelihood that any food consumed will be stored as fat. In other words, externally responsive people are literally turned on by the sight of food. To avoid gaining weight these people must be very careful about their food environment as well as their consumption. There is not yet conclusive evidence regarding whether or not this external responsivity is largely genetic or largely learned.[46] However, the insulin response that occurs following consumption of the artificial sweetener saccharin (see below) will eventually extinguish following repeated exposure to the sweet taste of the saccharin, which results in no ensuing calories.[47] Thus it is at least possible for the insulin response to be conditioned.

Stress-Induced Eating

Walk into any cocktail party and you will see the guests consuming a great many potato chips, pretzels, and hors d'oeuvres that they would not ordinarily eat. As the conversation flourishes, hands repeatedly dip into the bowls of peanuts and crackers.

This phenomenon has been likened to the well-established laboratory finding that rats repeatedly given a mild tail pinch consume excessive food, to the point that they become obese. In an experiment by Neil E. Rowland and Seymour M. Antelman, rats whose tails were pinched for 10 to 15 minutes, six times per day, for up to 5 days, gained an average of 63 grams (18 percent of their average initial weight). Control rats whose tails were not pinched gained an average of only 17 grams.[48] Further, just as obese humans tend to eat more palatable food than do the nonobese, tail-pinched rats sometimes demonstrate a tendency to prefer palatable, familiar foods, particularly if they are food deprived.[49] Some tail-pinched rats will go on eating binges, reminiscent of the eating binges of humans.[50]

Another mildly stressful laboratory paradigm that will induce overeating in rats is intermittent schedules of reinforcement.[51] Recall from Chapter 3 that such schedules will also induce excessive drinking (schedule-induced polydipsia, SIP). Work by Michael B. Cantor and his colleagues provides another similar example. These researchers showed that information-processing tasks (which can be thought of as resulting in intermittent reinforcement) will induce eating in humans.[52] They found that when humans work on a tracking task involving aiming a stylus at a rotating dot, they tend to consume snacks. When the task is made more difficult, the tendency to consume snacks increases.

Cantor believes that all of these phenomena, together called adjunctive behaviors (tail pinch–induced eating, SIP, schedule-induced overeating, and humans' overeating during an information-processing task), are similar and can be explained by a common mechanism. According to Cantor, all of these manipulations result in arousal of the organism, and this arousal results in eating.[53] Consistent with this hypothesis, fast music, loud noise, and loud music, which can all be described as increasing arousal, increase the rate of eating, amount eaten, and/or preference for sucrose.[54]

T. W. Robbins and P. J. Fray have proposed a hypothesis similar to Cantor's.[55] They feel that these sorts of manipulations induce anxiety and make organisms more responsive to external stimuli. The organisms eat because they have difficulty discriminating between the internal stimuli associated with anxiety and those associated with hunger, similar to Hilde Bruch's hypotheses about eating disorders based on her results with psychodynamic therapy.[56] Robbins and Fray also propose that eating reduces anxiety. They, as well as Cantor, have related stress-induced eating to Schachter's and Rodin's concepts of externality.[57] Both tail-pinched rats and organisms relatively sensitive to external stimuli are more likely to eat, given the presence of food, than are nontail-pinched rats or organisms relatively insensitive to external stimuli. How far these parallels may extend is a question for further research.

Attempts to explain stress-induced eating and to generalize from it have resulted in much published discussion among researchers. For example, John E. Morley and Allen S. Levine have postulated that opiates manufactured by the rats' own bodies are involved in stress-induced eating, because injections of naloxone, an opiate antagonist, eliminate stress-induced eating. This type of research may help to improve both our understanding and our treatments of some cases of overeating in humans.[58]

Learning

Bruch's theories regarding the effects of learning on overeating leading to obesity are based on her experience with the psychodynamic treatment of obesity. She has stated that food can come to stand for love or power, can express rage and hate, and can be a substitute for sex. She feels that these multiple and inappropriate (from an energy regulation perspective) uses of food arise from the learning that goes on in the early infant–caregiver interaction. The caregiver may give the infant food whenever the infant is disturbed for any reason, rather than merely when the infant appears hungry.

In this way, Bruch hypothesizes, the child learns to use food to satisfy many drives in addition to hunger, and obesity can be the result.[59]

Two experiments, one conducted with rats and one with humans, illustrate the increasing experimental interest in the effects of learning on food consumption and obesity. First is an experiment by Harvey P. Weingarten[60] that investigated learning of meal initiation in rats. Weingarten paired a light and tone combination with each meal. The light and tone lasted for 4.5 minutes. A meal, consisting of a liquid diet based on evaporated milk, was presented in a food cup during the last 30 seconds of the light and tone. Meals occurred six times per day for 11 days. During the second phase of the experiment, Weingarten gave the rats free access to a bottle with liquid food. In addition, once per day, he presented the light and tone combination followed by a liquid diet meal (available from the food cup).

Despite the fact that the rats were not food deprived when the light and tone combination was presented in the second part of the experiment, they reliably ate from the food cup. The light and tone had become a conditioned cue that elicited food consumption. (Similar findings have been obtained with preschool children.[61]) The rats compensated for their intake from the cup by decreasing the amount of food they consumed from the bottle. However, suppose, as might occur with humans, that conditioned cues are always present for food consumption. Food consumption might then occur largely independently of hunger and frequently enough for obesity to occur.

The second experiment was conducted by Marcie Greenberg Lowe[62] using human subjects. Lowe wished to study the possible role of learning in the overeating that sometimes occurs when people break a diet. Subjects were told that the experiment was concerned with the effects of hunger on taste perception. They were also told that in a first session they would practice making taste ratings and would make baseline ratings, and that then, after 4 hours, in a second session they would make another set of ratings. Finally, they were told that during the 4 hours between the first and second sessions half of the subjects would eat normally and the other half would eat nothing.

At the start of the first session, all of the subjects were required to eat a number of small snacks as part of the supposed practice ratings. It was at this point that subjects were told whether they were assigned to the normal food consumption or the food deprivation condition. Because the first session (45 minutes in length) began between 10 a.m. and 1 p.m., if a subject were assigned to the deprivation condition, the 4-hour deprivation period between sessions would mean going without lunch or postponing dinner. Each subject was then left alone with plentiful snacks to make the "baseline" ratings of the snacks. Actually the measure of interest was the amount of snacks consumed by the two different groups of subjects. There was no second session.

As expected, those subjects who thought that they would be returning for a second session with no intervening food consumption ate significantly more of the snacks than did the subjects who thought that they would be able to eat normally between the two sessions. In other words, the food-deprivation condition subjects responded to learned cues indicating future food deprivation by consuming additional amounts to compensate for that deprivation. According to Lowe, this may explain why dieters who break their diets may then overeat. They are anticipating returning to their diets.

dieting ↓ overeats

The research discussed in prior sections regarding the effects of learning on the cephalic phase insulin response, and on our preferences for highly caloric foods, also suggests that learning contributes to overeating. However, additional investigations of the effects of learning on meal initiation and termination are needed.[63]

Social Factors

Sometimes the mere presence of another person can change the amount of food that someone consumes. Two recent experiments illustrate these effects. Sharon Lee Berry and her colleagues[64] demonstrated that both male and female undergraduates eat more ice cream when they eat in groups than when they eat alone. Similarly, Barbara Edelman and her colleagues[65] showed that men eat more lasagna when they eat in groups than when they eat alone.

In still another experiment, Janet Polivy and her colleagues[66] investigated whether the eating behavior of a woman (the model) would affect the eating behavior of other women (the subjects). The model was actually an accomplice of the experimenter, but the subjects thought that she was another participant. The model told half the subjects that she was dieting and half the subjects that she was not dieting. The model ate with each subject individually after the experimenter had simultaneously instructed the model and the subjects to consume food until they were full. The model ate very little in the presence of half the subjects to whom she had said that she was dieting and half the subjects to whom she had said she was not dieting. She ate a lot in the presence of the other subjects. This research design therefore yielded four groups of subjects (Figure 10.2). There was an overall tendency for all the subjects to eat more when the model ate more. In addition, the subjects to whom the model had identified herself as dieting generally ate less than the subjects to whom the model had identified herself as nondieting.

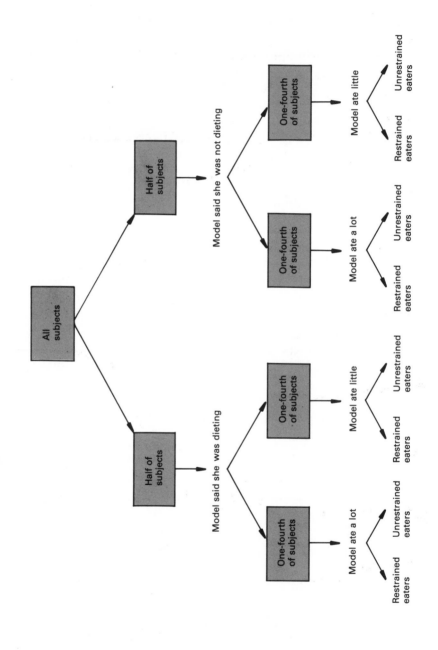

Clearly, amount of food consumed can be affected by the presence or absence of others. Such an effect is consistent with the research described in Chapter 6 in which organisms' food preferences and aversions are affected by observation of other organisms' food preferences and aversions. More research is needed to determine what aspects of someone's presence can affect amount of food consumed, and whether social factors can increase food consumption to the point that overeating occurs.

METHODS OF DECREASING OVEREATING AND OBESITY

There are probably more how-to books on weight loss than on any other do-it-yourself subject. Most of these books are ignorant of the research on the origins and the methods used to decrease overeating and obesity. Fortunately, many people with research training have investigated weight- loss techniques. The references list a few of the publications that provide scientifically based general information, written for educated readers, about weight loss. The rest of this chapter provides more specific information regarding methods of decreasing overeating and obesity. To evaluate these techniques properly, a brief introduction to relevant methodological issues will first be necessary.

Methodology

Many of the methodological issues discussed in Chapter 8 are applicable to all experimental research, including experimental research on decreasing overeating and obesity. But there are several issues of research design and data interpretation not discussed there that arise frequently in the research on obesity interventions. Excellent reviews by D. Balfour Jeffrey and by G. Terence Wilson have summarized these issues.[67]

For example, researchers testing a method for decreasing obesity are likely to find that some of the subjects drop out of the experiment or become unavailable for follow-up assessments. If these subjects are those for whom the method did not succeed, the results of the study may be biased.

Another relevant methodological issue is the use of follow-up assessment. Follow-up assessments must be conducted at long intervals following

FIGURE 10.2   *Design of Polivy, Herman, Younger, and Erskine's experiment.* (After J. Polivy, C. P. Herman, J. C. Younger, and B. Erskine, "Effects of a Model on Eating Behavior: The Induction of a Restrained Eating Style," *Journal of Personality* 47[1979]: 100–117.)

any attempt to decrease obesity in order to determine whether the effects of the manipulation prevent relapse, so common following weight loss.[68] Any method for decreasing obesity that results in only a temporary weight loss is unsatisfactory.

When researchers select subjects for an experiment comparing various weight-loss methods, or for an experiment that assesses only the effect of a single method, it is important that they keep in mind the subjects' motivation to lose weight. Subjects in these experiments are frequently volunteers or people attending a weight-loss clinic, and therefore they may be more motivated to lose weight than is the average person who needs to do so.

If a weight-loss method seeks to monitor and modify behavior as a means of modifying weight, reports of that behavior must be accurate. Frequently, studies use subjects' self-reports of their behavior, but self-reports may not be accurate.

In any attempt to change a behavior, it is important to repeatedly assess many different aspects of the patients' behavior. Thus if a manipulation has an adverse side effect, that side effect will be identified.

Finally, no examination of any method for decreasing overeating and obesity is complete without a determination of the cost-effectiveness of that method. An intervention may work very well but entail so much money or time that its use is impossible for most people.

Physiological Interventions

GASTRIC SURGERY.   The most drastic method for decreasing obesity is surgery. In gastric bypass surgery the lower part of the stomach is bypassed by first disconnecting it from the top part, and by then connecting the top part of the stomach directly to the intestine.[69] Bypass surgery is extremely successful in decreasing obesity. Several studies have shown average weight losses of more than 100 pounds.[70]

There can occasionally be some potentially dangerous side effects from this operation, with vomiting being the most common. Ulcers can also occur. In addition, major surgery of any kind always involves risk.[71] But there are also benefits from gastric bypass surgery in addition to the loss of weight. In general, patients appear to be better adjusted and happier after surgery. Patients report that, as a result of losing weight, they are now able to engage in physical activities that were previously impossible, they can wear a greater variety of attractive clothes, and they feel that they are more sexually appealing. Apparently elimination of obesity does not result in some underlying emotional problem's manifesting itself in some other way. In general the patients are better off psychologically.[72]

There is still the question about why bypass operations result in a loss of weight. At first it would seem that the weight loss must result from the decreased surface area of the gastrointestinal tract over which food can be absorbed. However, the weight loss can be explained by a significant postoperative reduction in food intake.[73] Therefore the question becomes, instead, why food intake decreases following the operation. One possibility is that gastrointestinal distention is now more apparent, and this serves as a satiety signal (see Chapter 2). In addition, perhaps the emotional changes and the expectations of improvements in the quality of living described above are at least partially responsible for the changes in postoperative food consumption. It is not yet know in these cases to what extent the emotional changes affect food consumption or to what extent food consumption affects the emotions, or whether both effects occur together. In any event, the benefits of this operation make it a viable choice for cases of severe obesity. Patients should be at least 100 pounds overweight and should have attempted (unsuccessfully) to lose weight using other, less drastic means. For other overweight persons, those for whom obesity is not life threatening, the potential dangers and side effects, as well as the cost, make gastric bypass surgery inadvisable.[74]

OTHER TYPES OF SURGICAL/MECHANICAL INTERVENTIONS. Three other types of surgical/mechanical interventions have been examined in attempts to decrease overeating and obesity: stomach banding, jaw wiring, and insertion of a balloon into the stomach. Stomach banding uses surgery to decrease the volume of the stomach. Although subsequent weight loss is often substantial, on the average better results are obtained with gastric bypass surgery.[75] Jaw wiring, by completely preventing the ingestion of solid food (liquids can still be ingested), usually results in weight loss. However, when the jaw wiring is removed, the weight most often returns.[76]

Use of a stomach balloon for weight control enjoyed recent, but fleeting, popularity. This procedure involves inserting a deflated balloon into the stomach. The balloon is then inflated and may be left thus in the stomach for many weeks.[77] Presumably this device was developed under the assumption that stomach distention will decrease food consumption. However, the data presented in Chapter 2 indicate that stomach distention is only likely to affect appetite if the distention is caused by a nutritive substance, a condition that the balloon does not satisfy. It is perhaps not surprising, then, that in an elaborate double-blind study, conducted by Reed B. Hogan and his colleagues, use of a stomach balloon was no more effective at inducing weight loss than was sham insertion of a balloon. Therefore use of the stomach balloon is no longer recommended except for research purposes.[78]

PHARMACOLOGICAL INTERVENTIONS. One commonly mentioned pharmacological agent in the decrease of overeating and obesity is amphetamine. The effects of amphetamine on appetite are described in Chapter 9. To review briefly, amphetamine does decrease food consumption, although the mechanism for this decrease has not yet been clearly established. It is clear, however, that side effects occur frequently with amphetamine, and some of them can be life threatening. Common side effects include increase in blood pressure, tachycardia, palpitations, and the danger of addiction. Further, weight loss with amphetamine is usually only temporary.[79] In summary, amphetamine does not appear to be a good solution for people who want to lose weight and is not recommended for that purpose.[80]

There are a larger number of other commercially available appetite-suppressing drugs. Although most of then are less addictive than amphetamine, they do, however, generally produce cardiovascular side effects. In addition, weight lost due to consumption of these drugs is frequently regained when the drug is stopped. Much research remains to be done on effective and safe pharmacological treatments for obesity.[81]

There have also been investigations of the usefulness of certain gut peptides, notably glucagon and CCK, as agents for appetite suppression. Glucagon and CCK are both produced during food digestion and may play a role in termination of feeding (see Chapter 2). Therefore it has been hypothesized that administration of either of these two gut peptides should suppress appetite. Experimental evidence tends to confirm this hypothesis. However, there are significant problems associated with using either glucagon or CCK to decrease overeating and obesity: There is not yet an oral, active form of either (therefore injections are necessary); the long-term efficacy of using either is unknown, particularly when preferred foods are available; and the long-term safety of using either is also unknown.[82]

There is one specific group of overeaters for whom a particular pharmacological approach may be useful. Overeaters who crave carbohydrates, including those suffering from SAD (see above), may have a deficit in the neurotransmitter serotonin. Therefore drugs that raise serotonin level should, and apparently do in many cases, alleviate carbohydrate craving and its associated depression.[83]

There is room for much more investigation and development of safe, effective pharmacological agents for decreasing overeating and obesity. Additional drugs could be developed that would reduce energy intake, reduce its absorption, reduce its storage, and increase its expenditure.[84] However, even if drugs with these effects were available, their use would have to be monitored very carefully. The potential for abuse, with the ensuing excessive weight loss, would be very high.

EXERCISE.   Exercise can be useful in decreasing obesity for at least two reasons. First, exercise uses calories. Second, as has been previously discussed, there is some evidence suggesting that under certain conditions exercise can elevate the metabolic rate for several hours following exercise; more total calories are burned than would be burned by the exercise alone. At least four other factors add to the attractiveness of exercise as a treatment method. First, when performed properly, exercise can also improve cardiovascular fitness and increase muscle tone. Second, evidence suggests that exercise helps to improve mood.[85] Third, exercise can help to prevent *osteoporosis* (loss of calcium from the bones in postmenopausal women).[86] Finally, exercise can increase the relative amounts of HDL cholesterol in men (but not in women), thus possibly decreasing their cardiovascular risk.[87] It is no wonder that many researchers and therapists have promoted exercise as a useful component of any treatment for obesity. The main drawback to using exercise as a treatment for obesity is the difficulty that patients have in adhering to an exercise program.[88]

Contrary to popular reports, however, exercise will not necessarily decrease the amount of food a person consumes. Some studies have reported decreases, but others have reported no change.[89] Judith Stern summarizes a review of the literature as follows: "The bulk of the evidence points to lower food intakes in sedentary obese individuals in comparison with those of normal weight individuals engaging in moderate or heavy physical activity."[90]

DIETS.   Just about every women's magazine at the checkout counter in the grocery store contains advice about how to lose weight safely, quickly, and/or permanently by using the latest diet. There are low-calorie diets, low-carbohydrate diets, low-fat diets, total fasts, and many others. But how well do any of these diets work? And how safe are they?

Johanna Dwyer, a professor of nutrition at Tufts University School of Medicine, performed nutritional analyses of 16 popular diets to determine their adequacy and safety.[91] She found that many of these diets were lacking in basic nutrients. Even worse, she found that three of the diets, the Scarsdale Diet, the Last Chance Refeeding Diet, and the Fasting Is a Way of Life diet, were dangerous to use, dehydration being just one of the many possible complications. One type of diet, the liquid protein diet, fortunately no longer popular, by 1978 was associated with 61 deaths. Liquid protein diets are extremely low in nutritional value and have been known to cause tachycardia and cardiac fibrillation. On the other hand, several diets were well balanced nutritionally and contained sound advice about behavioral techniques to help control food consumption (see the section below on behavior therapy). The conclusion from Dwyer's research is that diets are not to be undertaken lightly; they can result in serious medical complications. Even if a diet is unlikely to cause death, it may contain insufficient nutrients to promote good health.

Which diets work? It is important to keep in mind here that no magic is involved in losing weight. Calories from digested food do not disappear unless they are excreted, lost as heat, or used for metabolic or physical work. Weight can be lost as a result of diets, but it is necessary to use more energy than is taken in by eating fewer calories, or using more energy, or both. Further, a diet should cause weight to be lost from fat deposits, not from protein tissue.[92]

But knowing what is necessary for a diet to work and discovering a diet that results in an initial and permanent weight loss are two different things. If any diet were easily and reliably successful, that diet's fame would be widespread and lasting. Instead, we have a continual turnover of new diets. As yet there is no diet that is successful for most people over the long term.[93] Lack of initial weight loss may be due to noncompliance with the diet or to a decrease in metabolic rate as a result of the dieting. The weight loss may not last because the person may have increased appetite related to empty adipose cells, because the person may resume normal food consumption when the metabolic rate is still low, or because the person may simply resume the old food consumption and exercise behaviors that were responsible for the weight gain in the first place.

One method used by many dieters to try to decrease the number of calories consumed is the substitution of low-calorie foods and drinks for traditional ones. Frozen low-calorie entrees for busy people who are watching their calories, as well as products containing artificial sweeteners, are commonplace in American homes. Yet popularity aside, do they accomplish their purpose? Do people consume fewer total calories when they use low-calorie food and drink substitutes? In general, people who use artificial sweeteners tend to consume a lower-calorie diet than people who do not use artificial sweeteners. However, people who use artificial sweeteners also tend to be those who are heavier and who have a greater tendency to gain weight.[94] It is hard to tell what causes these correlations; experiments (in which the experimenter manipulates the only variable) are needed to identify the cause or causes. The experimental data that have been collected are not much help, however, because they are mixed; some studies show that human subjects consume fewer total calories when an experimenter introduces low-calorie foods and drinks into their meals, other studies show no difference, and still other studies show an increase in calorie consumption.[95]

The most comprehensive experiment was conducted by Richard W. Foltin and his colleagues.[96] In this experiment the subjects, all nondieters of normal weight, lived for 2 weeks in an enclosed, isolated suite of rooms. The subjects were continuously monitored and could only request food by using a computer terminal. On days 1–5 and 12–14 the subjects were given traditional foods. On days 6–11 they were given low-calorie versions of some of those foods. Except in a few rare instances, the subjects did not realize that they received some low-calorie food and drink substitutes. Nevertheless, when given the low-calorie substitutes they compensated by eating more, so that their total amount of ingested calories remained the same. However, when the traditional foods were reintroduced on days 12–14, consumption did not decrease, so that the subjects consumed more calories during this part of the experiment than when they were first exposed to the traditional foods during days 1–5. Certainly these data are not very encouraging with respect to the assistance low-calorie foods and drinks can provide with weight loss. However, it is not clear whether the results from this experiment would generalize to situations in which the subjects were obese dieters who knew they were consuming low-calorie items. The question of whether low-calorie food and drink substitutes can assist dieting does not yet appear to be resolved.

Several techniques may improve the success rate of a diet. One is to increase exercise, as discussed above. Another arises from research showing that rats given one meal per day store more of their calorie intake as fat than do rats that are given continual free access to food.[97] Consistent with these results, men who consumed a total of 2,500 calories per day in 17 snacks, as compared with men who consumed the same amount of calories in 3 meals, had lower total cholesterol as well as lower HDL cholesterol levels, possibly due to changes in their secretion of insulin.[98] Perhaps, then, if the daily number of calories allotted by a diet were comsumed in several smaller meals rather than one large meal, a diet might bring better, and healthier, results. Diets may also be assisted by various types of psychotherapeutic interventions (see below).

Reducing calories can have a number of effects in addition to weight loss. First, in men (but not in women) it can increase the relative amounts of HDL cholesterol.[99] Second, men who have had large weight fluctuations in early adulthood are twice as likely to die from coronary heart disease than are men whose weight during early adulthood stayed relatively constant.[100] Third, diets can cause nutritional deficiencies and even death (see above). Fourth, the bodies of people who have lost weight may be more likely to store any ingested food as fat, and dieters salivate more when exposed to food;[101] together, these last two findings suggest that dieting may result in abnormal cephalic phase reflexes (see Chapter 2). Fifth, as discussed above, the food deprivation of dieting can lower metabolic rate, and this lowered metabolic rate can persist even when the diet is over. Metabolic rate can decrease even further with repeated diets.[102] This means that to obtain a given rate of weight loss, as well as to maintain a weight loss, someone who has previously dieted must eat less than prior to dieting, essentially repeatedly dieting with all of dieting's ensuing effects. Finally, a history of dieting behavior, sometimes known as restrained eating, can make someone prone to bulimia (see Chapter 9) and to bouts of overeating in general.[103]

Psychotherapeutic Interventions

When an attempt to decrease overeating and obesity involves some sort of verbal rather than somatic means, it can be classified as psychotherapy.[104] Many different types of psychotherapy are used. The discussion here is divided into three parts: community and self-help groups, psychodynamic therapy, and behavior therapy.

COMMUNITY AND SELF-HELP GROUPS.   One approach that has been used in decreasing obesity is to surround the obese person with a large supportive group of people, many or all of whom are willing to help the obese person lose weight. These people need not be professionals; they may be trying to lose weight themselves. Indeed, many professionals believe that a supportive group and/or community is critical for permanent weight change to occur.[105]

An example of this type of approach is the Stanford Three Community Study, an extremely ambitious study conducted by members of Stanford University.[106] The purpose of the study was to find out if media information alone, or media information combined with individualized instruction, could change the food-consumption habits and weights of the members of a community. The project used three semirural towns in northern California, each with a population of approximately 12,000 to 15,000 people. The study focused on people aged 35 to 39, of whom there were approximately 3,000 to 4,000 in each town.

The researchers first collected baseline data on plasma cholesterol concentration, blood pressure, weight, and types of food intake from the residents of the three towns. One town was selected to serve as a control group. The other two towns were subjected to a media campaign: announcements and programs on television and radio, newspaper articles, and direct mailings that attempted to induce reductions in consumption of calories, cholesterol, saturated fats, alcohol, sugar, and salt. In one of these two towns people with a high risk of cardiovascular disease were also identified. A random sample of these high-risk people was then given intensive personal instruction on diet and on the behavior necessary to avoid cardiovascular disease, including advice on how to lose weight. Data were then collected on the same measures taken for the baselines, followed by another treatment phase, and finally by another collection of data. From the first data that were collected to the last, the project took approximately 2 years.

The results showed that the media campaign did result in improvements in saturated fat intake, plasma cholesterol, blood pressure, and overall measures of risk for cardiovascular disease. However, the only subjects who lost significant amounts of weight were those who received intensive personal instruction, and this significant weight loss had disappeared by the time of final data collection. Therefore the media campaign by itself was ineffective in reducing weight, and even personalized instruction had no lasting effect.

Another type of weight-loss approach involving a community is weight-loss competitions between people at different work sites, such as workers at different banks. Attrition in this type of competition is very small, as is the number of dollars expended to run these programs. Average weight loss in one set of such competitions, each lasting from 12 to 15 weeks, was about 12 pounds.[107] However, no follow-up assessments were reported.

More commonly used group methods of decreasing weight are self-help groups. These are groups consisting of people with a similar problem, in this case obesity. They meet to discuss common experiences, difficulties, and possible solutions. An example is Overeaters Anonymous (see the list of self-help groups on page 298). These organizations can have extremely high dropout rates. The people who stay in the group may be those who are losing weight.[108] A report published in 1970 showed that even among the participants remaining in one such group, only moderate amounts of weight loss were reported—an average of about 15 pounds in 16.5 months, out of an average need to lose 69 pounds.[109]

Richard B. Stuart and Christine Mitchell reviewed studies of weight loss in members of self-help groups.[110] Participants in most of the studies summarized in this review obtained a weight loss of approximately 1 pound per week, and there were indications that these weight losses were maintained. Results were better when behavioral self-management techniques, not just diet, were a part of the program (see below for a description of behavioral techniques). The authors point out that in addition to the weight-loss benefits, self-help groups can also provide emotional outlets and opportunities for socialization. Stuart and Mitchell conclude that "self-help group programs into which behavioral self-management techniques are incorporated may constitute the current treatment of choice for the mild to moderately overweight individual."[111]

PSYCHODYNAMIC THERAPY. Psychodynamic therapy involves long-term individual psychotherapy. Bruch's pioneering work in the use of psychodynamic therapy in the treatment of eating disorders has included the treatment of obesity. She has documented her work on many individual cases in her book on eating disorders.[112] Because psychodynamic therapists are not usually researchers as well, there is a great deal of objective evidence available regarding the efficacy of psychodynamic therapy. However, a study completed by Colleen S. W. Rand and Albert J. Stunkard[113] does provide some information about the success of psychoanalysis (included within the psychodynamic therapies) in treating obesity.

Rand and Stunkard mailed invitations to participate in their study to all 572 members of the American Academy of Psychoanalysis. Approximately half of the members indicated a desire to participate, and, of these, 104 reported that they were currently treating at least one obese patient. These 104 psychoanalysts were sent detailed questionnaires both for themselves and for their obese patients to complete. A total of 72 of the psychoanalysts returned the questionnaires, yielding data on 72 psychoanalysts and 34 obese patients. After 18 months, questionnaires were sent out again to the 72 psychoanalysts. This time 70 of the psychoanalysts returned them.

When the first questionnaires were completed, the patients had already been in treatment for an average of 31 months. Between the obese patient's entry into treatment and the completion of the first questionnaires, the patients were reported to have lost an average of 9.9 pounds. By the time of the final questionnaires, that number had risen to 20.9 pounds.

Rand and Stunkard point out that only two of the psychoanalysts reported actually encouraging their patients to lose weight. The emphasis of the therapists appears not to have been on the patients' weight but on the patients' underlying emotional conflicts that may have been responsible for the weight gain. As explained by Rand, "classical psychoanalytic theory considers obesity to be a symptom of underlying emotional disturbances arising from unsatisfactory experiences during infancy. Treatment of obesity without concurrent treatment of underlying psychopathology is felt to be futile and psychologically dangerous."[114] Rand believes that her study with Stunkard supports the idea that treatment of underlying emotional problems is sufficient for long-term weight loss.

Nevertheless, it should be pointed out that there are some difficulties with Rand and Stunkard's study. Their final sample comprised only 12 percent of the members of the American Academy of Psychoanalysis and only 67 percent of those psychoanalysts who first indicated that they would be interested in participating and had at least one obese patient. Psychoanalysts who were not part of the final sample may have been those who had obese patients who were not losing weight. Recall that the psychoanalysts who participated reported that their patients had already lost some weight by the time of the first questionnaire. In addition, there is no way of knowing whether the psychoanalysts who participated gave the questionnaires only to obese patients who were losing weight. Further, although Stunkard[115] believes that only people who have previously failed to lose weight arrive at an expensive therapist's office, the opposite may be true. People who have a weight problem and are willing to spend many months and a great deal of money to find out what is at the root of that problem may be much more highly motivated than the average overweight person. Finally, the weight measurements used were those reported on the questionnaires, and it is impossible to assess the accuracy of these measurements.

The conclusion that treatment of underlying emotional problems is sufficient for long-term weight loss is also in opposition to the conclusion to be drawn from the data on bypass surgery. The data on bypass surgery are consistent with other findings indicating that, at least in part, the emotional problems of obese people are a result, not a cause, of the obesity.[116] The data already presented on metabolic and dietary determinants of obesity also seem to dispel the conception that an underlying emotional problem is usually the prime cause of obesity. Added to this is the huge cost of long-term individual psychotherapies such as psychoanalysis. Clearly, support for the psychoanalytic treatment of obesity will have to await further research.

BEHAVIOR THERAPY.   At the other end of the research spectrum are weight-loss methods using behavior therapy (see Chapter 9 for an introduction to behavior therapy). Behavior therapists use principles of learning theory to induce behavior changes in their patients. Behavior therapists are therefore tied closely to the research literature. Many see themselves as at least part-time researchers who are committed to a scientific approach to therapy. Therefore it is not surprising that by far the greatest amount of published research on psychotherapeutic treatments for obesity concerns behavior therapy. Behavior therapy for obesity consists of a number of different techniques; some reviews of these methods are listed in a note for this chapter.[117] Here the more commonly used behavior therapy techniques will simply be summarized.

First, positive stimuli, such as the receipt of money or engaging in pleasant activities, are often made contingent on appropriate behaviors. For example, money can be paid for pounds lost, or going to the movies can be made contingent on going without dessert. Aversive stimuli, shock or illness, are also occasionally administered by a therapist. These are scheduled to follow inappropriate behaviors. For example, consumption of dessert could be followed by illness. Based on the information presented in Chapter 6, one would expect illness to be more effective than shock in decreasing food consumption. However, to date there have been no extensive comparative tests on the success of shock versus illness as an aversive stimulus for decreasing food consumption in the obese.

Stimulus-control techniques consist of controlling the stimuli that are likely to lead to overeating. For example, use of precommitment devices (discussed in the section on self-control in Chapter 7) can be taught to patients. Patients can learn to avoid situations in which they are likely to be tempted, for instance, by taking only a limited amount of money to the grocery store. People who have problems with tempting situations (as described by Schachter and Rodin, see above) may benefit especially from stimulus-control techniques.

Behavior therapists also teach their patients to relax their muscles. This response is thought to be incompatible with many instances of overeating, such as eating in anxiety-provoking situations. Patients are also taught to eat slowly, taking small bites, in an attempt to break up existing chains of inappropriate eating behaviors. Finally, an integral part of any behavior therapy weight-loss program is monitoring the relevant patient variables. Every attempt is made to obtain reliable, objective data. Teaching self-monitoring of variables such as weight, calories consumed, time spent eating, and the like is often a part of this process.

Generally either the therapist or some trusted person other than the patient is responsible for monitoring as well as delivering positive and aversive stimuli. But this is not always possible. In these cases, cognitive-behavior therapy is often used (see Chapter 9). In cognitive-behavior therapy the patient is responsible for thinking reinforcing and punishing thoughts following appropriate and inappropriate behaviors, respectively. The patient may also be taught by the therapist to change various attitudes, such as any feelings of helplessness. Gloria Rakita Leon[118] has been a proponent of these techniques. However, some behavioral scientists are uncomfortable with cognitive-behavior therapy for obesity, partly because of its lack of basis in laboratory learning theory and partly because of questions about its rate of success.[119]

Programs for decreasing obesity using behavior therapy usually incorporate a variety of techniques, sometimes including drugs, exercise, and nutrition information as well as the techniques described above. Consequently it is difficult to assess the effectiveness of any single behavioral technique. However, a great many studies have compared the efficacy of various types of behavior therapy program packages with one another, with no intervention, or with other types of weight-loss methods. A note for this chapter lists a selection of these studies.[120]

The general conclusion from these studies is that behavior therapy does result in short-term weight loss, in the range of 10 to 30 pounds over a period of several weeks or months. However, few experiments have examined the long-term efficacy of behavior therapy used for weight loss. The experiments that have been conducted seem to indicate that at best the weight is not regained. If behavior therapists really were successful at teaching their patients new eating behaviors, one might expect those patients who need to continue to lose weight to do so, but this does not occur. According to some researchers, weight loss does not continue because treatment is not continued long enough for the appropriate behaviors to be adequately learned.[121] Others have pointed out that the decreasing benefits seen with continued behavior therapy are consistent with the research on the decreasing metabolic rate that occurs with dieting.[122] In any case, more long-term assessments of the benefits of behavior therapy for weight loss are needed.[123]

CONCLUSION

No weight-loss program has proven consistent, safe, and successful for all obese people. Some people find success with some programs and some do not. Most likely, part of the reason for these differences is that there appears to be no single cause of overeating and obesity.[124] Some people may be obese because their metabolic rate is unusually low, some because they spend a lot of time around food and have a conditioned insulin response, some because they were overweight as children and now have a great many adipose cells, some because they get little exercise, and some because they live in a college dormitory where socialization always involves eating. One kind of weight-loss method will not necessarily result in the same weight loss for all of these people. Which method is used for reducing obesity should be adjusted to the individual.[125] Certain methods do seem more successful than others at decreasing weight. Bypass surgery, exercise, diets, self-help groups, and behavior therapy all work for at least some people. The case for drug therapy and psychoanalysis is not so strong.

Generally, however, the statistics on methods for decreasing obesity are depressing.[126] A survey of the literature showed that, in studies published between 1966 and 1976, the maximum percentage of body weight reported lost by dietary or behavioral methods was, on average, 8.9 percent. The decade from 1977 to 1986 showed no improvement; for those years the average maximum percentage of body weight lost was 8.5 percent.[127] It does not seem that all the research on how to decrease overeating and obesity has had any positive effects on actual weight lost by people participating in reducing programs. This is not really surprising. Our species evolved in an environment that featured repeated periods of food scarcity.[128] As a result, our bodies are designed to ingest large amounts of calories and to retain those calories.[129]

Therefore, while many researchers are calling for more experiments, it has been questioned whether all the time, money, and effort put into reducing mild to moderate (i.e., not life-threatening) obesity is worth the small number of pounds usually lost. In addition, weight-loss methods are sometimes medically unsafe, and they continue to focus our already too weight-conscious society on ever-elusive standards of thinness.[130] Finally, weight loss may result in a high probability of future weight gain.

Nevertheless, interest in weight loss seems unlikely to diminish unless the present fashion image changes so that more moderate, medically desirable weights become fashionable.

CHAPTER
11
❦
Alcohol Use and Abuse

The amount of alcohol people consume in the United States varies widely from individual to individual. According to the American Psychiatric Association, approximately 35 percent of adult Americans abstain from alcohol, about 55 percent consume fewer than three alcoholic drinks per week, with the remainder being moderate to heavy consumers of alcohol.[1] The purpose of this chapter is to try to explain why some people drink and some do not, and how excess drinking behavior can be changed.

Chapter 11

Excess Alcohol Consumption

The Problem

Why some people drink, why others do not, and how drinking behavior can be changed are questions of more than mere theoretical interest. Although there is some evidence that moderate alcohol consumption can decrease cardiovascular disease,[2] excess alcohol consumption represents one of the largest health problems in the United States. To begin with, excess alcohol consumption is associated in many ways with an increased probability of death, including:

1. An increased probability of all types of accidents, for example, automobile accidents.

2. Aggravation of other diseases already present, such as bleeding peptic ulcer.

3. A decreased probability of someone's detecting when he or she is sick or injured, for example, with a head injury.

4. An increased chance of suicide and of being a victim of homicide.

5. Death due to acute alcohol poisoning, as a result of the depressant effect of alcohol on the central nervous system, particularly in interaction with other drugs.

6. Death due to the effects of chronic alcoholism, for example, poor nutrition or cirrhosis of the liver.[3]

To illustrate how frequently some of these deaths associated with alcohol consumption occur, consider the following. Each year more people are killed in motor vehicle accidents than were killed in the Vietnam War, and approximately 50 percent of these accidents are caused by drunk drivers.[4] Approximately 3,000 drownings in the United States per year involve victims who have been drinking, these constituting approximately 60 percent of all drownings. According to a 1978 report, in North Carolina approximately 34 percent of suicide victims and approximately 70 percent of homicide victims had been drinking immediately prior to death.[5] Among people between 15 and 24 years of age, there are a total of about 10,000 alcohol-related deaths per year. Alcohol is considered the leading cause of death in that age group.[6]

The data do not prove that alcohol increases accidents, suicides, and homicides, but the high degree of association between alcohol and these events strongly suggests a causal relationship. In cases of death due to alcohol poisoning or cirrhosis of the liver, there is no doubt that alcohol plays a causative role. Add to these obvious physical health problems the toll that excess alcohol consumption also takes on mental health, both the mental health of the person who drinks and the mental health of his or her friends and family, and it is apparent that excess alcohol consumption causes a great many physical and mental problems.[7] It also causes monetary loss. For example, some colleges report that approximately 80 percent of the vandalism on campus is alcohol related.[8] In addition, approximately 15 percent of health costs in the United States result from alcoholism and alcohol-related disorders.[9] Overall, the total economic cost of alcohol-related problems in the United States has been estimated at $1,117 billion per year. This includes costs due to workdays lost, failed promotions, health care, accidents, crime, incarceration, and social welfare programs.[10]

Definitions

A person who consistently drinks too much, so that some of the problems described above occur, is described as an *alcoholic*. There is no precise criterion by which someone who drinks can be classified as either an alcoholic or a nonalcoholic. Many different definitions of alcoholism have been proposed.[11] In the 1950s E. M. Jellinek proposed his now classic descriptions of different types of alcohol consumption, shown in Figure 11.1. Jellinek saw alcoholism as a progressive, treatable disease that advances in phases, with later phases tending to follow earlier ones in a specific order. A person would be classified as an alcoholic at any phase after the prealcoholic phase, and different types of alcoholics are indicated in Figure 11.1 by the subsequent different phases. However, according to Jellinek, progression from one phase to the next does not always occur.[12]

More recently, alcoholics have been divided into those who are psychologically addicted, those who are physiologically addicted, and those who show signs of neurological disorder. Alcoholism appears to follow the above order of classification as the disease progresses, as in Jellinek's typology. However, again similar to Jellinek's typology, an alcoholic in one of the earlier phases need not progress to one of the more advanced phases.[13] In general usage, the term *alcoholism* encompasses a heterogeneous group of people.[14]

The American Psychiatric Association recognizes three main types of chronic alcohol abuse or dependence. "The first consists of regular daily intake of large amounts; the second, of regular heavy drinking limited to weekends; the third, of long periods of sobriety interspersed with binges of daily heavy drinking lasting for weeks or months."[15]

ADDICTIVE PHASES SUPERIMPOSED OVER SYMPTOMATIC DRINKING

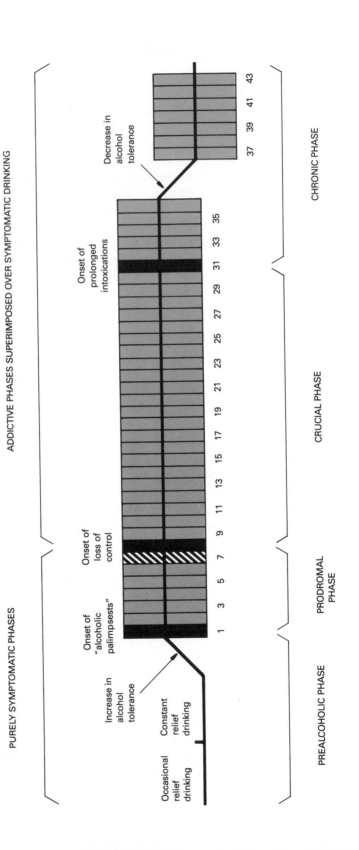

PURELY SYMPTOMATIC PHASES

Occasional relief drinking

Increase in alcohol tolerance

Constant relief drinking

Onset of "alcoholic palimpsests"

Onset of loss of control

Onset of prolonged intoxications

Decrease in alcohol tolerance

1 3 5 7 9 11 13 15 17 19 21 23 25 27 29 31 33 35 37 39 41 43

PREALCOHOLIC PHASE

PRODROMAL PHASE

CRUCIAL PHASE

CHRONIC PHASE

Prevalence

Estimates of the prevalence of alcohol use and alcoholism vary widely, partly because of the varying definitions of alcoholism and partly because of the difficulty in obtaining accurate assessments of people's drinking behavior.[16] However, the available data seem to indicate that approximately 13 percent of the American adult population have at some point in their lives satisfied the American Psychiatric Association's criteria for alcohol abuse or alcohol dependence; many more have had less serious problems with alcohol. Different groups of people demonstrate different prevalence rates of alcohol abuse. For example, males are from two to five times more likely than females to be heavy consumers of alcohol.[17]

Prevalence of alcohol also varies between different ethnic and cultural groups. One survey examined the prevalence of different levels of alcohol use among different groups in San Francisco. This survey found that approximately 10 percent of Chinese men in San Francisco would be classified as heavy drinkers and approximately 30 percent as abstainers. On the other hand, the survey found that of white men in San Francisco approximately 30 percent would be classified as heavy drinkers and approximately 15 percent as abstainers.[18] Another study in Sydney, Australia, found that 48 percent of men and 15 percent of women were heavy drinkers.[19] In both of these studies a heavy drinker was defined as someone who drinks "(a) . . . at least two or three times a month with modal quantity [the most frequently consumed amount] of five or more drinks on an occasion; [or] (b) those who drink at least three or four times a week, with any modal quantity and a range of five or more drinks; [or] (c) those who drink nearly every day or more often, with any modal quantity and a range of three or more drinks."[20] Someone who minimally satisfied this definition of a heavy drinker would not be classified as an alcoholic.

In general, Asian and Jewish populations are among those groups known to have low rates of alcoholism, and Irish Catholics, males, and people of low socioeconomic status are among those groups known to have very high rates.[21] Between 79 percent and 95 percent of college students consume alcohol.[22] However, virtually every group of substantial size contains both abstainers and heavy consumers of alcohol. Any way you add the figures, there are a great many people with drinking problems in the United States as well as in other countries.

FIGURE 11.1   *Jellinek's phases of alcoholism.* (After E. M. Jellinek, "Phases of Alcohol Addiction," *Quarterly Journal of Studies on Alcohol* 13[1952]:673–684.)

Chapter 11

THE EFFECTS OF ALCOHOL CONSUMPTION

To understand why people consume alcohol and how to decrease that consumption, it is necessary first to understand the effects of drinking alcohol. The description of these effects will be divided into two types: acute and long-term effects.

Acute Effects

In assessing the acute effects of alcohol consumption it is important to separate the actual physiological effects of the alcohol from any effects due solely to subjects' expectations following their consumption of alcohol. These two factors can be teased apart using the *balanced-placebo design* developed by G. Alan Marlatt and his colleagues (see Figure 11.2).[23] In this design, half of the subjects receive alcohol, and half receive a placebo. In each of these two groups of subjects, half are led to believe that they are consuming alcohol and half are led to believe that they are not. Elaborate precautions are taken to ensure that the subjects believe what they are supposed to believe. For example, if a subject is not supposed to consume alcohol but is supposed to think that he or she has consumed it (group C in Figure 11.2), the experimenter will go to great pains to mix the subject's "drink," with the subject observing, from clearly labeled bottles of vodka and tonic water. The liquid in all of the bottles, however, is actually tonic water. (For those groups of subjects that are supposed to consume alcohol, the bottles will contain tonic water premixed with vodka.) Subjects may be asked to rinse their mouths out with mouthwash prior to drinking to help prevent them from determin-

SUBJECT EXPECTS TO RECEIVE

		Alcohol	No alcohol
SUBJECT ACTUALLY RECEIVES	Alcohol	A	B
	No alcohol	C	D

FIGURE 11.2   *Balanced-placebo design.* (Adapted from W. H. George and G. A. Marlatt, "Alcoholism: The Evolution of a Behavioral Perspective," in *Recent Developments in Alcoholism*, vol. 1, ed. M. Galanter, New York: Plenum, 1983.)

ing whether or not alcohol is present. The group of subjects who consume no alcohol but think that they have will demonstrate any effects that might result from the belief that alcohol has been consumed uncontaminated by alcohol's physiological effects. The three other groups of subjects—those who consume no alcohol and do not think that they have (group D), those who consume alcohol and think that they have (group A), and those who consume alcohol but think that they have not (group B)—provide data useful for establishing a baseline, for simulating what usually happens in the real world, and for assessing the physiological effects of alcohol uncontaminated by expectations, respectively.

In general, experiments using balanced-placebo designs find that both expectations and alcohol itself influence behavior, although in different ways. Alcohol consumption by itself seems to interfere with information-processing tasks and with motor performance. It also appears to increase aggression. On the other hand, alcohol expectancies appear to result in increased sexual arousal to erotic stimuli.[24] People may use alcohol as an excuse for engaging in usually unacceptable behavior.[25] More detail on some of the acute effects of alcohol consumption is given in the following sections.

PHYSIOLOGICAL EFFECTS.   When alcohol (technically, *ethanol*) is consumed there are immediate bodily reactions. In the liver, the alcohol is metabolized into *acetaldehyde*, then into *acetic acid*, and finally into carbon dioxide and water. Some of the acetaldehyde in the liver is absorbed into the bloodstream. Acetaldehyde is a very reactive substance that affects most of the tissues in the body.[26]

The physiological effect of alcohol on the nervous system as a function of dose is biphasic. Like opiates, in low doses alcohol acts as a nervous system stimulant, but in high doses it acts as a depressant. Therefore many of alcohol's effects are dose dependent.[27] Some of the physiological effects of relatively large amounts of alcohol and acetaldehyde include *sleep apnea* (a disruption in breathing),[28] a decrease in the amount of *REM* (restful) *sleep,*[29] headaches,[30] and an inhibition of the synthesis of the male hormone *testosterone.*[31]

There are many additional changes in the neural system that are induced by alcohol consumption. For example, neural activation in the hippocampus, a part of the brain that is involved in memory, is inhibited by the presence of alcohol. This effect could be a physiological mechanism responsible for at least some of the acute cognitive impairments that accompany consumption of alcohol.[32]

AGGRESSION.   The physiological changes resulting from acute consumption of alcohol manifest themselves as various psychological symptoms as well. For example, the propensity for violent behavior appears to be in-

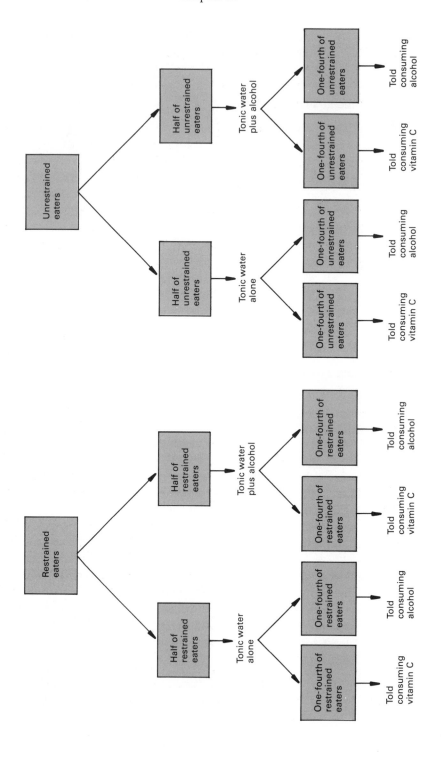

creased, contributing to the large number of deaths associated with alcohol consumption.[33] However, research has suggested that some of the increase in aggressive behavior associated with alcohol consumption may be due to consumers' expectations that alcohol will change their behavior, and not to the physiological effects of the alcohol itself.[34]

MEMORY.   One of the most investigated areas of alcohol's effects on psychological functioning is the acute effects of alcohol on memory. There is general agreement that alcohol consumption disrupts memory, although there is wide variation in the extent of this disruption, depending on the dose of alcohol and on the type of task used to test memory.[35] For example, alcohol disrupts the tendency of people to *construct* stories about some items for use in assisting memory of these items. Alcohol consumption does not, however, appear to disrupt the *use* of these stories for improving memory if these stories are provided for the person.[36] The characteristics of the subjects are also important in the degree to which alcohol disrupts memory. Middle-aged subjects retain less information when they perform memory tasks after alcohol consumption than do younger subjects.[37]

EATING.   Alcohol consumption can also affect eating behavior, depending on whether or not the subject is a restrained eater. (The concept of restrained versus unrestrained eating is discussed in Chapters 9 and 10.) Janet Polivy and C. Peter Herman conducted an experiment in which their female college student subjects were identified as either restrained or unrestrained eaters.[38] A balanced-placebo design was used. All of the subjects were given two capsules to take along with 15 ounces of liquid. For half of the subjects the liquid was tonic water. For the other half the liquid was tonic water mixed with an amount of vodka equivalent to about two drinks. Half of the women in each of these two groups were told that they were consuming vitamin C, and the other half were told that they were consuming alcohol. Subjects were then asked to make taste ratings of three different flavors of ice cream. The variable of interest was not the subjects' ratings, as the subjects thought, but the amount of ice cream that each subject ate.

Figure 11.3 shows the design of Polivy and Herman's experiment. The results demonstrated that when restrained eaters were given alcohol, they ate more than without alcohol only when they had been told that they had received alcohol, not when they had been told that they had received

FIGURE 11.3   *Design of Polivy and Herman's experiment on the effects of alcohol on eating.* (After J. Polivy and C. P. Herman, "Effects of Alcohol on Eating Behavior: Influence of Mood and Perceived Intoxication," *Journal of Abnormal Psychology* 85 [1976]:601–606.)

vitamin C. The opposite was true for unrestrained eaters. They ate more when they had been given alcohol only if they had been told that they had been given vitamin C, not if they had been told that they had been given alcohol. In other words, in restrained eaters, alcohol only affected eating behavior if the subjects knew that they had consumed it; in the unrestrained eaters, alcohol only affected eating behavior if the subjects did not know that they had consumed it. These results suggest that the amount of food consumed is dependent on both actual physiological state and expected physiological state.

MOOD.   Polivy and Herman also examined the subjects' moods during this experiment. The researchers found that subjects reported a greater elevation in mood if they were told they had received alcohol but had actually received vitamin C than if they were told they had received vitamin C but had actually received alcohol. Apparently, alcohol's reputation for elevating mood exceeds its actual physiological effect on mood.

CONCLUSION.   Consumption of alcohol only once can lead to a myriad of physiological and psychological effects. The consumption of large amounts of alcohol over long periods of time can lead to even more dramatic effects, some of them quite devastating.

Long-Term Effects

GENERAL PHYSIOLOGICAL EFFECTS.   The long-term consumption of at least several drinks per day can be extremely damaging to the body. For example, although moderate alcohol consumption (1–2 drinks per day), in comparison with abstention, can decrease cardiovascular risk, consumption of greater amounts of alcohol can result in increased cardiovascular risk and damage to the heart.[39] The more alcohol is consumed, the higher is HDL cholesterol (greater amounts of HDL cholesterol are associated with lower cardiovascular risk), but the higher also is blood pressure (higher blood pressure is associated with higher cardiovascular risk).[40]

In addition, the acetaldehyde and the excess hydrogen resulting from the metabolism of alcohol can eventually cause cirrhosis and hepatitis. Tolerance to and physical dependence on alcohol can also occur.[41] Physical dependence on alcohol can contribute to the loss of control that alcoholics feel when they cannot stop drinking after taking one drink (see Figure 11.1).[42] Further, physically dependent alcoholics can experience potentially dangerous withdrawal symptoms when their alcohol consumption decreases.[43] Finally, alcohol consumption by a pregnant woman can be extremely damaging to the fetus she is carrying (see Chapter 12).

LEARNED TOLERANCE.   Some researchers feel that tolerance to alcohol is learned, not simply a physiological reaction such as occurs with addiction and withdrawal. For example, Shepard Siegel[44] has proposed a model of drug tolerance similar to *Solomon's opponent process model.*[45] According to Siegel, when a drug causes a physiological response in the body, the body reacts by generating a compensatory, opponent-process physiological response, thus helping to maintain homeostasis. With repeated drug administrations, this compensatory response grows. It can also become conditioned to environmental stimuli present when the drug is usually administered and can therefore be generated by these stimuli alone, without the drug.

An experiment by A. D. Lê, Constantine X. Poulos, and Howard Cappell illustrates the application of this theory to alcohol consumption. Alcohol consumption results in a *hypothermic* physiological response (a decrease in body temperature). When the experimenters repeatedly injected rats with alcohol in a distinctive environment, this hypothermic response decreased; tolerance occurred. However, when alcohol was then administered in a new environment, the hypothermic response increased. Further, when the rats were given saline instead of alcohol in the environment usually associated with alcohol administration, they demonstrated *hyperthermia* (an increase in body temperature), direct evidence of a conditioned compensatory response.[46]

Other researchers have also argued that alcohol tolerance is learned, but for a different reason. According to these researchers, alcohol tolerance is always assessed by noting a subject's improvement in performance on a task while he or she is under the influence of alcohol, following repeated exposures to alcohol. But it appears that this improved performance only occurs if the subject repeatedly performs the task while under the influence of alcohol. If repeated practice performing the task and being under the influence of alcohol occur separately, there is no improvement in performance when subjects later try the task under the influence of alcohol (there is no evidence of tolerance). Therefore, contrary to the traditional interpretation, tolerance must arise from learning to perform a task while under the influence of alcohol, rather than from a diminished physiological effect of the alcohol.[47] Nevertheless, the hypothesis that learning is the major factor underlying alcohol tolerance remains controversial.[48]

EATING AND METABOLIC RATE.   Food intake and metabolism are also affected by long-term excess consumption of alcohol. Alcoholics' food intake is frequently inadequate. This inadequate food intake, added to decreased vitamin activation caused by the acetaldehyde and to irritation of the gastrointestinal tract directly caused by the presence of alcohol, can result in serious malnutrition.[49]

Despite the high number of calories contained in alcohol, consumption of large amounts does not necessarily result in weight gain. When a standard 2,200-calorie daily diet was supplemented by 2,000 calories of alcohol, subjects showed no consistent weight gain over a 4-week period. However, when the same 2,200-calorie daily diet was supplemented by 2,000 calories of chocolate, subjects gained an average of about 6.5 pounds in 2 weeks. The lack of weight gain when large amounts of alcohol are consumed may be due to excess energy released in the metabolism of alcohol.[50]

GENERAL COGNITIVE FUNCTIONS.   With repeated excess alcohol consumption, brain density decreases and other types of general brain damage occur.[51] Given these effects, damage to psychological functioning seems inevitable. Indeed, there are many psychological effects. Alcoholics tend to perform worse than nonalcoholics on many types of intellectual tasks, ranging from block design to perceptual-motor efficiency. However, there seems to be more damage with respect to performance, as opposed to verbal, IQ test subscales.[52] Responding on many of these tasks—for example, skill in forming nonverbal concepts—tends to improve if the alcoholic stops drinking.[53]

As yet there is no definitive evidence regarding how much of a history of alcohol consumption is necessary in order for these cognitive deficits to occur. It is possible that even social drinkers who never consume large amounts of alcohol may demonstrate some of these deficits. More research is needed to settle this issue conclusively.[54]

MEMORY.   One of the most investigated effects of long-term alcohol consumption, as well as of acute alcohol consumption, is impaired learning and memory functions. Even when learning and memory are assessed while the subject is sober, memory is impaired in chronic alcoholics.[55] When abstinent long-term alcoholics are provided with mnemonics, they are able to remember a list of noun pairs as well as are nonalcoholics. However, without mnemonics, abstinent chronic alcoholics, similar to people who have recently consumed alcohol, are less able to remember lists than are nonalcoholics.[56]

When someone has consumed alcohol excessively a number of times, amnesic blackouts can regularly accompany instances of alcohol consumption. Blackouts do not mean that the person becomes unconscious; rather, the person remains conscious but cannot remember what happened during the drinking bout. Jellinek saw the regular occurrence of such blackouts as the signal that the alcoholic had advanced to a more advanced phase of alcoholism (see Figure 11.1). However, research has shown that not all chronic alcoholics suffer blackouts.[57]

As described in Chapter 8, sometimes alcoholics develop an irreversible memory disorder, called Korsakoff's syndrome, in which they have trouble remembering certain kinds of recent events.[58] For example, one patient with Korsakoff's syndrome could not remember how to get to the greenhouse on the grounds of the psychiatric hospital where she was staying. She claimed that this was because she had just arrived at the hospital. Yet she had been living in the hospital for several weeks and had visited the greenhouse many times. Patients with Korsakoff's syndrome are able to recall rules for organizing information, however, and their recall of information can be facilitated by various kinds of cues.[59]

CONCLUSION.   The physical and psychological consequences of alcohol consumption are varied and often devastating. As a result, the Surgeon General has recommended that no one consume more than two drinks per day (except for pregnant women, who should abstain).[60] The next section discusses the possible causes of alcohol consumption, particularly excess consumption.

POSSIBLE CAUSES OF ALCOHOL CONSUMPTION

With a disorder as prevalent and as damaging as alcoholism, it is not surprising that many theories have been proposed to explain how alcoholism arises and, more generally, what causes people to consume alcohol. As in previous chapters, discussions of these theories are divided into two sections: genetic determinants and environmental determinants. These divisions are largely for convenience, because no behavior is or could be due entirely to genetic or to environmental factors (see Chapter 5).

Genetic Determinants

One influence of the genes on the course of alcoholism is evident in Korsakoff's syndrome: A certain genetic metabolic abnormality, along with a thiamine deficiency (common in alcoholics), can result in this memory-deficiency syndrome (see Chapter 8). But can the tendency to consume alcohol have a genetic component? This question has been examined in studies using both nonhuman and human subjects.

RESEARCH WITH NONHUMANS.   Most of the research with nonhumans conducted to investigate genetic determinants of alcoholism has involved breeding strains of rats and mice that have specific reactions to alcohol. (This kind of approach is described in Chapter 10.) The purpose of these breeding experiments has been to elucidate the mechanisms of alcohol preference and alcoholism. Researchers have hypothesized that if it proved possible to breed a nonhuman animal that behaved similarly to a human alcoholic, that animal might provide some clues about the physiological determinants of alcoholism.[61] The variety inherent in these nonhuman genetic models of alcoholism suggests that there may be a number of different ways in which the genes can affect alcohol consumption.

It has been possible to breed rats that prefer alcohol. Usually in these types of studies rats are given free access to food, to a solution of alcohol, and to water. In one study rats that showed the greatest preference for a 10-percent alcohol solution over water were bred together, as were those rats that showed the least preference. After 32 generations, on the average the rats descended from high-preference rats were consuming 1.6 times as much 10-percent alcohol solution as water, but the rats descended from low-preference rats were consuming 6.1 times as much water as 10-percent alcohol solution. In fact, the descendants of the high-preference rats were consuming an average of 17 percent of their total caloric intake in the form of alcohol, but this value was only 4 percent for the descendants of the low-preference rats.[62] Scaled to human proportions, the amounts consumed by the male descendants of the high-preference rats would be equivalent to four 8-ounce glasses of beer or 6 ounces of whiskey per day when consumed by a 165-pound man on a weight-maintenance diet of 3,000 calories per day.

One strain of high-preference rats has been bred for so many generations that their descendants sometimes obtain blood alcohol concentrations equivalent to four drinks consumed within 1 hour by a 160-pound man.[63] This consumption level would eventually result in physical dependence if it were maintained.[64] All of the high-preference strains of rats described above appear to be good candidates for a nonhuman model of alcoholism.

Marshall B. Waller and his colleagues took this kind of approach a step further.[65] They selectively bred rats to prefer alcohol, but instead of giving the rats free access to water, alcohol, and food, they delivered the alcohol solution and the water through an intragastric catheter. The rats were trained to lick from two tubes, each containing a different flavor of water. As they licked a particular tube, an equal amount of either plain water or alcohol solution, depending on the tube licked, was infused through the catheter. Despite the fact that the rats never tasted or smelled the alcohol, it was possible to breed rats that preferred to lick the tube with the taste associated with alcohol infusion. In fact the descendants of the high-preference rats regularly reached blood alcohol concentrations equivalent to that of a 160-pound man who has consumed approximately eight drinks in 1 hour.[66] Apparently alcohol consumption can be discriminated on the basis of its postabsorption effects alone. Because alcohol preference in this strain of rats cannot be due solely to a taste or smell preference, Waller and his colleagues believe that this strain should provide a good nonhuman model of alcoholism.[67]

In addition to breeding rats according to the rats' preference for alcohol, researchers have bred mice according to their *sensitivity* to alcohol. The result has been a strain of mice that sleep for a relatively long time folowing a large alcohol dose, and a strain of mice that sleep for a relatively short time following a large alcohol dose. Because these two groups of mice appear to metabolize alcohol similarly, researchers have hypothesized that the different sensitivities to alcohol are due to differences in the mice's central nervous systems.[68] Perhaps such inherited variations in central nervous system sensitivity play a role in the development and/or course of alcoholism in humans.

RESEARCH WITH HUMANS.   The research using human subjects to investigate a genetic basis for alcoholism can be divided into four types. The first type involves looking at people who do and do not have alcoholic relatives to see if there are any differences between these two groups. George E. Vaillant and Eva S. Milofsky took this approach in a large study that involved 456 Caucasian male subjects.[69] These subjects were followed for 33 years, from early adolescence until middle age. The subjects were originally part of another study, but they were subsequently followed by Vaillant and Milofsky for clues about the determinants of alcoholism.

Vaillant and Milofsky found that whether or not a subject became alcoholic was almost entirely predicted by whether or not he had alcoholic relatives and whether or not his family was of Mediterranean ethnicity. Someone was more likely to become alcoholic if his relatives were alcoholic, but less likely to become alcoholic if his family was of Mediterranean ethnicity (as compared with, for example, Northern European ethnicity). Other variables such as social class, IQ, and mental illness were nonpredictive. In fact, Vaillant and Milofsky showed that low social class and mental illness tend to follow alcoholism—they do not precede it. Therefore these common characteristics of alcoholics appear to be results, not causes, of alcoholism.

If social class, IQ, and mental illness can be eliminated as possible causes for alcoholism, what does tend to cause alcoholism to occur when there are alcoholic relatives and not to occur when Mediterranean ancestry is present? Alcoholic relatives and Mediterranean ancestry could be either salient environmental variables or genetic variables. Perhaps different rates of alcoholism among different cultures are due to different frequencies of genes for alcoholism. The aversive physiological reactions to alcohol ingestion frequently reported by some Asians (including a hot feeling in the stomach, palpitations, muscle weakness, dizziness, and flushing after only small amounts of alcohol consumption) are probably factors that at least contribute to the low consumption of alcohol among some Asians.[70]

Vaillant and Milofsky hypothesized that rates of alcoholism are low among some ethnic groups, for example, Italians and Jews (both considered Mediterranean in Vaillant and Milofsky's study), because those groups teach their young members how to use alcohol responsibly. However, perhaps those groups that can afford to incorporate alcohol use into daily family life are precisely the ones that have low frequencies of the genes for alcoholism. This hypothesis would be consistent with Vaillant and Milofsky's observation that some of the Irish subjects who had alcoholic relatives abstained from alcohol for life. Vaillant and Milofsky's study does not resolve these issues.

Marc A. Schuckit and Vidamantas Rayses also attempted to examine the determinants of alcoholism by comparing human subjects with and without alcoholic relatives.[71] First Schuckit and Rayses asked a sample of young men to tell them how much they and their relatives drank. The researchers chose 20 of these young men, who were not themselves alcoholic but who had an alcoholic parent or sibling, as the alcoholic-relative group. An additional 20 subjects without an alcoholic parent or sibling, matched to the first group on age, sex, race, marital status, and drinking history, were selected as the non-alcoholic-relative group. Each of the 40 subjects drank the equivalent of approximately two drinks over a 5-minute period. Schuckit and Rayses measured the blood acetaldehyde levels of the subjects. As Figure 11.4 shows, the subjects with alcoholic relatives had much higher levels of acetaldehyde than did the subjects with nonalcoholic relatives, comparable to results obtained by Marc A. Korsten and his colleagues with alcoholics and nonalcoholics.[72] Similarly, Henri Begleiter and his colleagues have found that during information-processing tasks sons of alcoholic fathers and nonalcoholic mothers show deficiencies in a particular brain wave (the P3 evoked potential), similar to deficiencies seen in abstinent adult alcoholics. These deficiencies are not shown by matched control subjects who are sons of nonalcoholic fathers and mothers.[73] There are additional differences in the brain activity of the offspring of alcoholic as compared with nonalcoholic parents.[74]

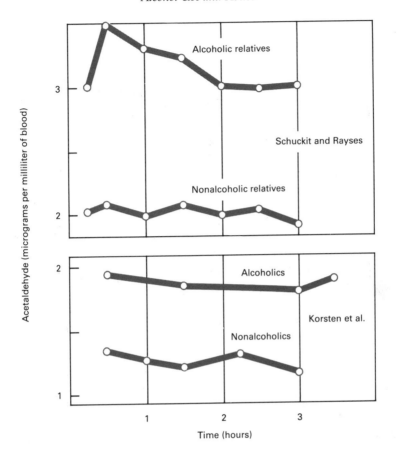

FIGURE 11.4   *Top curve: Acetaldehyde levels following alcohol ingestion by nonalcoholic male subjects with and without alcoholic relatives.* (After M. A. Schuckit and V. Rayses, "Ethanol Ingestion: Differences in Blood Acetaldehyde Concentrations in Relatives of Alcoholics and Controls," *Science* 203[1979]:54–55.)   *Bottom curve: Acetaldehyde levels following alcohol ingestion by nonalcoholics and alcoholics.* (After M. A. Korsten, S. Matsuzaki, L. Feinman, and C. S. Lieber, "High Blood Acetaldehyde Levels after Ethanol Administration: Difference Between Alcoholic and Nonalcoholic Subjects," *New England Journal of Medicine* 292[8][1975]:386–389.) Note that the method of alcohol administration in the study by Schuckit and Rayses and the study by Korsten and his colleagues differed so that only the relative, and not the absolute, values obtained in the two studies can be compared.

It appears that some of the physiological differences that are typically found between alcoholics and nonalcoholics are not due to long-term exposure to alcohol but may be due instead to some genetically determined physiological reactions. Further research is needed to determine whether these findings reflect causes or simply correlates of causes of alcoholism.

The second type of study using human subjects in the investigation of genetic determinants of alcoholism has been twin and adoption studies. (The logical basis for twin and adoption studies is described in Chapter 4.) Twin studies have shown that identical twins are more frequently concordant for the presence or absence of alcoholism than are same-sex fraternal twins. Adoption studies have shown that adopted children have a greater tendency to be alcoholic if their biological parents are alcoholic. Note, however, that the majority of alcoholic twins do not have an alcoholic co-twin, and that the majority of the biological children of alcoholics, whether or not they are adopted, are not themselves alcoholic. If someone has an alcoholic twin or an alcoholic biological parent, the chances are still better than 50 percent that that person will not become alcoholic.[75]

The third type of study investigating genetic determinants of alcohol consumption in human subjects has attempted to identify a particular gene that is present in alcoholics but not in nonalcoholics. The assumption is that, were such a gene to be found, that gene would be at least partly responsible for the development of alcoholism. In fact, a gene has recently been identified that was present in 77 percent of an alcoholic sample but in only 28 percent of a nonalcoholic sample. Therefore some researchers believe that this gene is likely to be involved in the origins of at least some cases of alcoholism. Other researchers stress caution until the results are replicated with a large group of subjects.[76]

Finally, researchers have approached the question of whether or not there is a genetic component to alcoholism by first determining whether certain personality types are associated with alcoholism, and then investigating whether those personality types have a genetic component. There are two basic personality types that have been associated with alcoholism. Alcoholics of the first type are sensitive, apprehensive, inhibited, pessimistic, and the like. They become alcoholics later in life and frequently experience loss of control once they start drinking. *Type I alcoholics* feel guilty about their alcoholism. They drink in order to relieve anxiety. Alcoholics of the second type are sensation seekers (see Chapter 5). They become alcoholics early in life, are unable to abstain, and frequently engage in aggressive behavior when drinking. Women alcoholics are mostly Type I, but both Type I and *Type II alcoholics* are found among men. Adoption studies appear to indicate that these two groups of personality traits, along with their associated drinking patterns, do indeed have a genetic component.[77]

The studies described here indicate that there is a genetic component in at least some types of alcoholism. However, the influence of the environment is not at all negligible.

Environmental Determinants

Many behavior therapists, such as G. Alan Marlatt, Peter E. Nathan, and G. Terence Wilson, have taken an entirely different approach to investigating the causes of alcoholism (see Chapter 9 for a definition of behavior therapy).[78] They have assumed that at least some of the behaviors associated with problem drinking and with alcoholism are learned behaviors rather than genetically determined involuntary behaviors. This contrasts with the concept of alcoholism as a progressive disease that was espoused by Jellinek (Figure 11.1). The behavior therapists' aim is not to define alcoholism but to describe drinking behavior, including the antecedents and consequences of that behavior. Accordingly it should then be possible to disrupt the antecedents and/or the consequences and thereby change the behavior. (Additional explanation of behavior therapy treatments for alcoholism are given in the section on treatment below.) Behavior therapists therefore focus on controlling the drinker's environment rather than on investigating the drinker by himself or herself.

Learned acquisition and maintenance of behavior within an environment, including the part of the environment that consists of other people, are the basics of social learning theory. Most behavior therapists now approach alcoholism from a social learning theory perspective.[79] Peter M. Miller and Richard M. Eisler have described how social learning theory applies to the investigation of substance abuse such as alcoholism:

> Within a social-learning framework, alcohol and drug abuse are viewed as socially acquired, learned behavior patterns maintained by numerous antecedent cues and consequent reinforcers that may be of a psychological, sociological, or physiological nature. Such factors as reduction in anxiety, increased social recognition and peer approval, enhanced ability to exhibit more varied, spontaneous social behavior, or the avoidance of physiological withdrawal symptoms may maintain substance abuse.[80]

Observations of what behavior actually occurs are critical to the behavior therapists' scientific approach to understanding alcoholism. For this reason, alcoholics' self-reports regarding how much they drink are often necessary; the alcoholic himself or herself is often the only person present or available for reporting on the alcoholic's drinking.[81] Research seems to indicate that whereas these reports are not always entirely accurate, they usually give a fair estimate of how much the alcoholic has been drinking.[82]

The original approach of behavior therapists, to focus only on observable behaviors, has recently been modified. This modified approach, which is called cognitive-behavior therapy (see Chapter 9), focuses on the cognitive processes that modify the relationship between the environment and the person's behavior. These processes include, for example, expectancies.[83] Expectancies were discussed with regard to Polivy and Herman's experiment above. Their experiment showed that the mood of their subjects following consumption of either an alcoholic or a nonalcoholic beverage was greatly influenced by whether or not the subjects had been led to believe that they had consumed alcohol.

Alcoholism and problem drinking may not consist entirely of learned behaviors, but experiments conducted within the behavior therapists' theoretical framework have uncovered several principles of learning that govern drinking behavior. The interpretation of tolerance as a learned behavior, described previously, is one example of the usefulness of this approach. The experiments and analyses coming out of the learning tradition have broadened our understanding of the factors that may be responsible for tolerance.[84] The next sections describe further examples of how a learning–environmental approach has increased our understanding of the determinants of problem drinking and alcoholism.

RESEARCH WITH NONHUMANS.   A nonhuman animal model of alcoholism has arisen out of experiments using the schedule-induced polydipsia phenomenon (SIP, described in Chapter 3).[85] Recall that when animals learn to respond to food delivered at regular intervals with water freely available, the animals often begin to drink huge amounts of water following the food deliveries. John L. Falk has been able to substitute alcohol solutions for the water.[86] This results in rats that consume enough alcohol to become physically dependent and have continuously high blood alcohol levels.

Drinking is not the only behavior whose probability increases following regularly scheduled presentations of food. If wheel turning or biting is possible, the probability that the rats will turn the wheel or bite also increases.[87] All of these types of behaviors are called adjunctive behaviors (see also Chapter 10). Falk has hypothesized that the food presentations create a high-drive situation for the animal and that when the food is removed, this heightened arousal is alleviated through behaviors that satisfy other drives—behaviors such as drinking, running, and biting. Falk has argued further that adjunctive behaviors following food delivery can be adaptive, because they result in the organism's giving up now-ineffective eating-related behaviors. Perhaps alcoholism is also partly based on adjunctive responses; alcoholic drinking may be partly a result of high drives that cannot be satisfied in other ways.[88]

Another type of situation in which high levels of motivation may increase consumption of alcohol in rats is crowded social conditions. Research with rat colonies has shown that when a (noncrowded) colony is raised in a highly enriched environment, a small number of animals will become extreme overconsumers of alcohol, similar to what happens in human societies. These voluntary overconsumers of alcohol in rat colonies represent virtually the only nonhuman models of social alcoholism.[89]

Additional experiments with rats show how the consequences of alcohol consumption can modify future drinking behavior. Specifically, rats learn to prefer flavors associated with low concentrations of alcohol, apparently due to the reinforcing calories provided by the alcohol.[90] In other words, alcohol can function as a food. Like sugar, alcohol is an excellent source of energy.[91] High concentrations deliver even more calories, but the high concentrations also generate aversive physical reactions. The consumption of these high concentrations is therefore not reinforcing for most rats. The findings with low concentrations of alcohol are similar to those from the experiments described in Chapter 6, in which food consumption accompanied by caloric intake resulted in an increase in preference for the food. The experiments reported in Chapter 6 were conducted with both human and nonhuman subjects, which lends support to the possibility that the results here are relevant for at least some cases of preference for alcohol in humans.

RESEARCH WITH HUMANS.   A great variety of learning research with humans has been conducted to determine the causes of alcoholism. One of the classic learning theories of alcoholism has been the *tension-reduction theory*. According to this theory people drink because they are tense and alcohol relieves tension. Although this theory seems plausible, alcohol reduces tension only in some people in certain circumstances; the tension-reduction theory is not widely applicable as an explanation of alcoholism.[92]

A social learning approach has also been used in research on excess drinking in humans. This type of research is concerned with the effects that the presence of others and other aspects of the environment have on drinking behavior. For example, John B. Reid related an incident that he observed while traveling on a plane.[93] He took a trip that combined three short flights 28, 18, and 35 minutes in length. During the first two legs of the journey, the flight attendants did not bring out the drink cart because they said that there was not enough time to take it around between takeoffs and landings; however, the passengers were told that they were free to order drinks directly from the flight attendants. Nevertheless, during the first leg only 4 out of 103 passengers ordered a drink, and during the second leg only 1 out of 86. In contrast, during the third leg, when the flight attendants did bring out the cart, 42 out of 97 passengers ordered a drink. Although it is not apparent which aspect or aspects of the situation affected drinking behavior in this case (drink availability, opportunity to interact with flight attendants, modeling of other passengers' behavior, etc.), it is clear that the environment

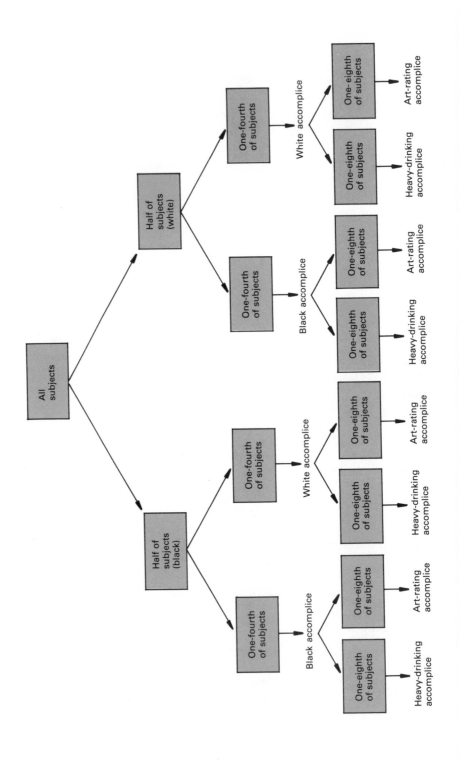

had a great deal to do with the amount of drinking that went on in this plane.

A more controlled study was performed by Donnie W. Watson and Mark B. Sobell.[94] These researchers first obtained a sample of 32 black and 32 white male nonalcoholics. The subjects were told that the experiment involved a comparison of racial differences in ratings of art objects and beers. Each subject participated in the experiment along with an experimental accomplice, whom the subject thought was another subject. For the "co-action" condition, half of the subjects rated the beers, as did a heavy-drinking accomplice. For the "control" observer condition, the other half of the subjects rated the beers while the accomplice rated the art objects. In half of the cases a subject was paired with an accomplice of the same race and in the other half, with an accomplice of the other race. Figure 11.5 gives the design of the experiment. The results showed that, independent of race, subjects drank more when they made their ratings accompanied by a heavy-drinking accomplice.

Many studies have found similar effects of modeling on alcohol consumption. Modeling might therefore be a helpful technique for treating excess alcohol consumption.[95] In agreement with the findings in modeling experiments, adolescent excessive drinking can be predicted to a large extent based on whether or not the adolescent's friends drink and whether or not the adolescent is involved in many social activities with peers. Adolescents whose friends drink and who are involved in many peer social activities are much more likely to drink excessively.[96]

The effect of alcohol availability on drinking can be explored from the perspective of economics, that is, using cost-benefit analyses (see Chapter 7). Clearly, if alcohol is not available there will be no alcoholics. But investigations of precisely how the price of alcohol, the number of places where it can be obtained, the laws governing drinking, and so on affect consumption have yielded somewhat inconsistent findings. Nonetheless it does appear that less hard liquor is consumed as its price increases[97] and that reduced physical availability of alcohol does decrease alcohol consumption. As a specific example, alcohol consumption decreased during Prohibition,[98] presumably as a result of the decreased availability of alcohol, the illegality of drinking it, or both.

Researchers have also investigated the effects of availability on alcohol consumption under controlled conditions in the laboratory. These experi-

FIGURE 11.5   *Design of Watson and Sobell's experiment on the effects of modeling on alcohol consumption.* (After D. W. Watson and M. B. Sobell, "Social Influence on Alcohol Consumption by Black and White Males," Addictive Behaviors 7[1982]:87–91.)

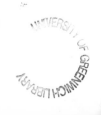

ments tend to confirm the principles of choice behavior described by the matching law in Chapter 7. Specifically, consumption of alcohol decreases as constraints on its consumption increase, and consumption of alcohol increases as the availability of alternative reinforcers decreases.[99] Perhaps some people who overconsume alcohol under natural conditions do so at least in part because they can easily obtain alcohol but not other types of reinforcers.

CONCLUSION.   There appear to be many different determinants of excessive alcohol consumption. Undoubtedly some causes have influenced some alcoholics more than others. Therefore some treatments might be more successful with some alcoholics than with others. In any case, the extensive and diverse literature on the etiology of alcoholism has helped generate an equally large and diverse literature on possible treatments for alcoholism.

TREATMENT OF ALCOHOLISM

There is no drug that cures alcoholism. The acute detrimental effects of alcohol are removed by removing the alcohol, sometimes while administering medication to alleviate the potentially life-threatening consequences of withdrawal. Many residential treatment programs for alcoholics include a period of "detoxification" for this purpose.[100] But actual treatment for alcoholism consists almost entirely of various forms of psychotherapy: group therapy or individual therapy. Therapy can be given in any of the treatment settings in which alcoholics are placed, on an inpatient or outpatient basis or in a halfway house. Alcoholics may participate in several different treatment programs at once. The following sections will first discuss several issues essential in treatment evaluation and selection, and then describe some of the particular treatments that have been employed for alcoholism.

Issues in Treatment Evaluation and Selection

LONG-TERM EFFECTS.   The first major concern that must be addressed in the evaluation of any treatment of alcoholism is whether the treatment results in a long-term removal of alcoholism. Relapses are frequent in alcoholism. Therefore for a treatment to be successful it must have continued success over long follow-up periods.[101]

The importance of posttreatment factors in the probability of a relapse was demonstrated in a study conducted by John W. Finney, Rudolf H. Moos, and C. Ronald Mewborn.[102] They found that if the patient's family was cohesive, participated together in recreational activities, and had a low level of conflict, the patient was more likely to have long-term success. Finney and his colleagues therefore concluded that family therapy should be helpful in obtaining long-term alleviation of alcoholism.

The concept of alcoholism as a disease, as espoused by Jellinek (see Figure 11.1), sees relapses as a result of the physiological craving for alcohol.[103] Behavior therapists, on the other hand, see relapses as a function of various environmental factors. Behavior therapists hypothesize that alcoholics relapse because they have previously learned that alcohol consumption is followed by various positive consequences. Further, these therapists feel that each time a relapse occurs the alcoholic learns that he or she is not cured. This self-perception then promotes further drinking. Therefore some behavior therapists have advocated planned relapses for their patients. In these cases the alcoholic is encouraged to briefly resume drinking (a *programmed relapse*), and then the therapist helps the alcoholic to stop again, teaching the patient how to cope with relapses in the future without the therapist.[104]

INPATIENT VERSUS OUTPATIENT TREATMENT.   A large number of studies have been conducted to determine whether inpatient treatment for alcoholism is superior to outpatient treatment. In particular, attention has been focused on the benefits of treatment by for-profit, inpatient, private institutions, many of which are quite expensive.[105] Research indicates that treatment is no more successful when it is inpatient, as opposed to outpatient, or when it is very, as opposed to less, intensive (except perhaps for seriously deteriorated alcoholics). The critical variable in treatment success appears to be the type of treatment used, not the setting within which it is offered. Therefore there would seem to be little justification for expending the large number of dollars required for treatment by an expensive, inpatient, private institution, especially when third-party reimbursement is involved.[106]

ABSTINENCE VERSUS CONTROLLED DRINKING.   The third major concern in evaluation of different treatments pertains to the goal of the treatment. Proponents of Jellinek's disease concept of alcoholism believe that in order for alcoholics to be cured and to stay cured they must avoid all alcohol forever.[107] This has been the approach adopted by the members of Alcoholics Anonymous (AA),[108] and there is evidence that for at least some alcoholics abstinence is essential for full recovery.[109] On the other hand, behavior therapists view alcohol consumption as at least in part a learned behavior, and they feel that if excessive drinking can be learned, so too can moderate drinking. Therefore the behavior therapists' position has been that at least some alcoholics can learn to drink socially.[110]

Mark and Linda Sobell brought the behavior therapists' view into sharp focus in their book *Behavioral Treatment of Alcohol Problems,* published in 1978.[111] In this book the Sobells described their use of *individualized behavior therapy* for the treatment of alcoholism. This type of therapy uses a variety of behavioral techniques to reduce alcohol consumption. The goal of the therapy—social drinking or abstinence—and the techniques used are chosen for each patient individually. The Sobells state that a goal of controlled drinking is easier for some patients to obtain than is a goal of abstinence.

There has been independent research support for the Sobells' position that some alcoholics can drink socially without reverting to alcoholism. Several reviews of the literature have reported successful social drinking by former alcoholics.[112] A RAND study published in 1980 followed the posttreatment progress of 780 males who had been treated for alcoholism, finding that 18 percent of the men were drinking without problems 4 years after treatment. Younger subjects and subjects who showed few symptoms of alcohol dependence at the time they were admitted to treatment were those most likely to maintain long-term drinking without problems.[113]

In 1982 Mary L. Pendery, Irving M. Maltzman, and L. Jolyon West published what appeared to be a devastating report on the outcome of the Sobells' approach.[114] Pendery and her colleagues followed up the progress of the patients whose controlled-drinking treatment formed the basis of the Sobells' book. At the time of this study, 10 years had elapsed since the subjects had been treated by the Sobells, and 7 years had elapsed since the last follow-up. Pendery and her coworkers found that of the 20 male subjects, only 1, a subject who had not shown symptoms of physical dependence on alcohol, was drinking without problems. Of the other 19 subjects, 8 were drinking excessively despite repeated aversive consequences, 6 were abstinent, 4 were dead for reasons related to alcohol consumption, and 1 could not be located (an earlier follow-up had shown that this subject was having severe problems resulting from excess alcohol consumption). Because of the physical dangers associated with excessive alcohol consumption, Pendery and her colleagues implied that by advocating controlled drinking that does not work for most patients, the Sobells had been promoting potentially life-threatening situations.

Finally, in reports to the media, Pendery and Maltzman accused the Sobells of having falsified their data so that it appeared that the controlled-drinking approach was more successful than it actually had been.[115] Needless to say, Pendery and her colleagues' article and the media reports touched off a flurry of commentaries and letters.[116] The issue of abstinence versus controlled drinking even made the pages of *The New York Times.*[117]

The Addiction Research Foundation appointed an outside committee to investigate the charges of fraud in the Sobells' work. While committee members did not reinterview the Sobells' subjects, they did go over the Sobells' original data. This committee found no evidence of fraud in the Sobells' research.[118] An investigating group organized by the Alcohol, Drug Abuse and Mental Health Administration also found no evidence of fraud, although their investigation was hampered by a lack of full cooperation from parties on both sides of the controversy. This group felt that at times the Sobells could have been more careful in preparing their results for publication.[119]

It should be emphasized that Pendery and her colleagues' study took place 10 years after the patients had been treated by the Sobells and 7 years after the Sobells' last follow-up—a long time to expect continued effect of treatment with no therapist-patient contact. The Sobells did have a control group consisting of patients who had been treated with the goal of abstinence. However, Pendery and her colleagues did not report follow-up data on the members of this group. It is possible that drinking would have caused even more of the control subjects to have suffered serious physiological consequences than occurred with the Sobells' patients trained as social drinkers. In fact, the Sobells presented data precisely of this nature in their 1984 response to Pendery and her colleagues' article (mortality rates 10 to 11 years after treatment were 20 percent for controlled-drinking subjects and 30 percent for control subjects).[120]

It should also be emphasized that the Sobells have never advocated controlled drinking as an alternative for everyone. No one disputes the fact that some alcoholics can learn to drink socially and some cannot. The challenge is to identify as precisely as possible those alcoholics who are likely to show success with controlled drinking. Perhaps more alcoholics could and would learn to be controlled social drinkers if more people in our society believed that this is a reasonable goal for at least some people.[121]

Psychotherapeutic Techniques

BLOOD ALCOHOL DISCRIMINATION TRAINING. A crucial aspect of controlled drinking training is that the drinker be aware of the amount of alcohol that he or she has consumed. Some researchers believe that careful monitoring of intake can help an alcoholic keep his or her level of intoxication low or moderate. One of the best ways to monitor intake is through monitoring *blood alcohol level (BAL)*, because BAL is a good indication of how much alcohol is actually entering the drinker's system. Research has shown that alcoholics seem to have difficulty discriminating their BALs using internal cues. However, they can learn to discriminate their BALs using external cues such as the score on a Breathalyzer machine. Discrimination training using such external cues may be helpful as part of those treatment programs that advocate controlled drinking.[122] To date there are no data on the long-term efficacy of BAL discrimination training by itself in decreasing drinking. Note the similarity between the BAL discrimination technique and the self-monitoring technique frequently used in behavior therapy for people who are obese (see Chapter 10).

MODIFYING THE FORM OF THE DRINKING RESPONSE.   Another technique that is used only by those who advocate controlled drinking is behavior therapy designed to modify the actual form (topography) of the alcoholic's drinking response. There appears to be a tendency for alcoholics to take large gulps rather than small sips of their alcohol. Alcoholics therefore tend to consume their alcohol faster than do nonalcoholics. The aim of topographic modification is to teach alcoholics to consume their alcohol much more slowly, in much the same way that therapists teach obese people to eat more slowly (see Chapter 10). Then, therapists reason, the probability that the alcoholic will consume excessive amounts of alcohol will be decreased. Alcoholics have made these changes in their drinking topography in experiments that have used experimenter instructions about the desired topography and in experiments using shocks following undesirable topography.[123] Again, the long-term success of this training in decreasing alcohol consumption is not yet known.

SKILL TRAINING.   Behavior therapists have reasoned that alcoholics' consumption of alcohol would be decreased if the alcoholics had alternatives to drinking in stressful situations. In other words, teaching patients how to cope with stressful situations might be helpful in decreasing alcohol consumption. This approach is known as *skill training,* and it emerges from the social learning orientation toward alcoholism.

For example, Stanton L. Jones, Ruth Kanfer, and Richard I. Lanyon used skill training with a group of alcoholics; they then compared the subsequent drinking of that group with the drinking behavior of a group of alcoholics who simply discussed the emotional aspects of their problems and a group who received no treatment. All three groups of subjects were simultaneously participating in a standard inpatient program.[124] The skill training

> focused on developing both general and specific strategies for dealing with the four general classes of potential relapse-precipitating events (anger and frustration, negative mood states, interpersonal pressure, and intrapersonal temptation). . . . Subjects discussed the nature of the problem situations, problem-solved for general strategies and specific tactics to use when dealing with that type of problem situation, the therapists modeled potentially effective responses, and the subjects rehearsed their chosen responses under the coaching of the therapists.[125]

Both the skills training and the discussion groups showed significantly less drinking than the no-treatment group at a follow-up conducted 11 to 14 months after the patients had been discharged.[126] Apparently some common aspect of skills training and discussion can be helpful in decreasing drinking.

SELF-CONTROL TRAINING. According to the definition presented in Chapter 7, self-control can be defined as the choice of a larger, more-delayed reinforcer over a smaller, less-delayed reinforcer. Impulsiveness is the reverse.[127] Alcoholics can be said to be impulsive in that they choose the smaller reinforcer of drinking now over the long-term larger reinforcers of avoiding the psychologically and physically hazardous consequences of drinking.[128]

Based on this analysis, impulsive drinking in alcoholics might be decreased by the following methods: making the larger reinforcer seem larger, making the smaller reinforcer seem smaller, making the time to the larger reinforcer seem shorter, or making the time to both reinforcers seem larger (thus resulting in a preference reversal and allowing precommitment; see Chapter 7). For example, in self-control training, patients can be taught to give themselves reinforcers immediately upon not drinking in certain situations.[129] This is a cognitive-behavior therapy approach.

There is as yet no long-term data on the relative success of this type of therapy. However, research has shown that alcoholics pressing a series of buttons for money are less affected by both immediate and delayed shock punishment of their button pressing than are nonalcoholics. It is therefore possible that alcoholics' operant behavior is less susceptible to contingencies than is nonalcoholics' behavior,[130] which would make self-control training less effective in alcoholics.

AVERSION THERAPY. Still another technique used by behavior therapists is *aversion therapy*. It actually comprises three different techniques. All have in common the administering of aversive consequences following drinking with the aim of decreasing future drinking. In one type of aversive conditioning, drinking is followed by illness (so as to establish taste aversions to alcoholic beverages; see Chapter 6); in another, by thoughts of illness (a procedure known as *covert sensitization*); and in a third, by shock.[131] There has been substantial basic and applied research relevant to the use and probability of success of these different types of aversion therapies in the treatment of alcoholism.

A number of experiments have been performed in which actual illness has followed drinking behavior. Illness has been induced by a number of different means, including putting the subjects in a rotating chair,[132] exposing them to a nauseating visual illusion,[133] or injecting them with drugs.[134]

251

Alternatively, taste aversions have been studied by observing those that occur when illness naturally follows food consumption. A. W. Logue, K. R. Logue, and Kerry E. Strauss conducted the latter type of study.[135] They interviewed 102 hospitalized alcoholics concerning their acquisition of taste aversions to all types of foods and drinks under natural conditions. As in other samples studied by Logue and her colleagues[136] (see Chapter 6), aversions were most likely to form when the illness followed (rather than preceded or accompanied) consumption of the food, and when an aversion did form, it was most likely to be an aversion to the taste of the food.

In general, research confirms that taste aversion therapy can be used successfully with many alcoholics.[137] About 15 percent of Logue and her colleagues' alcoholic subjects reported taste aversions to alcoholic beverages, even though in many of these cases the subjects had had strong preferences for the beverages and had drunk them frequently prior to forming the aversions. Experiments with rats also indicate that aversions to very familiar liquids can be conditioned if there are many taste–illness pairings and the illness is strong.[138] A report by Arthur N. Wiens and Carol E. Menustik summarized the results of 685 patients treated at one hospital using a taste aversion paradigm. Wiens and Menustik found that approximately 60 percent of the patients were continuously abstinent for 1 year following treatment and approximately 30 percent for 3 years following treatment.[139]

However, there have been reports that when taste aversion therapy consists of pairing a limited number of types of alcohol with illness, alcoholics will sometimes simply avoid the previously illness-paired drinks and consume other alcoholic drinks instead.[140] Consistent with these findings, Logue and her colleagues' study found that, unlike nonalcoholics, alcoholics reported very few instances in which taste aversions to any substance (alcohol or anything else) generalized to similar foods or drinks. They obtained comparable results with a sample of college students who were heavy drinkers. Alcoholics appear to show less generalization of their taste aversions than do nonalcoholics.[141]

Covert sensitization is similar to taste aversion learning, with the exception that the illness is induced by instructing the subjects to imagine that they are ill. This technique has several advantages over traditional taste aversion learning. No chemicals or devices are needed to induce illness. Illness can be induced anywhere and with no possible side effects. Vomiting is also more controllable and less likely to occur, which is certainly easier on the therapist. Ralph L. Elkins has reported significant success using covert sensitization.[142] He has even been able to show that, while imagining themselves ill, his patients undergo actual physiological changes indicative of autonomic distress, evidenced by such autonomic responses as altered galvanic skin response and respiration rate.[143]

Aversion therapy using illness, overt or covert, appears to have a high probability of decreasing alcohol consumption. However, such therapy will be assisted if therapists structure the conditioning sessions in line with principles discovered in basic learning experiments. For example, the patient should first taste the alcohol and then become ill; taste, not just smell or appearance, should be paired with illness; many pairings of a particular beverage with illness may be necessary for an aversion to form; and many beverages, rather than solely the patient's favorite beverage, should be paired with illness. Finally, therapists using overt illness should take into account findings with rats indicating that illness-induced aversions to alcoholic beverages are stronger when those beverages have a high congener content (that is, a high content of substances other than ethanol) and that aversions tend to be formed to the flavor, not the ethanol content, of the beverages.[144]

Based on the findings presented in Chapter 6, it would be expected that the shock pairings could be successful in conditioning the patients to simply not touch specific drinks. However, the illness pairings would be more likely to result in an actual decreased preference for alcohol per se by the patients. This hypothesis has been confirmed in several studies comparing the efficacy of pairing shock and illness with alcohol.[145]

DRUG THERAPY.   The drug *Antabuse* (*disulfiram*) is sometimes a component of treatments for alcoholism. This drug blocks the normal metabolism of alcohol. If someone has recently take Antabuse and then consumes alcohol, the acetaldehyde concentration is 5 to 10 times greater than if Antabuse had not been taken,[146] resulting in a profound physical reaction including "nausea, vomiting, tachycardia, marked drop in blood pressure, and other symptoms of massive autonomic arousal."[147] This reaction lasts as long as there is alcohol in the blood and can occur even if Antabuse has been ingested as much as 14 days earlier.[148] Thus alcoholics treated with disulfiram are exposed to a taste aversion paradigm each time that they drink alcohol. The success rate of patients treated with disulfiram has not been consistently high.[149] However, that may be because of a lack of compliance in taking the drug. George Bigelow and his colleagues required their subjects to first deposit a sum of money at a clinic. Each time a subject failed to return to the clinic to receive disulfiram, a portion of his or her deposit was sent to charity. The remainder was returned to the subject at the end of the study. Using this procedure, Bigelow and his colleagues found significant and consistent decreases in the drinking behavior of their subjects.[150] Note that this procedure was essentially a precommitment technique.

Another type of drug that could be used in treating alcoholism would be a drug that blocked the physical sensations accompanying intoxication.

Without these sensations, some alcoholics might no longer find drinking pleasurable and might therefore become abstinent. Such a drug has been identified, although so far it has been tested only in rats. This drug apparently inhibits the effects of alcohol on the brain, although BALs remain unaffected.[151] However, high doses of alcohol will still result in intoxication.[152] Therefore use of this drug might induce alcoholics to consume even more alcohol in order to attain an intoxicated state. Further, although this drug might be useful in preventing drunk driving, it would not remove or even meliorate any of the potentially lethal damage done to body tissues by a high BAL. Therefore if use of this drug in any way encouraged drinking (such as by someone at a party who ordinarily would have abstained in order to drive home safely), it could cause great harm. For all of these reasons this drug may never be developed for commercial use.[153]

ALCOHOLICS ANONYMOUS. *Alcoholics Anonymous (AA)* is a self-help group that was begun in 1935 when two alcoholics decided to meet together with other alcoholics to promote abstinence from alcohol. According to the beliefs of AA members, alcoholics have no control over their alcohol consumption and must therefore strive to abstain totally. Members go to meetings regularly and are always available to assist another member who is about to slip and drink alcohol. Membership in AA is anonymous and has become increasingly popular. In 1989 the total number of active members in AA was approximately 896,033 in the United States alone.[154]

Despite its popularity, statistics demonstrating the successfulness of AA over other treatments have been lacking. Finney, Moos, and Mewborn were unable to show any increased probability of long-term success for alcoholics if treatment was followed by AA membership, compared with treatment not followed by AA membership.[155] Similarly, Fredrick Baekeland, Lawrence Lundwall, and Benjamin Kissin, in a review of the literature, were unable to find any advantages to AA over treatment in a conventional clinic. They also point out that there may be great differences in the type of alcoholic who seeks treatment at AA, compared with those who seek treatment at a clinic. Such differences may hinder accurate treatment comparisons.[156] Even so, like the self-help groups for obesity described in the previous chapter, AA may serve a social function independent of decreasing alcohol consumption. Research is needed to obtain a more precise estimate of the benefits and efficacy of AA.[157]

HALFWAY HOUSES. A *halfway house* can be defined as "a transitional place of indefinite residence of a community of persons who live together under the rule and discipline of abstinence from alcohol and other drugs."[158] Typically, halfway houses are useful when an alcoholic does not need as much structure or supervision as would be obtained in a hospital but needs more than would be obtained by living at home. Most halfway houses follow the AA philosophy that alcoholics must completely avoid alcohol. Some halfway houses are privately operated, some are publicly operated, and some are operated by religious groups. Counselors in halfway houses interact with the residents in the house, and there may be house rules governing the residents' behavior.[159]

Many halfway houses lack the resources necessary to provide individualized therapy for alcoholics. More funding would improve this situation. Halfway houses could provide many opportunities for research concerning treatments of alcoholism.[160]

CONCLUSION

Progress has been made toward understanding both the genetic and the environmental determinants of alcohol use and abuse. There does appear to be a genetic component in at least some cases of alcoholism, and this may help explain why long-term success rates of treatment are generally low. This may also help explain why prevention of alcohol-related problems is still marginal.[161] Nevertheless, despite the existence of a probable genetic component in alcoholism, there are successful behavioral treatments, although they are not employed as often as they could be.[162] Excessive alcohol consumption is very expensive for our society not only monetarily but also medically and emotionally. Efforts to understand alcoholism and to develop successful treatments must continue.

Part V

APPLICATIONS TO EVERYDAY ISSUES AND PROBLEMS

This last part of the book consists of three chapters: applications of the psychology of eating and drinking to female reproduction, to smoking, and to cuisine and wine tasting. Most of us must face at least some of the problems and issues discussed in these chapters at one time or another in our lives. However, the study of these topics is valuable for another reason: The subject matter of each of the three chapters is best understood by drawing on themes and results discussed in several of the preceding chapters. In other words, the last three chapters in this book provide an excellent example of the benefits of taking an interdisciplinary approach to the psychology of eating and drinking.

CHAPTER
12

❧

Eating, Drinking, and Female Reproduction

In mammalian reproduction, the female produces an egg that is fertilized and nurtured within her body until the fetus is capable of surviving in the outside world. However, even after birth, for periods ranging from weeks to years, young mammals continue to depend mainly on their mothers for food in the form of milk produced by their mothers' bodies. The present chapter concerns the ways in which the psychology of eating and drinking impacts on mammalian reproduction, in particular with respect to the female's role as the ultimate provider of food to the young during pregnancy and immediately after birth. The material presented here will focus on the species of mammal of greatest concern to most of us: humans.

The early nutritive relationship between a mother and her offspring is critical to the survival of the offspring. For an infant to survive, the infant's mother must obtain adequate food for herself until the infant is old enough to be weaned. Thus survival of the woman results in survival of her offspring as well. Conception should not occur unless there is a high probability that there will be sufficient food to sustain the woman and her offspring throughout pregnancy and lactation. Therefore women's bodies should have evolved such that their reproductive functions and their eating and drinking behavior are closely related. For example, one would predict that women should store more fat on their bodies than do men, thus enabling women not only to survive but to reproduce during the frequent periods of food scarcity that occurred throughout our evolutionary history. The data are consistent with this prediction; the average percentage of total body weight that consists of fat is 27 percent for young women but is 15 percent for young men.[1] Further evidence supporting this evolutionary approach to understanding women's eating and drinking behavior and their reproductive functions will occur repeatedly throughout the present chapter.

THE MENSTRUAL CYCLE

The menstrual cycle plays an essential role in human reproduction. There are a number of physical changes that occur during the menstrual cycle, and they have a variety of outcomes, including the release of an egg and preparation of the uterine lining for the implantation and subsequent growth of the embryo and fetus (see Figure 12.1). However, in addition to ovulation, the menstrual cycle also frequently involves changes in the woman's consumption of food. There can be influence in the other direction as well: What a woman consumes can affect the menstrual cycle.

Influence of the Menstrual Cycle on What Is Consumed

Many women experience cravings for particular foods, notably high-carbohydrate, high-calorie, and/or chocolate foods, in the part of the menstrual cycle just prior to menstruation.[2] If these cravings are regularly accompanied by a number of other symptoms, such as marked irritability, lack of energy, and sleep disturbances, the woman is said to suffer from *premenstrual syndrome* (PMS) or *late luteal phase dysphoric disorder* (see Figure 12.1 for a description of the *luteal phase*).[3] There has been much discussion about what causes these food cravings.

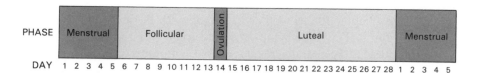

PHASE: Menstrual | Follicular | Ovulation | Luteal | Menstrual

DAY: 1 2 3 4 5 6 7 8 9 10 11 12 13 14 15 16 17 18 19 20 21 22 23 24 25 26 27 28 1 2 3 4 5

FIGURE 12.1 *A normal menstrual cycle.* The first day of menstruation is counted as day 1 of a cycle. During the follicular phase, in this example days 6–13, a follicle containing an egg develops in the ovary. At the time of ovulation, here occurring on day 14, the follicle ruptures, thus releasing the mature egg and allowing conception to occur. During the subsequent luteal phase (days 15–28 in this figure), the follicle, which has remained in the ovary, becomes the corpus luteum and secretes several hormones that prepare the uterine lining for implantation of the fertilized egg (should conception occur). If conception does not occur, as in the present example, menstruation and a new cycle begin. (Adapted from M. P. Warren, "Reproductive Endocrinology," in *Handbook of Behavioral Medicine for Women,* eds. E. A. Blechman and K. D. Brownell, New York: Pergamon, 1988.)

One explanation of the food cravings is based on the fact that basal metabolic rate is significantly higher during the luteal phase of the menstrual cycle. Consistent with this greater expenditure of calories, women consume more calories during the luteal phase,[4] similar to organisms' consuming more calories under any conditions in which their energy expenditure has increased (see Chapters 2 and 10). Data discussed in Chapter 6 suggest that people learn to prefer high-calorie foods when they are food deprived, but they do not prefer these foods when they are satiated. Thus the higher energy expenditure during the luteal phase could cause a woman to consume more calories and to show an increased preference for high-calorie foods (such as chocolate).

Nevertheless, there is evidence that the increased number of calories consumed by women during the luteal phase is sometimes greater than the increased energy expenditure that they experience at that time. When comparisons have been made between the follicular and the luteal phases (see Figure 12.1 for a description of the *follicular phase*), energy expenditure has been found to be from 8 percent to 20 percent higher during the luteal phase, but total number of calories consumed has been found to be from 20 percent to 30 percent higher during the luteal phase.[5] Therefore removal of an energy deficit cannot be the sole explanation of the food cravings present during this time. Another possible explanation is that, by consuming food in excess of energy usage during the luteal phase, some food is likely to be stored in the woman's body. Then, if conception should occur, the woman's and her offspring's chances of survival will be increased.

Still another explanation is related to the carbohydrate craving seen in people with seasonal affective disorder (SAD) and in obese carbohydrate cravers (see Chapter 10), as well as in people with PMS. Similar to people suffering from SAD, whose symptoms tend to be worst in the winter, and similar to obese carbohydrate cravers, whose symptoms tend to be worst at certain times of the day, PMS sufferers experience cyclical symptoms. Further, carbohydrate craving can be suppressed by drugs that increase the level of the neurotransmitter serotonin in the brain. Therefore Wurtman and Wurtman have hypothesized that PMS as well as SAD and obesity due to carbohydrate craving are caused or aggravated by insufficient levels of serotonin in the brain. When people with these three disorders ingest carbohydrates, their serotonin levels increase, as do their feelings of well-being.[6] Additional research is needed to determine to what degree serotonin deficiency, increased energy expenditure, a need for increased energy storage, and/or some as yet undiscovered factor are responsible for the food cravings seen during the luteal phase of the menstrual cycle.

The menstrual cycle may affect food consumption indirectly by means of the changes that it induces in olfactory sensitivity. Around the time of ovulation, mucus secretions in a woman's body, including those around the cervix and those around the olfactory epithelium (see Chapter 4 for general discussion of olfaction), become thinner. This increases the probability of conception, but it also increases olfactory sensitivity.[7] It is not known whether this heightened sensitivity makes women's food preferences and aversions more exaggerated. Perhaps the increased olfactory sensitivity induces women to consume more of their preferred foods around the time of ovulation, once again increasing the probability of survival of the woman and any infant she might conceive.

Influence of What Is Consumed on the Menstrual Cycle

A woman needs approximately 50,000 to 80,000 calories in order to produce a full-term baby.[8] Given this large energy requirement, it is not surprising that inadequate food will disrupt the menstrual cycle and inhibit ovulation. This fact was noted in Chapter 9, where it was pointed out that anorexics do not menstruate.

For many years the critical variable in food-deprivation-induced amenorrhea was thought to be the woman's percentage of body fat. A certain amount of body fat is necessary in order for the hormones to function properly. If a woman's body has less than that amount of fat, menstruation will not occur. Therefore when women lose weight, at some point their menstrual cycles cease.[9] More recently, Jill E. Schneider and George N. Wade have stated that general availability of fuel (of which fatty acids that can be mobilized from adipose tissue are only one component), and not percentage of body fat, is the critical variable. Experiments with hamsters have shown that even when a female hamster has a high percentage of body fat, if a chemical is used to prevent the hamster's utilization of fatty acids, even brief food deprivation will inhibit reproductive functioning.[10] Exercise may also be involved in menstrual regularity, given that women who are exercising a great deal sometimes have lower hormonal levels, or even amenorrhea, as well as fewer premenstrual symptoms.[11] However, it is not known whether exercise is exerting an effect that is independent of the effects of inadequate food consumption and low percentage of body fat, or if exercise is exerting its effect by inducing an energy deficit and/or by decreasing the percentage of body fat.[12]

It is possible that all three factors—amount of food consumed, amount of stored fat, and exercise level—play a role in menstrual regularity. Yet, even if we assume that all three are involved, we do not known what level of any of these three factors is needed before fertility is impaired. Obviously, if a woman eats so little or exercises so much or becomes so thin that she has no menstrual cycles, reproduction cannot occur. However, perhaps somewhat decreased food consumption or stored fat or somewhat increased exercise can impair, without completely eliminating, fertility. There is some experimental evidence supporting this possibility. For example, one experiment gave six hamsters 50 percent of their usual food intake for 4 days (the length of one estrous cycle). Despite the fact that the food deprivation was only partial and that it lasted for only 4 days, one of the hamsters did not ovulate at all and the number of eggs released by each of the other hamsters decreased from a mean of 11 to a mean of 9.[13]

Perhaps not only anorexics, but also chronic dieters and women who regularly eat little breakfast and lunch in order to consume a large dinner, may be at risk for impaired fertility. Recall from Chapter 10 that dieting can lower metabolic rate, even after the diet is over, so that it is necessary for a woman who has dieted to continue to consume little food if the weight loss is to be maintained. Some 60 percent of American women try at least one weight-reduction diet each year, and approximately one-third of American women between the ages of 19 and 39 (the prime reproductive years) diet at least once per month.[14] Keep in mind that the repeated, purposive food deprivation of many American women may not only inhibit fertility and the woman's available energy supply but also make it very difficult for the woman to obtain sufficient amounts of essential nutrients such as iron. As discussed in Chapters 9 and 10, the fact that our current female fashion image is so thin can result in many health problems for women.

PREGNANCY

Additional physical changes take place in a woman's body once conception has occurred. Once again, many of these changes are directed at survival of the fetus: The fetus must get adequate nutrition—either from what the woman eats, or from what is stored in her body, or both. However, although many foods and drinks that a woman consumes during pregnancy have positive effects on the embryo and fetus, others can do severe damage.

Food Preferences and Aversions

Some women develop food cravings during pregnancy. When these cravings are for high-calorie foods it is possible to invoke the energy deficit explanation used to explain high-calorie food cravings during the luteal phase of the menstrual cycle. As in the luteal phase of the menstrual cycle, metabolic rate is high during pregnancy.[15] The fetus imposes additional caloric requirements on the pregnant woman. Therefore one would expect the pregnant woman to show an increased preference for high-calorie food.

However, some food cravings during pregnancy are not for high-calorie foods. In some cases pregnant women crave such items as clay and earth. This phenomenon, known as pica, is thought to be the result of specific hungers for minerals such as iron (see Chapter 6), which women need more of during pregnancy than at any other time in their lives.[16]

It is possible that other types of changes in food preferences may occur in pregnant women as well. The self-selected diet of pregnant rats contains a much higher percentage of protein than does the self-selected diet of non-pregnant rats.[17] In addition, hormonal changes during pregnancy apparently affect rats' neural processing of taste stimuli,[18] which could, in turn, affect food preferences. Perhaps future research will reveal similar effects in pregnant women.

During pregnancy there are changes in the digestive tract. For example, increased amounts of the gut peptide cholecystokinin (CCK; see Chapter 2) are released, particularly during the first trimester. The increased CCK contributes to the sleepiness felt by women at this time and, because it inhibits gastric emptying, also contributes to the nausea and vomiting experienced by over 25 percent of women during the first trimester.[19] This may explain why some women find high-fat foods aversive at this time: High-fat foods pass more slowly through the digestive tract than do low-fat ones.[20] It is also possible that the nausea and vomiting become accidentally paired with specific foods, so that taste aversions occur. Recall from Chapter 6 that taste aversions are strong, can last for years, and can form even though the person knows that his or her illness was not caused by the food to which the person develops an aversion. Unfortunately, there has been no detailed study of taste aversion learning in pregnant women.

Weight Gain

A major concern of many pregnant women is weight gain. There is fear that too much weight will be gained and that not all of that weight will be lost once the baby has been born. On average, women gain 33 pounds during pregnancy, of which about 9 pounds consist of stored fat.[21] A weight gain of 24 to 28 pounds is advised if someone is of normal weight at the start of pregnancy—somewhat more if the woman is initially underweight and somewhat less if the woman is initially overweight.[22] Research has found that women frequently name pregnancy as a factor responsible for an increase in weight during their lifetimes. Among one sample of 197 women who had given birth, 168 reported a net weight gain during their childbearing years.[23] However, given that most women (and men) gain weight as they age,[24] one wonders how many of these women would still have shown a net weight gain even if they had never been pregnant.

Nevertheless, despite the higher metabolic rate present during pregnancy, women's fat stores increase even during the first trimester. This increase cannot be attributed to greater food consumption during that time period; instead, it is probably another effect of the increased CCK release during the first trimester.[25] Clearly, for evolving human females, a tendency to store consumed food as fat, particularly at a time when food consumption is sometimes inhibited by nausea, would have increased the probability of survival of the mother and her infant.

Even though in developed countries there may be less need for women to store fat during pregnancy in order to successfully reproduce, women are advised not to curtail their food intake during pregnancy and to gain a minimum of 15 to 20 pounds even if overweight at the start of pregnancy.[26] Not only could an illness in which food consumption was decreased make fat stores useful to the woman and her fetus, but it is known that when pregnant women consume limited amounts of food there can be fetal damage.[27] A historical study of 300,000 men who had been conceived but not yet born, or who had just been born, at the time of the Dutch famine of 1944–1945 provides just one example of such damage. The study showed that extreme

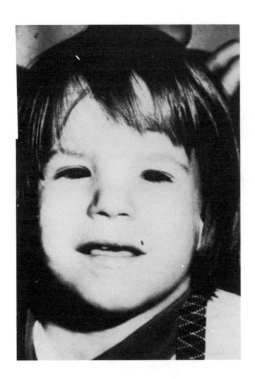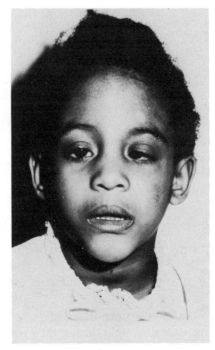

FIGURE 12.2 *Physical appearance of three children with FAS syndrome.* (Reprinted with permission from A. P. Streissguth, S. Landesman-Dwyer, J. C. Martin, and D. W. Smith, "Teratogenic Effects of Alcohol in Humans and Laboratory Animals," *Science* 209[1980]:353–361. Copyright 1980 by the American Association for the Advancement of Science.)

food deprivation during the first part of pregnancy tended to result in high obesity rates (possibly due to interference with hypothalamic development; see Chapter 2); on the other hand, extreme food deprivation during the last part of pregnancy and the first few months of life tended to result in low obesity rates (possibly due to interference with adipose cell development).[28] Dieting is also not advisable during pregnancy because if a woman's preexisting fat stores are metabolized, toxins contained in that fat, such as pesticides, can be released into her bloodstream and thus passed to the fetus.[29]

Fetal Alcohol Syndrome

One of the more striking and tragic long-term effects of excess alcohol consumption occurs when pregnant women drink excessively. A number

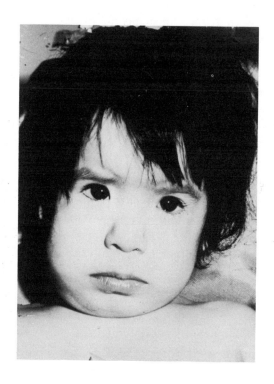

of specific physiological and behavioral changes occur in the fetuses of such women, and together these changes are known as *fetal alcohol syndrome (FAS)*.[30] First, the facial appearance of a child born with FAS is different from that of a normal child. The head circumference and nose are smaller, the nasal bridge is lower, and the upper lip is thinner than that of a non-FAS infant. The FAS infant also has folds of skin at the inside corners of the eyes that are absent in normal infants. These external physical characteristics remain as the FAS child ages (Figure 12.2). FAS infants are smaller than non-FAS infants, and this growth deficiency persists after birth. The brains of FAS infants are smaller and less ridged than the brains of non-FAS infants. As FAS infants age, it becomes apparent that they are permanently mentally retarded. FAS infants also tend to be hyperactive and irritable and to show poor coordination. Approximately 1 out of every 750 infants born in the United States shows clear evidence of this disorder.[31]

The description of FAS is noncontroversial. However, the cause of FAS and the level of alcohol consumption that is safe for a pregnant woman are controversial. Women who tend to drink a lot of alcohol during pregnancy may also tend to do other things that are not beneficial for the fetus, such as not eating properly, smoking cigarettes, and taking drugs. One of these other behaviors correlated with drinking could actually be responsible for the low birth weights and FAS seen in children of women who drink during pregnancy. Further, reports of drinking behavior may be inaccurate. For both of these reasons it may be difficult to isolate precisely what is responsible for FAS—alcohol ingestion or some other factor.[32] However, the weight of the evidence now suggests strongly that alcohol is directly responsible.[33]

Experiments with animals have supported the direct involvement of alcohol consumption in FAS. For example, an experiment with monkeys has shown that alcohol ingested during pregnancy can cut off circulation to the fetus, a possible mechanism for FAS.[34] Another experiment, this one with mice, has shown that alcohol ingested during pregnancy can result in pups with facial deformities resembling those seen in FAS.[35] The results of the experiment with mice seem particularly ominous for humans because the facial malformations occurred when alcohol was given at the equivalent of the third week of a human pregnancy, a time before most women are even aware that they are pregnant.

However, both of these experiments used doses of alcohol that would rarely be ingested by humans under natural conditions. In the experiment with monkeys the dose was equivalent to injecting a 120-pound woman, directly into the vein, with about 18 ounces of 80-proof whiskey over a 1- to 2-minute period.[36] In the experiment with mice the dose was equivalent to a 120-pound woman's consuming six drinks each in two sessions, with 4 hours between the two drinking bouts.[37] Nevertheless, the arteries and veins in isolated human umbilical cords have been shown to contract and spasm when exposed to a concentration of alcohol equivalent to that in the blood of a pregnant woman 30 minutes after having ingested one to one-and-a-half drinks of 100-proof whiskey.[38]

Because of this sort of evidence the Surgeon General and the National Institute on Alcohol Abuse and Alcoholism have recommended that women consume no alcohol during pregnancy.[39] Some small or moderate level of alcohol consumption is unlikely to have any effects on the fetus, but because that level is unknown many people have thought it wise to recommend total abstinence during pregnancy. Others worry that attempts at abstinence might result in dangerous binges or in undue anxiety.[40] However, it should be pointed out that whereas the harmful effects of substantial alcohol consumption during pregnancy are easy to see in the fetus, consumption of smaller amounts may result in more subtle but still harmful effects that might be difficult to discern in research studies. In addition, it has recently been shown that women metabolize alcohol differently from men, so that much smaller amounts of alcohol are necessary for a woman to attain a blood alcohol level concentration comparable to that of a man of the same size.[41] Clearly women who might become pregnant or who are pregnant must be extremely cautious in their consumption of alcohol.

Other Substances Potentially Harmful to the Fetus

There are many other substances in addition to alcohol whose consumption during pregnancy can be harmful to the growing fetus. For example, studies using both female nonhuman animals and female humans have shown that caffeine consumption can result in various reproductive disorders, such as miscarriages and stillbirths. There is also some evidence that caffeine consumption may sometimes be linked to birth defects in animals.[42] Thus pregnant women should probably avoid consumption of caffeine. As still another example, Chapter 8 discussed how mental retardation can result if a fetus is exposed to the toxic chemical methylmercury through consumption by a pregnant woman of contaminated fish. Pregnant women must eat and drink with caution, and this is one of the reasons that medical attention and nutritional counseling early in pregnancy are so important.

LACTATION

Women who choose to breast-feed are well aware of the importance of this task for the survival of their infants: "The overriding concern of all mothers, once they have established that their newborn baby is alive and well, is the establishment of a successful feeding relationship."[43] There are actually many aspects of the breast-feeding relationship that are important for the future health of the infant as well as the mother.

Effects of Breast Feeding on the Infant

Breast milk is specifically designed to meet the needs of growing infants. Although it can be contaminated with potential toxins, such as the caffeine mentioned above as well as other drugs,[44] breast milk, unlike formula, is never mixed at the wrong concentration with unsanitary water. Further, it is possible that substances present in breast milk as a result of particular foods and drinks consumed by breast-feeding women influence infants' food preferences. Recall that this is one of the mechanisms by which rat pups learn to eat the safe, nutritious food that adult rats have learned to prefer. Advantages could accrue to children were such a mechanism inherent in the breast-feeding relationship (or disadvantages, depending on what were the resulting food preferences). However, there have been no detailed studies of this possibility.

Although it is difficult to conduct controlled experiments on the relationship between breast-feeding and infant obesity, infants who are breast-fed appear to be less likely to become obese. This may be because, with a bottle, caregivers are more likely to try to persuade the infant to consume a certain number of ounces even though the infant is not that hungry.[45] However, although infant obesity may be influenced by whether or not an infant is breast-fed, it is important to remember that the tendency for infants to become obese is also influenced by differences in energy expenditure that are present early in the first year of life and by whether or not the infants' biological parents are obese (see Chapter 10).[46]

Even when infants are breast-fed, there are times when nutrition is inadequate due to insufficient breast milk or to the infant's not feeding for an appropriate length of time. Just as was described above for pregnancy and in Chapter 8, severe undernutrition during early childhood can result in developmental damage, including low IQ scores.

Suckling provides benefits to the infant in addition to simply the ingestion of milk. Suckling triggers the release of gut peptides that improve digestion and the utilization of ingested fuel, as well as inducing sleepiness. This is one of the reasons that use of a pacifier is advisable, unless parents intend for a child to breast- or bottle-feed continuously—unlikely in the American culture.[47]

Many factors are involved in the timing of weaning.[48] For example, weaning occurs around the time when lactose intolerance is developing (see Chapter 5) and when the infant can begin to consume many types of solid foods. Lactose intolerance and the ability to consume solid foods both help to ensure that the infant will cease drinking mother's milk, so that the woman is then available for the nurturing of a subsequent child (but not until the first child can ingest food independently).

Effects of Breast Feeding on the Mother

Lactating women need even more calories and other nutrients per day than do pregnant women. Specifically, lactating women need approximately 765 to 980 calories more than before they became pregnant.[49] Therefore lactating women should, and do, consume more calories than nonpregnant women.[50] Lactating rats, like pregnant rats, have been shown to select a higher proportion of protein in their diets than nonlactating, nonpregnant rats.[51] As with pregnant women, such effects have not been investigated in lactating women.

Many women see the lactation period as a time to lose the weight accumulated during pregnancy. Lactating women are indeed better able to lose weight from their hips and abdomen, where weight is deposited during pregnancy, but from where it is traditionally difficult to lose weight. However, suckling an infant seems to decrease the heat generated by the muscles and to increase energy storage in certain parts of the lactating woman's body. It also makes the woman sleepy. This sleepiness, and the consequently decreased activity level, may be adaptive for the survival of the infant in that it tends to keep the mother nearby.[52] All of these suckling effects decrease the woman's energy usage, thus meliorating the caloric drain of the production of milk. This could help explain the fact that most women who have given birth do not lose sufficient weight to return to their prepregnant weight.

CONCLUSION

Many aspects of female reproduction ensure that the result is a healthy child and a mother who is healthy enough to produce another child. The present chapter demonstrates clearly, perhaps more than any other chapter, how the psychology of eating and drinking is tied intimately to survival and to inclusive fitness (Chapter 1). We cannot survive, and we cannot reproduce, unless we eat and drink properly. Therefore natural selection has resulted in a variety of mechanisms to ensure that appropriate eating and drinking behavior will meet the unusual nutritional requirements of conception, pregnancy, and lactation. Natural selection has not provided for every modern-day adverse contingency, such as the harm that can be caused to a fetus if the woman carrying it consumes caffeine—we did not evolve in an environment in which such toxins were common. Further, some of the adaptations that are present, such as the tendency of pregnant and lactating women to store fat, although useful in the environment in which we evolved, are not as necessary, and can even cause weight problems, in our society in which lack of food is not a problem for most people. As research continues, the resulting data will make it easier for parents and their physicians to ensure the health of the mothers and their offspring.

CHAPTER
13

☙

Smoking: Weight Loss and Weight Gain

Approximately 54 million people in the United States smoke cigarettes. This huge number is tragic because smoking is responsible for more disease and death in the United States than is any other preventable behavior. Over 350,000 deaths per year are attributed to smoking. Smoking increases the risks of contracting coronary heart disease, respiratory disease, and cancer. In addition, millions of dollars are spent on cigarettes that could be spent on something else, extra days are lost from work, and health care costs are increased. When people stop smoking (and many cannot do so even when they actively participate in specially designed programs), they may suffer withdrawal symptoms from their addiction to nicotine.[1]

With all of these adverse consequences, why do people start smoking, and if they do smoke, why do they not all quit? There are many factors, most of which are beyond the scope of the present text. However one factor that is within the purview of this book is weight gain. In one study, some people (approximately 10 percent of males and 5 percent of females) had started smoking because they had thought that by doing this they would lose weight. In addition, some smokers (47 percent of the males and 59 percent of the females in this study) continued to smoke because they feared gaining weight if they stopped, and subjects (most often women) who had stopped and then had gained weight had sometimes resumed smoking in order to counteract the weight gain.[2] In other words, weight loss and gain appear to play a significant role in smoking behavior. This means that, although behavioral and other techniques can be helpful in making ex-smokers out of smokers, and in preventing people from ever starting to smoke in the first place,[3] these techniques could be assisted by a thorough understanding, and ultimately, control of the relationship between smoking and weight.[4]

The present chapter will examine to what extent smoking does indeed affect weight, and what factors might be responsible for any such effects.

EFFECTS OF SMOKING ON BODY WEIGHT

People who begin smoking cigarettes, on the average, lose weight. In addition, on the average, smokers weigh less than nonsmokers.[5] These findings do not only apply to humans; rats given nicotine also lose weight.[6] There is therefore substantial evidence that smoking of tobacco or nicotine exposure alone decreases weight (as opposed to smoking of marijuana, which increases food consumption and can cause weight gain).[7] The question then becomes: What causes this weight decrease?

Decrease in Total Calories Consumed

One possible explanation is that smoking decreases the total number of calories consumed. In humans this could be due to changes in appetite, changes in hand activity, changes in oral activity, and so on.[8] Given that rats are usually exposed to nicotine by means of a needle, not a cigarette, it is not possible to explain any decreases in rats' food consumption as a function of exposure to nicotine as being due to changes in hand activity or oral activity. Keep in mind, however, that, in rats or in humans, more than one mechanism could be responsible for any decrease in food consumption seen as a function of smoking or nicotine exposure.

Some evidence with rats indicates that the weight loss is indeed due to a decrease in the total amount of food consumed. Rats chronically exposed to smoke and rats given injections of nicotine decrease the amount of food that they consume (as well as having a suppressed growth rate). In addition, exposure to smoke or nicotine raises these rats' blood glucose levels, thus, perhaps, making them less hungry and less likely to eat (see Chapter 2). However, when hamsters are chronically exposed to smoke, although their weights decrease, the amount of food that they consume does not change.[9]

If smoking decreases the total number of calories consumed, then one would expect that the more someone smokes, the less inclined that person should feel to eat. However, a study by Joan B. Beckwith, using 766 20- to 30-year-old women, demonstrated that the extent to which these women felt compelled to eat was not significantly correlated with their level of smoking.[10]

Decrease in Sweet Foods Consumed

Another possible explanation of the decrease in weight that accompanies smoking is that smoking and exposure to nicotine decrease consumption of sweet foods.[11] According to this explanation, the total number of calories consumed does not change when a person starts smoking, but the proportion of calories that come from sweet foods decreases. Recall from Chapter 10 that consumption of palatable foods can lead to obesity, and the taste of sweet can lead to increased storage of consumed food as fat.

Neal E. Grunberg and David E. Morse[12] examined the number of cigarettes consumed per person in the United States as a function of the amount consumed per person of each of 41 different foods over the years from 1964 to 1977. They found significant negative correlations between the number of cigarettes smoked and the amount of sugar consumed. In other words, in years in which a large number of cigarettes were consumed per person, less sugar was consumed per person and vice versa (see Figure 13.1).

Grunberg and Morse's data are correlational and therefore do not prove that smoking decreases sugar consumption; some third variable could be causing the variations in both number of cigarettes smoked and amount of sugar consumed. However, laboratory data demonstrating that smoking and nicotine exposure in both humans and rats decrease consumption of sweet foods, while not changing consumption of other foods, tend to confirm the hypothesis that weight decrease in smokers is due to a decreased consumption of sweet foods.[13]

One possible explanation for the decrease in consumption of sweet foods by smokers is a decreased preference for the taste of sweet. Another possible explanation comes from work on preference for different brands of ciga-

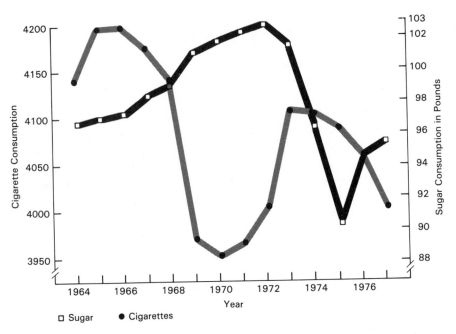

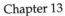

FIGURE 13.1   *Number of cigarettes consumed per person and number of pounds of sugar consumed per person during the years 1964 to 1977. (After N. E. Grunberg and D. E. Morse, "Cigarette Smoking and Food Consumption in the United States," Journal of Applied Social Psychology 14[1984]:310–317.)*

rettes. A smoker's rated pleasantness of a particular brand or rated satisfaction provided by a particular brand is highly correlated with the smoker's perceived sweetness of the brand.[14] Perhaps smokers consume fewer sweet foods than nonsmokers because their desire for the taste of sweet is satisfied by the cigarettes themselves.

Increase in Energy Expenditure

Finally, perhaps smoking results in decreased weight because it increases energy expenditure.[15] If this were so, and smokers ate the same amount as nonsmokers, then smokers would weigh less than the nonsmokers.

Some evidence supports this possibility.[16] For example, one experiment examining energy usage found that smokers' metabolic rates were 10 percent higher during a 24-hour period when they smoked than during a 24-hour period when they abstained from smoking.[17] This greater metabolic rate was not due to an increase in basal (i.e., resting) metabolic rate, but was apparently due to nicotine's affecting the body in such a way that total energy usage was increased. For example, perhaps smokers' metabolic rates increase more than those of nonsmokers when they consume the same amounts of food (recall that food consumption can increase metabolic rate; see Chapter 10). This raises a possible problem with the experiment. Food consumption under the two conditions of smoking and nonsmoking was not controlled or even measured. Perhaps smokers consume more food than nonsmokers and it is for this reason that smokers have a higher metabolic rate. However, there is absolutely no evidence that more food is consumed by smokers than by ex-smokers (in fact, evidence discussed above and below indicates that if there is any difference in amount consumed by smokers and ex-smokers, the smokers consume less food). A more serious problem with this research is that, because chronic smokers were used, we do not know if the metabolic rate observed in the smokers when they were smoking, which was greater than when they were not smoking, was also greater than before they ever started smoking. It is possible that starting smoking does not change metabolic rate, but that stopping smoking decreases it.

Another laboratory finding consistent with the hypothesis that smoking increases energy expenditure, and that as a result weight decreases, comes from research with rats. Rats chronically exposed to smoke have increased brown adipose tissue as well as decreased growth rate.[18] Recall from Chapter 10 that thermogenesis is thought to be a function of the brown adipose tissue. Perhaps an increase in brown adipose tissue is the cause of higher energy expenditure in smokers.

Conclusion

There does not appear to be any firm evidence supporting the hypothesis that the decreased weight in smokers is due to decreased total calorie consumption. On the other hand, there is some evidence supporting both the hypothesis that smoking results in decreased consumption of sweet foods and that smoking results in an increased metabolic rate. However, all of these hypotheses deserve further research.

EFFECTS OF STOPPING SMOKING ON BODY WEIGHT

Many people who stop smoking gain weight. In one study the average subject who remained abstinent from cigarettes for 6 months gained 9 pounds.[19] However, there are individual differences in whether or not weight is gained.[20] By examining what types of people do and do not gain weight when they stop smoking, and under what conditions there is a weight gain, it may be possible to obtain some clues as to what can cause a weight gain to occur. There is a large variety of possibilities.

Nicotine

One hypothesis is that the weight gain is somehow a function of the removal of nicotine. Some evidence supports this hypothesis. For example, heavier smokers are more likely to gain weight when they stop smoking than are moderate or light smokers.[21] In addition, when people stop smoking, the more they chew nicotine gum, the less likely they are to gain weight.[22] These studies by themselves, however, do not tell us why it is that nicotine removal affects weight gain. Perhaps nicotine removal affects appetite, metabolic rate, food preferences, or activity level (see below). In a study by Janet Gross, Maxine L. Stitzer, and Janelle Maldonado,[23] ex-smokers who chewed nicotine gum reported smaller increases in hunger and food consumption following cessation of smoking than did ex-smokers who chewed placebo gum. Unfortunately, data on the possible mechanisms by which nicotine removal could affect weight gain are very limited.

Relapse

A number of studies have indicated that some of the individual differences in weight gain in ex-smokers are related to how successful a particular ex-smoker is at abstaining from smoking. People who manage to remain abstinent for a long period of time are more likely to gain weight than people who remain abstinent for only a short period of time.[24] Thus successful cessation of smoking does seem to come with a sometimes unwelcome consequence—weight gain. Nevertheless, even in successful ex-smokers, a weight gain is not inevitable, as will be described in some of the sections below.

Increase in Total Calories Consumed

Another possible explanation for the weight gain that sometimes accompanies cessation of smoking is that those ex-smokers who gain weight have increased the total number of calories that they consume.[25] The data are mixed on whether such an increase does or does not occur.

In one experiment, the weights and food intake of 95 smokers were repeatedly measured. Two weeks after stopping smoking, these subjects were consuming significantly more than they had consumed when they were smoking. In addition, it appeared that the more food a subject consumed in the first few weeks after stopping smoking, the more likely that subject was to gain weight.[26] Another experiment, this one with rats, also obtained increases in total caloric consumption, as well as body weight, when nicotine exposure was discontinued.[27] Finally, a study by Bonnie Spring and her colleagues directly measured food intake. This study found that, over a period of 4 weeks, overweight female smokers who had stopped smoking on the average consumed 300 more calories per day than when they had been smoking, gaining 3.5 pounds.[28]

On the other hand, in one intensive study of a single subject who stopped smoking, the subject gained almost 8 pounds without any increase in total food consumption.[29] Further, Judith Rodin[30] found that, among middle-aged smokers who stopped smoking, those who gained weight had not consumed more total calories than those whose weights remained stable.

It would appear that many cases of weight gain following cessation of smoking may be due to increased food consumption, but some may not. For those cases in which food consumption does increase, it is useful to consider some possible causes of those increases:

1. Stress results in adjunctive behavior. Many smokers are under stress and for them smoking can serve as an adjunctive behavior.[31] In these subjects, when smoking ceases, another adjunctive behavior, such as snacking, must substitute for smoking (see Chapter 10 for more discussion of adjunctive snacking's leading to weight gain). Further, independent of whatever other sources of stress may exist, cessation of smoking by itself can also result in stress, thus leading to adjunctive snacking and weight gain.

2. People who smoke have a high oral drive,[32] and they must continue to satisfy that drive in some way if they stop smoking. Therefore their food consumption increases.

3. People use their hands when they smoke and need a substitute hand activity if they stop. Therefore they use their hands in increased feeding behavior.[33]

4. People who eat more after stopping smoking and therefore gain weight are those people whose history indicates that they are likely to have weight and eating-pattern problems.[34]

5. Food consumption is increased following cessation of smoking due to disruptions in insulin level.[35]

All of these possible explanations require a great deal more research before they can be unequivocally accepted.

Increase in Sweet Foods Consumed

Perhaps the weight gain that many people experience when they stop smoking is due not to an increase in the total amount of calories consumed but instead to an increase in the amount of sweet foods consumed.[36] If this were so, a greater proportion of consumed calories could be stored as fat (see Chapter 10).

A number of studies have found increased consumption of sweet foods among recent ex-smokers as compared to when these subjects were still smoking. For example, one study showed increased consumption of sucrose (but not other sugars) in subjects who had stopped smoking 2 weeks earlier.[37] In another study, ex-smokers who gained weight also tended to consume an increased proportion of their diets as sugar (although their total consumed calories did not increase).[38] Finally, an experiment with rats showed that when nicotine exposure was terminated, the rats' consumption of sweet foods increased.[39] What could be responsible for this increase in preference for sweet foods? Insulin level and substitution for the sweetness previously provided by cigarettes, both mentioned above, are possibilities. In addition, if ex-smokers are experiencing stress, not only could the total number of calories consumed be increased (see above), but the number of calories consumed that consist of palatable (such as sweet) foods could increase as well (see Chapter 10).

Decrease in Metabolic Rate

Perhaps ex-smokers who gain weight do so not because they consume more of all or of certain foods but because they use fewer calories. This could occur, for example, if their metabolic rates decreased when they stopped smoking. Then if their food intake did not also decrease when they stopped smoking, these ex-smokers would gain weight.[40] As discussed above, one experiment has shown that, when energy usage was measured during two 24-hour periods, one when a habitual smoker was smoking and one when the smoker abstained, on the average metabolic rate was 10 percent higher when the subject was smoking. Once again, the greater metabolic rate that occurs when people are smoking may be due to the effects of nicotine on the sympathetic nervous system,[41] thus helping to explain the lower weight gain of ex-smokers who use nicotine gum. If indeed the weight gain following smoking cessation is due to the effects of lowered metabolic rate, this could help to explain the fact that ex-smokers with a history of weight problems are more likely to gain weight than ex-smokers without such a history.[42] Perhaps ex-smokers with a history of weight problems also have a history of frequent dieting, making them more prone to low metabolic rates and thus weight gain (see Chapter 10).

Decrease in Activity Level

Activity level may also play a role in whether or not someone gains weight when he or she stops smoking. There is no evidence that a decrease in activity level is responsible for the weight gain seen in ex-smokers. However, there is evidence that those ex-smokers who engage in relatively more aerobic exercise are less likely to gain weight.[43] As discussed in Chapter 10, exercise appears to be a useful strategy for weight control, even in ex-smokers.

Summary

Some people do gain weight when they stop smoking, and in some cases this may be due to increased consumption of food, particularly sweet food. However, a decrease in metabolic rate that occurs following cessation of smoking probably also results in weight gain in some people. It is not yet clear precisely what role nicotine plays in the weight gain that can occur following smoking cessation. Future research will undoubtedly continue to pursue these issues.

CONCLUSION

The widespread opinion that smokers weigh less than nonsmokers and that ex-smokers risk weight gain is an accurate one. However, not every person who stops smoking will gain large numbers of pounds. Not only are there individual differences in weight gain that are a function of characteristics of individual subjects, but particular behaviors such as use of nicotine gum and aerobic exercise can help to prevent a weight gain (if such a gain is not desired). Researchers are beginning to understand the many complex factors responsible for these findings—such as types of foods consumed, metabolic rate, and stress. Ultimately, these research results can be used to help free smokers from feeling that they must keep smoking, or resume smoking, in order not to gain excess weight.

CHAPTER
14

❦

Cuisine and
Wine Tasting

$\mathbf{M}$uch of this book has been concerned with understanding how and why people choose certain foods and drinks. The purpose of the present chapter is to use the principles described in previous chapters to understand two disciplines of interest to specialists in the psychology of eating and drinking, as well as of interest to all lovers of good food and drink: cuisine and wine tasting.

CUISINE

According to Elisabeth Rozin, cookbook writer and culinary historian, a particular cuisine consists of several parts: the foods that are used, the techniques that are employed to modify the foods, the flavorings that are added to the foods, and any special cultural constraints that restrict what types of food may be eaten or how foods may be prepared.[1] Although the behavior of animals other than humans may demonstrate certain elements of cuisine, such as the salting of sweet potatoes by monkeys described in Chapter 1, cuisine with all of its characteristics appears to be a uniquely human enterprise.

Determinants of Cuisine

Many principles are responsible for the characteristics of any given cuisine. One is simply the foods that are available to a particular cultural group.[2] Blueberries are not likely to be a staple part of an Algerian diet.

Of the foods that are available, those that will be eaten will tend to be those that humans find inherently preferable, for example, sweet and salty foods, but not bitter foods. However, there may be exceptions; preferences may be acquired for inherently aversive foods such as chili pepper (see below) and coffee (see Chapter 6). Metabolic and sensory constraints will also affect the foods included in a cuisine. An example of such a constraint, lactose intolerance, was discussed in Chapter 5. If most of a population is lactose intolerant, unfermented milk is unlikely to be a part of that population's cuisine. As another example, although fava beans are toxic for some people, they may increase resistance to malaria. Therefore in populations in which resistance to malaria is more useful than the toxicity of fava beans is damaging (which occurs in various Mediterranean populations), fava beans should be, and are, a part of that population's cuisine.[3]

The technology available to a particular cultural group is also an important determinant of that group's cuisine. Until fermentation was discovered, no cuisine could contain alcoholic beverages.

Another important factor in the determination of any cuisine is the nutrition provided by the cuisine: The only cultures that survive are those that obtain and consume foods that are basically nutritionally balanced. There are many different ways of doing this. One way is by the combination of foods eaten. In the Northeastern United States a typical, nutritionally complete meal might consist of a piece of chicken, some salad, and a baked potato. But in Mexico, a nutritionally complete meal might consist of corn tortillas, beans, and tomatoes. Mexicans in the past, and very occasionally in the present, have sometimes ensured their protein intake by including insects and worms (both high in protein) in their cuisine.[4] Another way to ensure a nutritionally complete cuisine is by the treatment of the particular foods eaten. The treatment of corn with an alkali solution, prior to consumption of the corn, is a Native American practice that appears to have increased in prevalence because it significantly enhances the nutritional value of the corn.[5]

As described in Chapter 7, the amount of energy required to prepare food, or the money required to purchase it, will also affect the content of a cuisine. If a group of 10 people living at a subsistence level must walk 50 miles through a desert in order to obtain grain, and then spend several days working to make a single loaf of bread from that grain, bread will not be a part of that group's cuisine.

Other people's food preferences and practices (i.e., food cultural beliefs) can also affect cuisine (see Chapter 6). For example, children and adults prefer foods at breakfast and dinner that they have learned to identify as breakfast foods and dinner foods, respectively.[6] As another example, the laws of *kashrut*, which determine the kosher food practices of Jews, are passed from generation to generation. The cultural traditions of *kashrut* are so strong that they can affect the consumption of foods that appear not to be kosher, but actually are. The principles of contiguity and similarity from traditional association theory (see Chapter 6) can help to explain such cases.[7] To illustrate, a kosher Jew may have difficulty eating a mock-turkey and cheese sandwich even though the mock turkey is made out of tofu (kosher Jews cannot consume meat and milk in the same meal). Perhaps one of the best examples of how food cultural beliefs can affect someone's cuisine occurs when a person moves from one culture to another. Such cross-cultural changes often result in people's, particularly young people's, acquiring the food-preference pattern of the new culture.[8]

Finally, an important factor influencing the form cuisines take is neophobia (see Chapter 6). Humans as well as other species have a tendency to fear new foods. This may be why most cuisines have a number of *flavor principles*, characteristic flavorings, around which the cuisine revolves. These flavorings are added to many of the dishes in the cuisine and serve to identify dishes as belonging to a particular tradition.[9] For example, it is possible to take hamburger, a substance not present in Asian cuisines, add soy sauce, rice wine, and ginger root to it, and end up with a hamburger that tastes Chinese. E. Rozin describes the flavor principles of many different cuisines in her unusual and fascinating cookbook, *Ethnic Cuisine: The Flavor-Principle Cookbook*.[10]

Examples of Cuisines

Table 14.1 shows some of E. Rozin's flavor principles for different cuisines. Note that cultures that are in close geographical proximity tend to have overlapping flavor principles. For example, soy sauce is common to Japanese, Chinese, and Korean cuisines, and olive oil is common to many

TABLE 14.1
Flavor Principles in Different Cuisines

Cuisine	Flavor Principles
China	Soy sauce, rice wine, and ginger root
Peking	+ miso and/or garlic and/or sesame
Szechuan	+ sweet-sour-hot
Canton	+ black bean–garlic
Japan	Soy sauce, sake, and sugar
Korea	Soy sauce, brown sugar, sesame, and chile
India	Curry
Northern India	Cumin, ginger, garlic + variations
Southern India	Mustard seed, coconut, tamarind, chile + variations
Central Asia	Cinnamon, fruit, nut
Middle East	Lemon, parsley
West Africa	Tomato, peanut, chile
Northeastern Africa	Garlic, cumin, mint
Morocco	Cumin, coriander, cinnamon, ginger + onion and/or tomato and/or fruit
Greece	Olive oil, lemon, oregano
Southern Italy and Southern France	Olive oil, garlic, parsley, and/or anchovy
Italy, France	Olive oil, garlic, basil
Provence	Olive oil, thyme, rosemary, marjoram, sage
Spain	Olive oil, onion, pepper, tomato
Northern and Eastern Europe	Sour cream, dill or paprika or allspice or caraway
Normandy	Apple, cider, calvados
Northern Italy	Wine vinegar, garlic
Mexico	Tomato, chile

Source: Adapted from E. Rozin, *Ethnic Cuisine: The Flavor-Principle Cookbook*, Brattleboro, VT: The Stephen Greene Press, 1983.

Mediterranean cuisines. According to E. Rozin, flavor principles are the most important factor in identifying any ethnic cuisine.

All of this can be seen at work in the creation of Cajun cuisine. The Cajuns are a group of people who live in an area of Louisiana close to New Orleans (see Figure 14.1). The word *Cajun* comes from Acadian, for

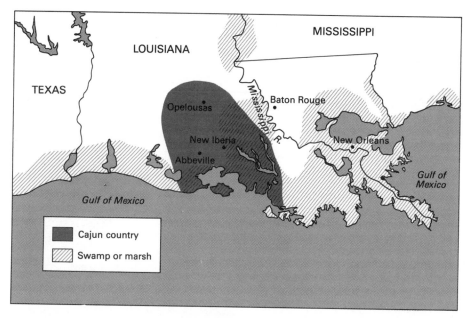

FIGURE 14.1   *Approximate locations of Cajuns.* (After B. Greene, "Cajun Country," *Cuisine* [September 1979]:42–54.)

Cajuns were originally from Nova Scotia (Acadia), French Canada. They were transported involuntarily to Louisiana by British soldiers in the eighteenth century.[11] The area where they arrived has also been inhabited by, among others, the French, Native Americans, and blacks brought there as slaves.

The Cajuns' new location, the bayou, was near the ocean and filled with swamps, lakes, and islands. Seafood was plentiful, particularly oysters, crawfish (a larger variety of the crayfish), and crab. Chili peppers also grew well in the area.

The various groups of people in the area all had their own unique cooking techniques. Both the Cajuns and the French were familiar with the French cooking technique of a *roux*. This is a sauce base that is made by combining melted butter and flour. The blacks used a slow-tempered cooking fire along with a heavy iron pot.

The combination of all these ingredients and techniques, including okra (used by the blacks) and a powder made from sassafras leaves (used by the Native Americans), resulted in the now-famous Cajun dish called gumbo. This particular dish, more than any other, is identified with Cajun cooking

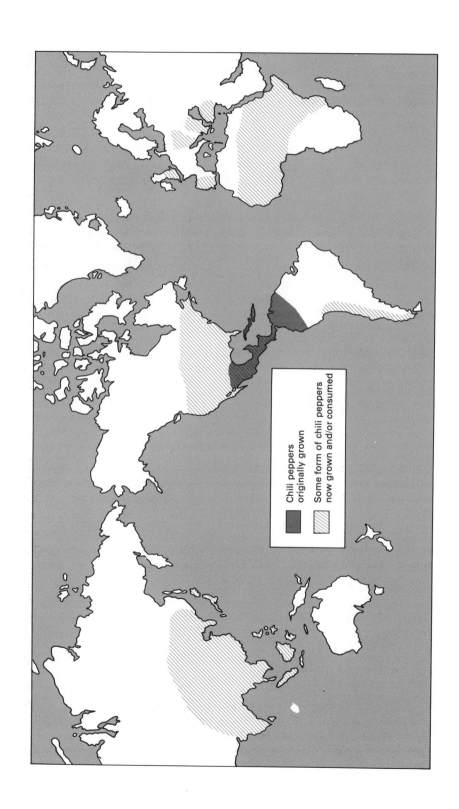

Chili peppers
originally grown

Some form of chili peppers
now grown and/or consumed

because it represents the unique mixture of other cuisines that is Cajun cooking. Cajun cooking is quite different from Creole cuisine in nearby New Orleans; Creole cooking is almost identical to French cooking except that local ingredients are used instead of traditional French ingredients.[12]

Examples of Flavor Principles

THE PREFERENCE FOR CHILI PEPPER.   By studying a single food preference, the preference for chili pepper, it is possible to examine many potential mechanisms for the origins of flavor principles, and thus for the formation of cuisines. The preference for eating chili pepper is of particular interest for several reasons. First, although chili peppers were originally grown only in the New World, they are now grown and consumed around the globe (Figure 14.2). Chili pepper is now one of the most widely consumed spices in the world.[13] The market for chili peppers has even been a subject of discussion in the *Wall Street Journal*.[14] Second, most humans initially find the consumption of chili pepper to be aversive. Third, the physical effects of chili pepper in the mouth are similar to effects of being burned; there is a sensation of pain, and the skin temperature is raised. As a result, chili pepper is sometimes sold as a powder for hikers and skiers to apply to their feet to keep them warm in cold weather. Fourth, humans are the only omnivores that regularly eat chili pepper; the preference for chili pepper is one of the few differences between the real-world food preferences of humans and rats. In the early twentieth century Appalachian women took advantage of the rat's aversion to chili pepper: They kept rats from eating their wallpaper by mixing the wallpaper paste with chili pepper.[15] However, although rats exposed to chili pepper will not eat it, they can learn to prefer chili pepper if they are exposed to other rats that have consumed it (using the demonstrator–observer paradigm described in Chapter 6).[16] Further, chimpanzees that are gradually exposed to chili pepper through contact with humans can acquire a preference for it.[17] Thus chili peppers have quickly be-

FIGURE 14.2   *Map of the world showing the locations in which chili pepper was originally grown and the locations where it is now consumed.* (After F.W. Moore, "Food Habits in Non-Industrial Societies," in *Dimensions of Nutrition*, ed. J. Dupont, Boulder, CO: Colorado Associated University Press, 1970; F. Rosengarten, *The Book of Spices*, Wynnewood, PA: Livingston Publishing, 1969; P. Rozin, "Psychobiological and Cultural Determinants of Food Choice," in *Appetite and Food Intake*, ed. T Silverstone, Berlin: Dahlem Konferenzen, 1976.)

come a part of a great many cuisines, despite their being initially aversive to all species and despite their causing physical effects similar to those of being burned. There must therefore be some powerful factor or factors responsible for the acquired preference for chili pepper.

There are many possible reasons why humans learn to prefer chili pepper. Initially, they probably sample it because of social pressure (similar to the ways in which chimpanzees and rats come to prefer chili pepper). Later, they may come to like it because of the large amounts of vitamins A and C that it contains, the increase in salivation and gastric movement that it engenders, which assists in the digestion of starchy foods, or the "zest" that it adds to a meal. Another possibility is that the pain that accompanies consumption of chili pepper is enjoyed because it seems dangerous but is actually safe ("thrill seeking"; see sensation seeking in Chapter 5).[18] There is some desensitization that occurs with frequent exposure to *capsaicin*, the active ingredient in chili peppers. In other words, with frequent exposure some of the sensory reactions to capsaicin decrease.[19] However, this effect is small and therefore cannot explain the increase in liking for chili pepper that comes from exposure.[20] Finally, the aversive reaction on first tasting chili pepper may be followed by, and even overwhelmed by, a positive, opponent reaction.[21] This hypothesis has received some support in experiments with another widely consumed but initially aversive substance, coffee.[22] Little or no empirical evidence supports a variety of other explanations as to why people come to prefer chili pepper, such as that chili pepper helps to preserve food, that it masks the odors and tastes of spoiled food, and that it causes sweating and thus cooling (resulting in relief in hot climates).[23]

There are many ways by which people may come to prefer chili pepper. It is possible that different mechanisms may be responsible for the chili pepper preference in different people. Paul Rozin[24] has elegantly compiled and summarized most of the available information on this ubiquitous and perplexing flavor principle.

THE PREFERENCE FOR CHOCOLATE. Chocolate has long been a popular food in many countries. This is despite the fact that it, like chili pepper, originated in the New World and that it has only been available to most of the world for the past several hundred years. In fact, it was only after chocolate was brought to Europe that it was manufactured with sugar and milk into the form of chocolate with which we are most familiar today: milk chocolate.[25] There are probably many reasons for chocolate's popularity. One reason is undoubtedly the fact that chocolate is usually consumed mixed with sugar, thus engaging our largely inherited preference for sweet tastes (see Chapter 5) and arousing strong sensual and pleasurable sensations.[26] Another reason is that chocolate is high in fat. Recall from Chapter 6 that we learn to prefer foods that are high in calories and that fat contains more calories per gram than do carbohydrates or protein. One ounce of milk chocolate contains 520 calories, as well as significant amounts of calcium, potassium, magnesium, vitamin A, and vitamin B₃, all essential nutrients.[27] However, chocolate also contains caffeine. One ounce of bittersweet chocolate contains about one-third the amount of caffeine as a cup of tea.[28] Chapter 8 discussed the fact that caffeine can induce physiological dependence and is a stimulant. Chocolate also has a smooth, pleasant texture and melts at body temperature, thus adding to its appeal. Given all these characteristics of chocolate, it is not surprising that it is so preferred and has become a part of so many cuisines.

Examples of Cultural Constraints

THE SACRED COW.   The principles of optimal foraging theory (described in Chapter 7) have been used to explain the origins of cultural constraints on cuisine. In particular, optimal foraging theory has been used to explain the prohibition against eating cows by the Hindus in India.[29] At first this prohibition appears counterproductive, because many people in India do not have sufficient food. However, research by Marvin Harris has contended that the sacred cow of India is actually greatly beneficial to India's economy for the following reasons.[30]

According to Harris, oxen (castrated male cattle) are essential to the Indian agricultural system, providing the power necessary to till the soil. It is difficult for oxen to be shared by a group of farmers because, as a result of the monsoon rains, all of the crops tend to become ready for harvesting at once. Therefore most farmers need their own oxen. Oxen also provide transportation. But in order to get oxen, cows are necessary.

During droughts, cows may become temporarily infertile. However, if they are not kept alive there will not be any cows to produce oxen. At such times, the local Indian government provides homes for infertile cows. A farmer can reclaim his cow from one of these homes when the cow shows signs of regaining her fertility. Thus, during droughts, the burden of supporting nonproductive cows falls frequently on the government, not on the individual farmer.

At other times, when there is little food to give the farm animals (e.g., in the spring, when it is hot and dry in India), cattle are allowed to wander along the roads. Although it may appear that the cattle are being permitted to wander freely because they are "sacred," actually they are eating the grass along the road so that their owners do not have to feed them. Further, if a farmer's choice does come down to either feeding the cows or feeding the oxen, the oxen are usually fed, thus protecting the farmer's present survival, though perhaps sacrificing future survival. Generally the food that is given to cattle consists mostly of the parts of plants that humans cannot eat. Cattle also provide dung, which is very important in India both as cooking fuel and as fertilizer. In some parts of India virtually 100 percent of the dung is utilized for these purposes. It has been calculated that to replace India's oxen with tractors, fertilizer, coal, and family transportation would result in an expenditure so large (billions of dollars) that international monetary relations would be in disarray for years.

Finally, statistics on the relative number of cows versus male cattle show that more cows die than oxen, perhaps because of differential amounts of neglect. In any case, when a cow does die, it can only be touched by a member of the lowest Indian caste, the untouchables. A member of this caste will take the carcass, consume the meat, and use the hide for leather. This provides a sort of welfare system for some of India's poorest people.

For all of these reasons Harris believes that the treatment of the cow as sacred in India is actually beneficial to the country's economy. His theory of how this behavior may have arisen is the following. By 300 B.C. there were between 50 million and 100 million people living in India. At that time there were a great many droughts and floods. Because of the reasons given above, people who protected their cattle survived and people who did not protect them died. Therefore a cultural trait of food choice that maximized survival came to predominate.

Harris sums up his beliefs regarding the effects of food economics on cultural behavior in this quotation:

> Human society is neither random nor capricious. The regularities of thought and behavior called culture are the principal mechanisms by which we human beings adapt to the world around us. Practices and beliefs can be rational or irrational, but a society that fails to adapt to its environment is doomed to extinction. Only those societies that draw the necessities of life from their surroundings without destroying those surroundings, inherit the earth.[31]

Harris, along with others, believes that eating is so crucial to the survival of a species that how a culture obtains food can determine many of its cultural characteristics.[32] The necessity of obtaining food optimally can even determine the food-consumption relationships among various species.[33] Because humans evolved in an environment with a frequently inadequate food supply,[34] it is not surprising that cuisines, as well as other aspects of culture, often reflect optimal solutions in terms of maximizing survival.[35]

CANNIBALISM.   One type of food that is rarely, if ever, present in a cuisine is the flesh of conspecifics. It has been difficult to document the existence of human societies in which cannibalism has been a regular occurrence, as opposed to occasional instances in which there was no other means of survival. When these latter instances have occurred, they have been perceived by the societies within which they occurred as regrettable acts, as antisocial behavior, rather than as accepted practice.[36] Some researchers feel that, prior to 1900, there may have been some societies that engaged in regular cannibalism, but accurate, complete records from that time are difficult to obtain. In any case, the present and prior existence of cannibalism remains controversial.[37]

As discussed in Chapter 6, rats are also unlikely to consume members of their own species. It is not surprising that cannibalism is at most a rare occurrence in rats as well as humans. Species in which cannibalism occurred regularly might be inclined to augment their food supply by hastening the death of members of that species, thus decreasing the probability of survival of that species. Thus, once again, it appears that a cultural constraint on cuisine has as its basis the survival of the species.

The prohibition against consuming conspecifics can extend to other species closely associated with one's own species. Chapter 6 described research indicating that a rat is unlikely to consume mice if the rat has been raised with a mouse. Humans generally do not consume the members of other species with which they live and which they consider to possess human traits, species such as cats and dogs. At first, the fact that dogs are eaten by the Oglala, a Native American population in South Dakota, would appear to contradict this general principle. However, the Oglala consume the dogs only as part of certain special ceremonies and only if the dogs have never been given names by their owners. Further, although the Oglala consider dogs to possess certain human characteristics, dogs never live inside and are neither groomed nor trained.[38] Thus, although the Oglala might appear to provide an exception to the rule that humans do not consume closely associated species, in actuality there are a number of respects in which this tribe disassociates itself from dogs.

WINE TASTING

As an example of what can be accomplished with the unified approach to psychology that has been used in this book, consider an analysis of wine-tasting behavior. What is involved in evaluating wines, or any food or drink for that matter? What factors affect these evaluations?

First it will be helpful to describe the wine-tasting procedure. The *oenophile* (wine lover) begins wine tasting by simply looking at the wine. The wine is then swirled in the glass to increase its aroma and bouquet, which are smelled in the next step. Finally the wine is tasted in small sips. It is rolled over the tongue and bits of bread and/or cheese may be taken between sips. Some wine tasters spit out the sips of wine without swallowing them.[39]

Each of these steps is performed separately, quietly, and with as little distraction as possible. This separation and isolation in the wine-tasting process permit more attention to be focused on each of the steps. Sensory thresholds are lower under these conditions. Receiving rewards for accurate judgments or competing with other tasters also appears to lower thresholds; under these conditions people give more sensitive, accurate judgments.[40] However, the absolute thresholds probably do not change. As described by *signal detection theory*,[41] what changes is more likely the motivation to give accurate answers. A factor that does affect the taste and smell thresholds in wine tasting is the temperature of the wine. When wine is very cold it is harder to smell. Most people who taste wine without distractions and with the wine at the appropriate temperature can become skilled at discriminating between various types of wine.[42]

The senses of vision and touch, as well as smell and taste, are critical to wine tasting. The visual judgment of a wine includes judging both its color and its appearance (for example, whether it is cloudy).[43] To judge the odor of a wine, wine tasters pay attention to both the wine's *aroma*, which consists of the odors arising from the type of grape used in making the wine, and the wine's *bouquet*, which consists of the odors derived from fermentation, processing, or aging.[44] As described in Chapter 4, calling the various odors by specific names may help in their identification. For example, many people call the aroma of the Sauvignon blanc grape a spicy smell.[45] In judging the taste of the wine, the wine is rolled around on the tongue so that all of the taste receptors can be stimulated. To assess the touch of the wine, a wine taster notes any astringency on the tongue, as well as whether the wine feels full or thin. The wine feels thin when there is a low alcohol content and full when there is a high alcohol content.[46]

There are several psychological processes that may make accurate wine tasting difficult. First is *habituation*. The sensory cells that taste and smell the wine may not fire as readily after the taster's initial samples of wine (see Chapter 4). This is why wine tasters may take bites of bread between sips and why they taste slowly. They are trying to keep their sensory cells at a constant level of sensitivity. Spitting out the wine may also assist in this regard, but the main purpose of spitting it out is to prevent the ingestion of alcohol, which can strongly affect the tasters' behavior (see Chapter 11).[47]

Another problem that may arise in wine tasting concerns the effects of one sense on another, also known as *stimulus errors*. For example, if a wine appears cloudy a taster may be more likely to judge its taste as below par. This is probably because that taster has encountered cloudy wine before and it tasted poorly. However, since quality of appearance and of taste are not always related, it is important to remove such cross-modality effects. One way that this has been done has been to drink the wine out of a glass painted black, so that it is impossible to see the wine. Then the merits of the wine's taste can be judged by themselves.[48]

A third wine-tasting problem has to do with the words used to describe what is seen, smelled, tasted, and felt. Terms such as "fruity," "pale yellow," and "woody" are used frequently. However, there is no guarantee that the same word used by two different people has the same meaning for both of them. In addition, over time the use of certain words may change.[49]

Memory is also very important in wine tasting. A taster needs to compare wines to absolute standards developed from previous tastings. In addition, if too large a series of wines is tasted during one session, those tasted in the middle are likely to suffer in terms of the taster's subsequent memory of them. People tend to remember the beginning and end of a long series of items better than they do the middle. These are known as the *primacy* and *recency effects*.[50] A rating form may help a taster to remember what has been tasted.[51]

Wine tasters must also watch out for *contrast effects*. A poor wine tasted following another poor wine may be rated better than if it had followed an outstanding wine (see the discussion of incentive contrast in Chapter 6). Judgments of value tend to be relative, and that fact should be taken into account when evaluating wine ratings.[52]

Finally, many wine tasters tend to show a *central tendency* in making their ratings.[53] That is, they tend not to use the high or low points of rating scales; their judgments tend to stay around the middle of the scales. For this reason, some psychologists have argued that judgments should not be made using fixed scales, such as scales ranging from 1 to 10. Instead, they argue, subjects should be told to assign any number they want to the item being judged. There is then no upper limit to the scale being used, and subjects' ratings are not constrained.[54]

This illustration of wine tasting and the principles behind it draws on the areas of sensation, perception, learning, cognitive, and social psychology. This sort of interarea approach can be useful in understanding all eating and drinking behaviors.

Chapter 14

CONCLUSION

Cuisine and wine tasting, two expressions of our love for food and drink, illustrate many of the principles covered in previous chapters. They are excellent examples of the advantages accruing from taking an interdisciplinary approach to the psychology of eating and drinking. Our enjoyment of food and drink will continue to be enhanced by this type of approach, which takes into account all of the senses, past experiences, genes, and current circumstances, including companions. The psychology of eating and drinking has much to tell us based on findings obtained from many different fields, both the findings from past research and those from research yet to be conducted.

Clinics and Self-Help Organizations

T his is a partial list; it is not meant to be complete.

Taste and Smell Disorders

The Smell and Taste Center
Department of Otolaryngology
5th Floor, Ravdin Building
3400 Spruce Street
Hospital of the University of Pennsylvania
Philadelphia, PA 19104
(215) 662-2797 or (215) 662-6580

Taste and Smell Clinic
UConn Health Center
Farmington, CT 06032
(203) 679-2459

Eating Disorders

American Anorexia/Bulimia Association
133 Cedar Lane
Teaneck, NJ 07666
(201) 836-1800

BASH Treatment and Research Center for Eating and Mood Disorders
6125 Clayton Avenue, Suite 215
St. Louis, MO 63139
(800) 762-3334 or (314) 768-3794

Overeaters Anonymous
World Service Office
4025 Spencer Street, Suite 203
Torrance, CA 90503
(213) 542-8363

Alcohol Abuse

Alcoholics Anonymous
175 Fifth Avenue
New York, NY 10010
(212) 683-3900

Notes

Chapter 1: Introduction

1. J. Z. Young, "Influence of the Mouth on the Evolution of the Brain," in *Biology of the Brain*, ed. P. Person, Washington, DC: American Association for the Advancement of Science, 1968, p. 21.

2. J. Owen, *Feeding Strategy*, Chicago: University of Chicago Press, 1980, pp. 7–9.

3. J. Le Magnen, *Hunger*, Cambridge, Great Britain: Cambridge University Press, 1985, pp. 1–2.

4. A. Roosevelt, "The Evolution of Human Subsistence," in *Food and Evolution: Toward a Theory of Human Food Habits*, eds. M. Harris and E. B. Ross, Philadelphia: Temple University Press, 1987, p. 565.

5. J. A. Michener, *Alaska*, New York: Fawcett Crest, 1988, p. 65.

6. W. Shakespeare, "Twelfth Night," in *The Complete Works of William Shakespeare*, ed. W. A. Wright, Garden City, NY: Garden City Books, 1623/1936, p. 707.

7. H. Gleitman, *Psychology*, New York: W. W. Norton, 1981, p. 1.

8. D. P. Barash, *Sociobiology and Behavior*, New York: Elsevier, 1977.

W. D. Hamilton, "The Genetical Evolution of Social Behaviour. I," *Journal of Theoretical Biology* 7(1964):1–16.

W. D. Hamilton, "The Genetical Evolution of Social Behaviour. II," *Journal of Theoretical Biology* 7(1964):17–52.

J. Maynard Smith, "Optimization Theory in Evolution," *Annual Review of Ecology and Systematics* 9(1978):31–56.

9. A. W. Logue, "Taste Aversion Learning in Humans and Other Species," in *Evolution and Learning*, eds. R. C. Bolles and M. D. Beecher, Hillsdale, NJ: Lawrence Erlbaum Associates, 1988.

10. V. G. Dethier, *To Know a Fly*, Oakland, CA: Holden-Day, 1962.

11. Ibid.

12. W. J. Davis, "Motivation and Learning: Neurophysiological Mechanisms in a 'Model' System," *Learning and Motivation* 15(1984):377–393.

13. J. C. Bednarz, "Cooperative Hunting in

Harris' Hawks (*Parabuteo Unicinctus*)," *Science* 239(1988):1525–1527.

14. E. M. Blass and M. H. Teicher, "Suckling," *Science* 210(1980):15–22.

15. H. Kalmus, "The Sense of Taste of Chimpanzees and Other Primates," *The Chimpanzee* 2(1970):130–141.

16. A. Jolly, *The Evolution of Primate Behavior*, New York: Macmillan, 1972.

17. J. van Lawick-Goodall, *In the Shadow of Man*, New York: Dell, 1971.

18. M. Kawai, "Newly-Acquired Pre-Cultural Behavior of the Natural Troop of Japanese Monkeys on Koshima Islet," *Primates* 6(1965):1–30.

19. van Lawick-Goodall, *In the Shadow of Man*.

20. M. P. Ghiglieri, "The Social Ecology of Chimpanzees," *Scientific American* 252(6)(1985):102–104, 109–113.

21. K. A. Houpt and T. R. Houpt, "The Neonatal Pig: A Biological Model for the Development of Taste Preferences and Controls of Ingestive Behavior," in *Taste and Development*, ed. J. M. Weiffenbach, Bethesda, MD: U.S. Department of Health, Education, and Welfare, 1977.

22. Ibid.

23. S. A. Barnett, *The Rat: A Study in Behavior*, Chicago: Aldine, 1963.

24. J. J. Wurtman and R. J. Wurtman, "Sucrose Consumption Early in Life Fails to Modify the Appetite of Adult Rats for Sweet Foods," *Science* 205(1979):321–322.

25. Barnett, *The Rat: A Study in Behavior*.

Chapter 2: Hunger

1. C. Bernard, *Les Phénomènes de la Vie* (Paris, c. 1878), cited in W. B. Cannon, "Organization for Physiological Homeostasis," *Physiological Reviews* 9(1929):399–431.

2. Ibid., p. 400.

3. Cannon, "Organization for Physiological Homeostasis."

4. W. B. Cannon and A. L. Washburn, "An Explanation of Hunger," *The American Journal of Physiology* 29(1912):441–454.

5. W. B. Cannon, "Hunger and Thirst," in *The Foundations of Experimental Psychology,* ed. C. Murchison, Worcester, MA: Clark University Press, 1929.

6. E. Stellar, "The Physiology of Motivation," *Psychological Review* 61(1954):5–22.

A. J. Stunkard and S. Fox, "The Relationship of Gastric Motility and Hunger: A Summary of the Evidence," *Psychosomatic Medicine* 33(1971):123–134.

7. Ibid.

8. E. M. Bobroff and H. R. Kissileff, "Effects of Changes in Palatability on Food Intake and the Cumulative Food Intake Curve in Man," *Appetite* 7(1986):85–96.

J. D. Davis and G. P. Smith, "Analysis of Lick Rate Measures the Positive and Negative Feedback Effects of Carbohydrates on Eating," *Appetite* 11(1988):229–238.

T. A. Spiegel, E. E. Shrager, and E. Stellar, "Responses of Lean and Obese Subjects to Preloads, Deprivation, and Palatability," *Appetite* 13(1989):45–69.

9. M. Teghtsoonian, E. Becker, and B. Edelman, "A Psychophysical Analysis of Perceived Satiety: Its Relation to Consummatory Behavior and Degree of Overweight," *Appetite* 2(1981):217–229.

10. H. D. Janowitz and M. I. Grossman, "Some Factors Affecting the Food Intake of Normal Dogs and Dogs with Esophagostomy and Gastric Fistula," *American Journal of Physiology* 159(1949):143–148.

11. H. D. Janowitz and F. Hollander, "Effect of Prolonged Intragastric Feeding on Oral Ingestion," *Federation Proceedings* 12(1953):72.

I. Share and E. Martyniuk, "Effect of Prolonged Intragastric Feeding on Oral Food Intake in Dogs," *American Journal of Physiology* 169(1952):229–235.

12. N. E. Miller and M. L. Kessen, "Reward Effects of Food via Stomach Fistula Compared with Those of Food via Mouth," *Journal of Comparative and Physiological Psychology* 45(1952):555–564.

13. J. A. Deutsch, "Dietary Control and the Stomach," *Progress in Neurobiology* 20(1983):313–332.

14. P. M. Brala and R. L. Hagen, "Effects of Sweetness Perception and Caloric Value of a Preload on Short Term Intake," *Physiology and Behavior* 30(1983):1–9.

B. J. Rolls, M. Hetherington, and L. J. Laster, "Comparison of the Effects of Aspartame and Sucrose on Appetite and Food Intake," *Appetite* 11 Supplement(1988): 62–67.

T. B. Van Itallie, M. U. Yang, and K. P. Porikos, "Use of Aspartame to Test the "Body Weight Set Point" Hypothesis," *Appetite* 11 Supplement(1988):68–72.

15. Brala and Hagen, "Effects of Sweetness Perception."

N. Geary, "Carbohydrate's Effect on Hunger and Obesity: Commentary on Geiselman and Novin (1982)," *Appetite* 6(1985):60–63.

P. J. Geiselman, "Sugar-Induced Hyperphagia: Is Hyperinsulinemia, Hypoglycemia, or Any Other Factor a 'Necessary' Condition?" *Appetite* 11 Supplement(1988):26–34.

J. Rodin, J. Wack, E. Ferrannini, and R. A. DeFronzo, "Effect of Insulin and Glucose on Feeding Behavior," *Metabolism* 34(1985):826–831.

M. G. Tordoff and M. I. Friedman, "Drinking Saccharin Increases Food Intake and Preference—IV. Cephalic Phase and Metabolic Factors," *Appetite* 12(1989):37–56.

16. J. R. Brobeck, "Food Intake as a Mechanism of Temperature Regulation," *Journal of Biology and Medicine* 20(1948):545–552.

17. F. S. Kraly and E. M. Blass, "Increased Feeding in Rats in a Low Ambient Temperature," in *Hunger: Basic Mechanisms and Clinical Implications,* eds. D. Novin, W. Wyrwicka, and G. A. Bray, New York: Raven Press, 1976.

18. D. G. Fleming, "Food Intake Studies in Parabiotic Rats," *Annals New York Academy of Sciences* 157(1969):985–1003.

19. J. Mayer, "The Glucostatic Theory of Regulation of Food Intake and the Problem of Obesity," *Bulletin of the New England Medical Center* 14(1952):43–49.

20. Ibid.

21. G. C. Kennedy, "The Role of Depot Fat in the Hypothalamic Control of Food Intake in the Rat," *Proceedings of the Royal Society of London,* 140B(1953):578–592.

Mayer, "The Glucostatic Theory."

J. Mayer, "Regulation of Energy Intake and the Body Weight: The Glucostatic Theory and the Lipostatic Hypothesis," *Annals New York Academy of Sciences* 63(1955):15–43.

22. R. E. Keesey, "A Set-Point Analysis of the Regulation of Body Weight," in *Obesity,* ed. A. J. Stunkard, Philadelphia: W. B. Saunders, 1980.

J. Le Magnen, "Interactions of Glucostatic and Lipostatic Mechanisms in the Regulatory Control of Feeding," in *Hunger: Basic Mechanisms and*

Clinical Implications, eds. D. Novin, W. Wyrwicka, and G. A. Bray, New York: Raven Press, 1976.

Y. Oomura, "Significance of Glucose, Insulin, and Free Fatty Acid on the Hypothalamic Feeding and Satiety Neurons," in *Hunger: Basic Mechanisms and Clinical Implications*, eds. D. Novin, W. Wyrwicka, and G. A. Bray, New York: Raven Press, 1976.

23. S. Ritter, "Glucoprivation and the Glucoprivic Control of Food Intake," in *Feeding Behavior: Neural and Humoral Controls*, eds. R. C. Ritter, S. Ritter, and C. D. Barnes, New York: Academic Press, 1986.

24. H. A. Guthrie, *Human Nutrition*, Saint Louis: C. V. Mosby, 1975.

25. J. P. Flatt, "The Difference in the Storage Capacities for Carbohydrate and for Fat, and Its Implications in the Regulation of Body Weight," in *Human Obesity*, eds. R. J. Wurtman and J. J. Wurtman, New York: New York Academy of Sciences, 1987.

Y. Schutz, "Nutrient Ingestion and Body Weight Regulation," in *Low-Calorie Products*, eds. G. G. Birch and M. G. Lindley, New York: Elsevier, 1988.

26. L. A. Campfield and F. J. Smith, "Functional Coupling between Transient Declines in Blood Glucose and Feeding Behavior: Temporal Relationships," *Brain Research Bulletin* 17(1986):427–433.

E. Scharrer and W. Langhans, "Control of Food Intake by Fatty Acid Oxidation," *American Journal of Physiology* 250 (*Regulatory Integrative Comparative Physiology* 19)(1986):R1003–R1006.

M. G. Tordoff and M. I. Friedman, "Hepatic Control of Feeding: Effect ofGlucose, Fructose, and Mannitol Infusion," *American Journal of Physiology* 254 (*Regulatory Integrative Comparative Physiology* 23)(1988):R969–R976.

27. C. T. Dourish, W. Rycroft, and S. D. Iversen, "Postponement of Satiety by Blockade of Brain Cholecystokinin (CCK-B) Receptors," *Science* 245 (1989):1509–1511.

R. W. Foltin and T. H. Moran, "Food Intake in Baboons: Effects of a Long-Acting Cholecystokinin Analog," *Appetite* 12(1989):145–152.

N. Geary and G. P. Smith, "Selective Hepatic Vagotomy Blocks Pancreatic Glucagon's Satiety," *Physiology and Behavior* 31(1983):391–394.

B. G. Hoebel, "Neurotransmitters in the Control of Feeding and Its Rewards: Monoamines, Opiates, and Brain-Gut Peptides," in *Eating and Its Disorders*, eds. A. J. Stunkard and E. Stellar,

New York: Raven Press, 1984.

W. Langhans, U. Zieger, E. Scharrer, and N. Geary, "Stimulation of Feeding in Rats by Intraperitoneal Injection of Antibodies to Glucagon," *Science* 218(1982):894–896.

G. P. Smith and J. Gibbs, "The Effect of Gut Peptides on Hunger, Satiety, and Food Intake in humans," in *Human Obesity*, eds R. J. Wurtman and J. J. Wurtman, New York: New York Academy of Sciences, 1987.

28. A. Weller, G. P. Smith, and J. Gibbs, "Endogenous Cholecystokinin Reduces Feeding in Young Rats," *Science* 247(1990):1589–1591.

29. L. D. Lytle, "Control of Eating Behavior," in *Nutrition and the Brain*, vol. 2, eds. R. J. Wurtman and J. J. Wurtman, New York: Raven Press, 1977.

G. P. Smith, "Gut Hormone Hypothesis of Postprandial Satiety," in *Eating and Its Disorders*, eds. A. J. Stunkard and E. Stellar, New York: Raven Press, 1984.

30. A. W. Hetherington and S. W. Ranson, "Hypothalamic Lesions and Adiposity in the Rat," *Anatomical Record* 78(1940):149–172.

31. A. W. Hetherington and S. W. Ranson, "The Spontaneous Activity and Food Intake of Rats with Hypothalamic Lesions," *American Journal of Physiology* 136(1942):609–617.

32. P. Teitelbaum, "Disturbances in Feeding and Drinking Behavior after Hypothalamic Lesions," in *Nebraska Symposium on Motivation*, ed. M. R. Jones, Lincoln: University of Nebraska Press, 1961.

33. B. G. Hoebel and P. Teitelbaum, "Hypothalamic Control of Feeding and Self-Stimulation," *Science* 135(1962):375–377.

34. J. Mayer and N. B. Marshall, "Specificity of Gold Thioglucose for Ventromedial Hypothalamic Lesions and Hyperphagia," *Nature* 178(1956):1399–1400.

35. B. K. Anand and J. R. Brobeck, "Localization of a 'Feeding Center' in the Hypothalanus of the Rat," *Proceedings of the Society for Experimental Biology and Medicine* 77(1951):323–324.

36. P. Teitelbaum and A. N. Epstein, "The Lateral Hypothalamic Syndrome: Recovery of Feeding and Drinking after Lateral Hypothalamic Lesions," *Psychological Review* 69(1962):74–90.

37. J. F. Marshall and P. Teitelbaum, "Further Analysis of Sensory Inattention Following Lateral Hypothalamic Damage in Rats," *Journal of Comparative and Physiological Psychology*

86(1974):375–395.

38. Hoebel and Teitelbaum, "Hypothalamic Control of Feeding."

39. Stellar, "The Physiology of Motivation."

40. T. L. Powley, "The Ventromedial Hypothalamic Syndrome, Satiety, and a Cephalic Phase Hypothesis," *Psychological Review* 84(1977):89–126.

A. Sclafani and A. Kirchgessner, "The Role of the Medial Hypothalamus in the Control of Food Intake: An Update," in *Feeding Behavior: Neural and Humoral Controls*, eds. R. C. Ritter, S. Ritter, and C. D. Barnes, New York: Academic Press, 1986.

41. S. F. Leibowitz, "Hypothalamic Neurotransmitters in Relation to Normal and Disturbed Eating Patterns," in *Human Obesity*, eds. R. J. Wurtman and J. J. Wurtman, New York: New York Academy of Sciences, 1987.

42. W. Wyrwicka, *Brain and Feeding Behavior*, Springfield, IL: Charles C. Thomas, 1988.

43. J. R. Stellar and E. Stellar, *The Neurobiology of Motivation and Reward*, New York: Springer-Verlag, 1985.

44. S. P. Grossman, D. Dacey, A. E. Halaris, T. Collier, and A. Routtenberg, "Aphagia and Adipsia after Preferential Destruction of Nerve Cell Bodies in the Hypothalamus," *Science* 202(1978):537–539.

45. E. M. Stricker, "The Central Control of Food Intake: A Role for Insulin," in *The Neural Basis of Feeding and Reward*, eds. B. G. Hoebel and D. Novin, Brunswick, ME: Haer Institute for Electrophysiological Research, 1982.

46. M. R. Rosenzweig and A. L. Leiman, *Physiological Psychology*, Lexington, MA: D. C. Heath, 1982.

47. R. D. Myers and M. L. McCaleb, "Feeding: Satiety Signal from Intestine Triggers Brain's Noradrenergic Mechanism," *Science* 209(1980):1035–1037.

48. S. P. Grossman, "The Biology of Motivation," *Annual Review of Psychology* 30(1979):209–242.

Powley, "The Ventromedial Hypothalamic Syndrome."

49. Stellar and Stellar, *The Neurobiology of Motivation and Reward*.

50. Ibid.

J. Le Magnen, *Hunger*, Cambridge, Great Britain: Cambridge University Press, 1985.

51. Powley, "The Ventromedial Hypothalamic Syndrome."

H. P. Weingarten and T. L. Powley, "Ventromedial Hypothalamic Lesions Elevate Basal and Cephalic Phase Gastric Acid Output," *American Journal of Physiology* 239(1980):G221–G229.

52. Le Magnen, *Hunger*.

M. Saito, Y. Minokoshi, and T. Shimazu, "Brown Adipose Tissue After Ventromedial Hypothalamic Lesions in Rats," *American Journal of Physiology* 248(1985):E20–E25.

53. Le Magnen, *Hunger*.

Stellar and Stellar, *The Neurobiology of Motivation and Reward*.

54. Powley, "The Ventromedial Hypothalamic Syndrome."

55. Ibid.

P. E. Sawchenko, "Anatomic Relationships between the Paraventricular Nucleus of the Hypothalamus and Visceral Regulatory Mechanisms: Implications for the Control of Feeding," in *The Neural Basis of Feeding and Reward*, eds. B. G. Hoebel and D. Novin, Brunswick, ME: Haer Institute for Electrophysiological Research, 1982.

Sclafani and Kirchgessner, "The Role of the Medial Hypothalamus."

56. Ibid.

57. J. E. Cox and T. L. Powley, "Intragastric Pair Feeding Fails to Prevent VMH Obesity or Hyperinsulinemia," *American Journal of Physiology* 240(1981):E566–E572.

58. D. A. Booth, F. M. Toates, and S. V. Platt, "Control System for Hunger and Its Implications in Animals and Man," in *Hunger: Basic Mechanisms and Clinical Implications*, eds. D. Novin, W. Wyrwicka, and G. A. Bray, New York: Raven Press, 1976.

59. Ibid., p. 133.

60. G. Collier, "The Dialogue between the House Economist and the Resident Physiologist," *Nutrition and Behavior* 3(1986):9–26.

Leibowitz, "Hypothalamic Neurotransmitters."

61. W. Van Vort and G. P. Smith, "Sham Feeding Experience Produces a Conditioned Increase of Meal Size," *Appetite* 9(1987):21–29.

62. P. M. Fedorchak and R. C. Bolles, "Nutritive Expectancies Mediate Cholecystokinin's Suppression-of-Intake Effect," *Behavioral Neuroscience* 102(1988):451–455.

63. L. L. Birch, L. McPhee, S. Sullivan, and S. Johnson, "Conditioned Meal Initiation in Young Children," *Appetite* 13(1989):105–113.

64. J. A. Hogan, "Homeostasis and Be-

haviour," in *Analysis of Motivational Processes,* eds. F. M. Toates and T. R. Halliday, London: Academic Press, 1980.

65. G. H. Collier and C. K. Rovee-Collier, "An Ecological Perspective of Reinforcement and Motivation," in *Handbook of Behavioral Neurobiology,* vol. 6, eds. E. Satinoff and P. Teitelbaum, New York: Plenum, 1983.

Hogan, "Homeostasis and Behaviour."

R. E. Keesey and T. L. Powley, "The Regulation of Body Weight," *Annual Review of Psychology* 37(1986):109–133.

N. Mrosovsky and D. F. Sherry, "Animal Anorexias," *Science* 207(1980):837–842.

66. Hogan, "Homeostasis and Behaviour."

67. H. Bruch, *Eating Disorders,* New York: Basic Books, 1973.

68. H. F. Harlow, "The Nature of Love," *American Psychologist* 13(1958):673–685.

69. Bruch, *Eating Disorders.*

70. A. Thomas, S. Chess, and H. G. Birch, "The Origin of Personality," *Scientific American* 223(2)(1970):102–109.

71. Bruch, *Eating Disorders.*

72. G. A. Lucas and W. Timberlake, "Interpellet Delay and Meal Patterns in the Rat," *Physiology and Behavior* 43(1988):259–264.

73. J. E. R. Staddon, "Obesity and the Operant Regulation of Feeding," in *Analysis of Motivational Processes,* eds. F. M. Toates and T. R. Halliday, London: Academic Press, 1980, p. 105.

Chapter 3: Thirst

1. E. F. Adolph, "Water Metabolism," *Annual Review of Physiology* 9(1947):381–408.

N. Kleitman, "The Effect of Starvation on the Daily Consumption of Water by the Dog," *American Journal of Physiology* 81(1927):336–340.

2. D. Engell, "Interdependency of Food and Water Intake in Humans," *Appetite* 10(1988):133–141.

S. Lepkovsky, R. Lyman, D. Fleming, M. Nagumo, and M. M. Dimick, "Gastrointestinal Regulation of Water and Its Effect on Food Intake and Rate of Digestion," *American Journal of Physiology* 188(1957):327–331.

3. Lepkovsky et al., "Gastrointestinal Regulation of Water."

4. H. A. Guthrie, *Introductory Nutrition,* Saint Louis: C. V. Mosby, 1975.

5. E. M. Stricker and J. G. Verbalis, "Hormones and Behavior: The Biology of Thirst and Sodium Appetite," *American Scientist* 76(3)(1988):261–267.

6. B. J. Rolls and E. T. Rolls, *Thirst,* New York: Cambridge University Press, 1982.

7. J. T. Fitzsimons, "Drinking by Rats Depleted of Body Fluid without Increase in Osmotic Pressure," *Journal of Physiology* 159(1961):297–309.

P. J. D. Russell, A. E. Abdelaal, and G. J. Mogenson, "Graded Levels of Hemorrhage, Thirst and Angiotensin II in the Rat," *Physiology and Behavior* 15(1975):117–119.

8. Rolls and Rolls, *Thirst.*

9. J. T. Fitzsimons, "Thirst," *Physiological Reviews* 52(1972):468–561.

10. Rolls and Rolls, *Thirst.*

11. Ibid.

12. K. Oatley, "Dissociation of the Circadian Drinking Pattern from Eating," *Nature* 229(1971):494–496

13. Engell, "Interdependency of Food and Water Intake in Humans."

14. Rolls and Rolls, *Thirst.*

15. R. S. Weisinger, "Conditioned and Pseudoconditioned Thirst and Sodium Appetite," in *Control Mechanisms of Drinking,* eds. G. Peters, J. T. Fitzsimons, and L. Peters-Haefeli, Berlin: Springer-Verlag, 1975.

16. F. M. Toates, "Homeostasis and Drinking," *Behavioral and Brain Sciences* 2(1979):95–139.

17. J. L. Falk, "The Nature and Determinants of Adjunctive Behavior," *Physiology and Behavior* 6(1971):577–588.

18. T. F. Doyle and H. H. Samson, "Schedule-Induced Drinking in Humans: A Potential Factor in Excessive Alcohol Use," *Drug and Alcohol Dependence* 16(1985):117–132.

19. W. B. Cannon, "The Physiological Basis of Thirst," *Proceedings of the Royal Society, London* 90(1917-1918):283–301.

W. B. Cannon, "Hunger and Thirst," in *The Foundations of Experimental Psychology,* ed. C. Murchison, Worcester, MA: Clark University Press, 1929.

20. E. F. Adolph, *Physiology of Man in the Desert,* New York: Hafner, 1969.

21. Rolls and Rolls, *Thirst.*

22. N. E. Miller, R. I. Sampliner, and P. Woodrow, "Thirst-Reducing Effects of Water by Stomach Fistula vs. Water by Mouth Measured by Both a Consummatory and an Instrumental Response," *Journal of Comparative and Physiologi-*

cal Psychology 50(1957):1–5.

23. R. T. Bellows, "Time Factors in Water Drinking in Dogs," *American Journal of Physiology* 125(1939):87–97.

24. M. F. Montgomery, "The Role of the Salivary Glands in the Thirst Mechanism," *American Journal of Physiology* 96(1931):221–227.

F. R. Steggerda, "Observations on the Water Intake in an Adult Man with Dysfunctioning Salivary Glands," *American Journal of Physiology* 132(1941):517–521.

25. Fitzsimons, "Thirst."

Rolls and Rolls, *Thirst.*

26. B. Andersson, "Polydipsia Caused by Intrahypothalamic Injections of Hypertonic NaCl-Solutions," *Experientia* 8(1952):157–158.

B. Andersson, "The Effect of Injections of Hypertonic NaCl-Solutions into Different Parts of the Hypothalamus of Goats," *Acta Physiologica Scandinavica* 28(1953):188–201.

B. Andersson and S. M. McCann, "A Further Study of Polydipsia Evoked by Hypothalamic Stimulation in the Goat," *Acta Physiological Scandinavica* 33(1955):333–346.

27. B. Andersson and S. M. McCann, "Drinking, Antidiuresis and Milk Ejection from Electrical Stimulation within the Hypothalamus of the Goat," *Acta Physiologica Scandinavica* 35(1955):191–201.

28. P. Teitelbaum, "Disturbances in Feeding and Drinking Behavior after Hypothalamic Lesions," in *Nebraska Symposium on Motivation,* ed. M. R. Jones, Lincoln: University of Nebraska Press, 1961.

P. Teitelbaum and A. N. Epstein, "The Lateral Hypothalamic Syndrome: Recovery of Feeding and Drinking after Lateral Hypothalamic Lesions," *Psychological Review* 69(1962):74–90.

29. Rolls and Rolls, *Thirst.*

30. Rolls and Rolls, *Thirst.*

Russell, Abdelaal, and Mogenson, "Graded Levels of Hemorrhage."

31. Rolls and Rolls, *Thirst.*

32. I. Kupfermann, "Hypothalamus and Limbic System II: Motivation," in *Principles of Neural Science,* 2nd ed., eds. E. R. Kandel and J. H. Schwartz, New York: Elsevier, 1985.

33. Stricker and Verbalis, "Hormones and Behavior: The Biology of Thirst and Sodium Appetite."

34. Toates, "Homeostasis and Drinking."

35. Falk, "The Nature and Determinants of Adjunctive Behavior."

36. F. S. Kraly, "Physiology of Drinking Elicited by Eating," *Psychological Review* 91(1984):478–490.

F. S. Kraly, "Histamine: A Role in Normal Drinking," *Appetite* 6(1985):153–158.

37. B. J. Rolls and P. A. Phillips, "Aging and Disturbances of Thirst and Fluid Balance," *Nutrition Reviews* 48 (1990):137–144.

38. Kraly, "Physiology of Drinking Elicited by Eating."

Chapter 4: Taste and Smell

1. F. A. Geldard, *The Human Senses,* New York: John Wiley & Sons, 1972.

2. T. Engen, *The Perception of Odors,* New York: Academic Press, 1982.

3. C. Pfaffmann, M. Frank, and R. Norgren, "Neural Mechanisms and Behavioral Aspects of Taste," *Annual Review of Psychology* 3(1979):283–325.

4. J. G. Beebe-Center, "Standards for Use of the Gust Scale," *The Journal of Psychology* 28(1949):411–419.

5. J. Garcia, F. R. Ervin, and R. A. Koelling, "Learning with Prolonged Delay of Reinforcement," *Psychonomic Science* 5(1966):121–122.

6. Pfaffmann et al., "Neural Mechanisms and Behavioral Aspects of Taste."

7. Ibid.

M. Cabanac, "Physiological Role of Pleasure," *Science* 173(1971):1103–1107.

8. J. E. Steiner, "Facial Expressions of the Neonate Infant Indicating the Hedonics of Food-Related Chemical Stimuli," in *Taste and Development,* ed. J. M. Weiffenbach, Bethesda, MD: United States Department of Health, Education and Welfare, 1977.

9. W. R. Uttal, *The Psychobiology of Sensory Coding,* New York: Harper & Row, 1973.

10. Ibid.

11. H. Henning (1916), cited in Geldard, *The Human Senses.*

12. Geldard, *The Human Senses.*

L. M. Bartoshuk, "Taste," in *Stevens' Handbook of Experimental Psychology,* 2nd ed., vol. 1, eds. R. C. Atkinson, R. J. Herrnstein, G. Lindzey, and R. D. Luce, New York: John Wiley & Sons, 1988.

13. Ibid.

14. Uttal, *The Psychobiology of Sensory Coding.*

15. Bartoshuk, "Taste."

16. C. Pfaffmann, "Gustatory Afferent Impulses," *Journal of Cellular and Comparative Psychology* 17(1941):243–258.

17. C. Pfaffmann, "Gustatory Nerve Impulses in Rat, Cat and Rabbit," *Journal of Neurophysiology* 18(1955):429–440.

18. Bartoshuk, "Taste."

19. Pfaffmann et al., "Neural Mechanisms and Behavioral Aspects of Taste."

20. Ibid.

21. K. Arvidson and U. Friberg, "Human Taste: Response and Taste Bud Number in Fungiform Papillae," *Science* 209(1980):807–808.

22. Bartoshuk, "Taste."

V. F. Castellucci, "The Chemical Senses: Taste and Smell," in *Principles of Neural Science*, 2nd ed., eds. E. R. Kandel and J. H. Schwartz, New York:Elsevier, 1985.

D. V. Smith, "Brainstem Processing of Gustatory Information," in *Taste, Olfaction, and the Central Nervous System*, ed. D. W. Pfaff, New York: Rockefeller University Press, 1985.

23. V. G. Dethier, "Other Tastes, Other Worlds," *Science* 201(1978):224–228. D. H. McBurney and J. F. Gent, "On the Nature of Taste Qualities," *Psychological Bulletin* 86(1979):151–167.

24. L. Bartoshuk, "Separate Worlds of Taste," *Psychology Today* 14(4)(1980):48–63.

25. L. M. Beidler, "Anion Influences on Taste Receptor Response," in *Olfaction and Taste II*, ed. T. Hayashi, Oxford, Great Britain: Pergamon, 1967.

26. Uttal, *The Psychobiology of Sensory Coding.*

27. Bartoshuk, "Taste."

28. Ibid.

29. Ibid.

30. L. M. Bartoshuk, G. P. Dateo, D. J. Vandenbelt, R. L. Buttrick, and L. Long, "Effects of Gymnema Sylvestre and Synsepalum Dulcificum on Taste in Man," in *Olfaction and Taste: Proceedings of the Third International Symposium*, ed. C. Pfaffman, New York: Rockefeller University Press, 1969.

K. Kurihara, Y. Kurihara, and L. M. Beidler, "Isolation and Mechanism of Taste Modifiers; Taste-Modifying Protein and Gymnemic Acids," in *Olfaction and Taste: Proceedings of the Third International Symposium*, ed. C. Pfaffman, New York: Rockefeller University Press, 1969.

R. M. Warren and C. Pfaffmann, "Suppression of Sweet Sensitivity by Potassium Gymnemate," *Journal of Applied Physiology* 14(1959):40–42.

31. G. Borg, H. Diamant, B. Oakley, L. Strom, and Y. Zotterman, "A Comparative Study of Neural and Psychophysical Responses to Gustatory Stimuli," in *Olfaction and Taste II*, ed. T. Hayashi, Oxford, Great Britain: Pergamon, 1963.

32. Bartoshuk, "Separate Worlds of Taste."

Bartoshuk et al., "Effects of Gymnema Sylvestre and Synsepalum Dulcificum."

G. J. Henning, J. N. Brouwer, H. van der Well, and A. Francke, "Miraculin, the Sweetness-Inducing Principle from Miracle Fruit," in *Olfaction and Taste: Proceedings of the Third International Symposium*, ed. C. Pfaffman, New York: Rockefeller University Press, 1969.

Kurihara et al., "Isolation and Mechanism of Taste Modifiers."

33. Bartoshuk, "Taste."

L. M. Bartoshuk, "Bitter Taste of Saccharin Related to the Genetic Ability to Taste the Bitter Substance 6-n-Propylthiouracil," *Science* 205(1979):934–935.

H. Kalmus, "Inherited Sense Defects," *Scientific American* 186(5)(1952):64–70.

34. Ibid.

35. J. E. Amoore, *Molecular Basis of Odor,* Springfield, Illinois: Charles C. Thomas, 1970.

Engen, *The Perception of Odors.*

36. J. E. Amoore, "Olfactory Genetics and Anosmia," in *Handbook of Sensory Physiology*, vol. 4, New York: Springer-Verlag, 1971.

37. J. E. Amoore, J. W. Johnston, and M. Rubin, "The Stereochemical Theory of Odor," *Scientific American* 210(2)(1964):42–49.

Uttal, *The Psychobiology of Sensory Coding.*

38. W. S. Cain, "Olfaction," in *Stevens' Handbook of Experimental Psychology*, 2nd ed., vol. 1, eds. R. C. Atkinson, R. J. Herrnstein, G. Lindzey, and R. D. Luce, New York: John Wiley & Sons, 1988.

39. Cain, "Olfaction."

Engen, *The Perception of Odors.*

40. J. R. Mason, L. Clark, and T. H. Morton, "Selective Deficits in the Sense of Smell Caused by Chemical Modification of the Olfactory Epithelium," *Science* 226(1984):1092–1094.

41. Cain, "Olfaction."

42. Ibid.

43 M. M. Mozell and D. E. Hornung, "Peripheral Mechanisms in the Olfactory Process," in *Taste, Olfaction, and the Central Nervous System*, ed. D. W. Pfaff, New York: Rockefeller University Press, 1985.

44. Cain, "Olfaction."

45. G. M. Shepherd, "Are There Labeled Lines in the Olfactory Pathway?" in *Taste, Olfaction, and the Central Nervous System*, ed. D. W. Pfaff, New York: Rockefeller University Press, 1985.

46. P. Booth, M. B. Kohns, and S. Kamath, "Taste Acuity and Aging: A Review," *Nutrition Research* 2(1982):95–109.

B. J. Cowart, "Development of Taste Perception in Humans: Sensitivity and Preference throughout the Life Span," *Psychological Bulletin* 90(1981):43–73.

B. J. Cowart, "Relationships between Taste and Smell across the Adult Life Span," in *Nutrition and the Chemical Senses in Aging: Recent Advances and Current Research Needs*, eds. C. Murphy, W. S. Cain, and D. M. Hegsted, New York: New York Academy of Sciences, 1989.

D. A. Stevens and H. L. Lawless, "Age-Related Changes in Flavor Perception," *Appetite* 2(1981):127–136.

47. L. M. Bartoshuk, "Taste: Robust Across the Age Span?" in *Nutrition and the Chemical Senses in Aging: Recent Advances and Current Research Needs*, eds. C. Murphy, W. S. Cain, and D. M. Hegsted, New York: New York Academy of Sciences, 1989.

48. A. N. Gilbert and C. J. Wysocki, "The Smell Survey," *National Geographic* 172(October 1987):514–525.

49. B. J Cowart, "Relationships between Taste and Smell."

J. C. Stevens, L. M. Bartoshuk, and W. S. Cain, "Chemical Senses and Aging: Taste versus Smell," *Chemical Senses* 9(1984):167–179.

50. R. L. Doty, P. Shaman, S. L. Applebaum, R. Giberson, L. Siksorski, and L. Rosenberg, "Smell Identification Ability: Changes with Age" *Science* 226(1984):1441–1443.

51. C. J. Wysocki and A. N. Gilbert, "National Geographic Smell Survey: Effects of Age are Heterogenous," in *Nutrition and the Chemical Senses in Aging: Recent Advances and Current Research Needs*, eds. C. Murphy, W. S. Cain, and D. M. Hegsted, New York: New York Academy of Sciences, 1989.

52. R. L. Doty, "Influence of Age and Age-Related Diseases on Olfactory Function," in *Nutrition and the Chemical Senses in Aging: Recent Advances and Current Research Needs*, eds C. Murphy, W. S. Cain, and D. M. Hegsted, New York: New York Academy of Sciences, 1989.

53. Engen, *The Perception of Odors.*

54 H. B. Hubert, R. R. Fabsitz, M. Feinleib, and K. S. Brown, "Olfactory Sensitivity in Humans: Genetic versus Environmental Control," *Science* 208(1980):607–609.

55. W. S. Cain, "To Know with the Nose: Keys to Odor Identification," *Science* 203(1979):467–470.

M. D. Rabin and W. S. Cain, "Odor recognition: Familiarity, Identifiability, and Encoding Consistency," *Journal of Experimental Psychology: Learning, Memory, and Cognition* 10(1984):316–325.

56. W. S. Cain, "To Know with the Nose."

57. S. S. Schiffman and Z. S. Warwick, "Use of Flavor-Amplified Foods to Improve Nutritional Status in Elderly Persons," in *Nutrition and the Chemical Senses in Aging: Recent Advances and Current Research Needs*, eds. C. Murphy, W. S. Cain, and D. M. Hegsted, New York: New York Academy of Sciences, 1989.

58. Doty et al., "Smell Identification Ability."

Chapter 5: Genetic Contributions to Food Preferences

1. M. Dowd, "'I'm President,' So No More Broccoli!" *The New York Times* (March 23, 1990):A14.

J. Nisbet, "22 Celebs Bellyache about the Worst Food They Were Ever Asked to Eat," *Moneysworth* (March 1980):14–15.

C. Trillin, "Crescent City, Fla.: Just Try It," *The New Yorker* (May 31, 1982):68, 70–73.

2. J. Brody, *Jane Brody's Nutrition Book*, New York: W. W. Norton, 1981.

U. S. Department of Health and Human Services, *The Surgeon General's Report on Nutrition and Health: Summary and Recommendations* (DHHS Publication No. 88-50211), Washington, DC: U. S. Government Printing Office, 1988.

3. D. M. H. Thomsom, "Meeting Report: The Psychology of Food," *Appetite* 13(1989):229–232.

4. J. Money and A. A. Ehrhardt, *Man and Woman, Boy and Girl*, Baltimore, MD: Johns Hopkins University Press, 1972.

5. M. A. Einstein and I. Hornstein, "Food Preferences of College Students and Nutritional Implications," *Journal of Food Science* 35(1970):429–436.

H. L. Meiselman, "The Role of Sweetness in the Food Preference of Young Adults," in *Taste and Development*, ed. J. M. Weiffenbach, Bethesda,

MD: U.S. Department of Health, Education, and Welfare, 1977.

H. L. Meiselman, W. Van Horne, B. Hasenzahl, and T. Wehrly, *The 1971 Fort Lewis Food Preference Survey*, Natick, MA: United States Army Natick Laboratories, 1972.

H. L. Meiselman, D. Waterman, and L. E. Symington, *Armed Forces Food Preferences*, Natick, MA: United States Army Natick Development Center, 1974

D. R. Peryam, B. W. Polemis, J. M. Kamen, J. Eindhoven, and F. J. Pilgrim, *Food Preferences of Men in the U.S. Armed Forces*, Chicago: Quartermaster Food and Container Institute for the Armed Forces, 1960.

6. E. D. Capaldi, J. P. Bradford, J. D. Sheffer, and R. J. Pulley, "The Rat's Sweet Tooth," *Learning and Motivation* 20(1989):178–190.

C. Pfaffmann, "Biological and Behavioral Substrates of the Sweet Tooth," in *Taste and Development*, ed. J. M. Weiffenbach, Bethesda, MD: U.S. Department of Health, Education, and Welfare, 1977.

7. Pfaffmann, "Biological and Behavioral Substrates."

Brody, *Jane Brody's Nutrition Book.*

8. S. M. Garn and W. R. Leonard, "What Did Our Ancestors Eat?" *Nutrition Reviews* 47(1989):337–345.

M. Konner, "What Our Ancestors Ate," *The New York Times Magazine* (June 5, 1988):54–55.

9. M. Konner, "What Our Ancestors Ate."

P. Rozin, "The Selection of Foods by Rats, Humans, and Other Animals," in *Advances in the Study of Behavior*, vol. 6, eds. J. S. Rosenblatt, R. A. Hinde, E. Shaw, and C. Beer, New York: Academic Press, 1976.

P. Rozin, "Human Food Selection: The Interaction of Biology, Culture and Individual Experience," in *The Psychobiology of Human Food Selection*, ed. L. M. Barker, Westport, CT: AVI Publishing, 1982.

10. Brody, *Jane Brody's Nutrition Book.*

11. H. A. Guthrie, *Introductory Nutrition*, St. Louis: C. V. Mosby, 1975.

12. J. A. Desor, O. Maller, and R. E. Turner, "Taste in Acceptance of Sugars by Human Infants," *Journal of Comparative and Physiological Psychology* 84(1973):496–501.

13. N. W. Jerome, "Taste Experience and the Development of a Dietary Preference for Sweet in Humans: Ethnic and Cultural Variations in Early Taste Experience," in *Taste and Development*, ed. J.

M. Weiffenbach, Bethesda, MD: U.S. Department of Health, Education, and Welfare, 1977.

14. R. R. Bell, H. H. Draper, and J. G. Bergan, "Sucrose, Lactose, and Glucose Tolerance in Northern Alaskan Eskimos," *The American Journal of Clinical Nutrition* 26(1973):1185–1190.

G. J. Mouratoff, N. V. Carroll, and E. M. Scott, "Diabetes Mellitus in Eskimos," *The Journal of the American Medical Association* 199(1967):107–112.

15. J. E. Steiner, "Facial Expressions of the Neonate Infant Indicating the Hedonics of Food-Related Chemical Stimuli," in *Taste and Development*, ed. J. M. Weiffenbach, Bethesda, MD: U.S. Department of Health, Education, and Welfare, 1977.

16. Steiner, "Facial Expressions of the Neonate," pp. 174–175.

17. T. M. Field, R. Woodson, R. Greenberg, and D. Cohen, "Discrimination and Imitation of Facial Expressions by Neonates," *Science* 218(1982):179–181.

18. H. J. Grill and R. Norgren, "Chronically Decerebrate Rats Demonstrate Satiation but Not Bait Shyness," *Science* 201(1978):267–269.

19. Jerome, "Taste Experience and the Development of a Dietary Preference."

20. Guthrie, *Introductory Nutrition.*

21. J. E. R. Staddon, *Adaptive Behavior and Learning*, Cambridge, Great Britain: Cambridge University Press, 1983.

22. G. K. Beauchamp and M. Moran, "Dietary Experience and Sweet Taste Preference in Human Infants," *Appetite* 3(1982):139–152.

23. J. J. Wurtman and R. J. Wurtman, "Sucrose Consumption Early in Life Fails to Modify the Appetite of Adult Rats for Sweet Foods," *Science* 205(1979):321–322.

24. M. Frank, "The Distinctiveness of Responses to Sweet in the Chorda Tympani Nerve," in *Taste and Development*, ed. J. M. Weiffenbach, Bethesda, MD: U.S. Department of Health, Education, and Welfare, 1977.

25. R. Coopersmith and M. Leon, "Enhanced Neural Response to Familiar Olfactory Cues," *Science* 225(1984):849–851.

26. J. A. Desor, L. S. Greene, and O. Maller, "Preferences for Sweet and Salty in 9- to 15-Year Old and Adult Humans," *Science* 190(1975):686–687.

27. Wurtman and Wurtman, "Sucrose Consumption Early in Life."

28. A. W. Logue and M. E. Smith, "Predictors of Food Preferences in Humans," *Appetite*

7(1986):109–125.

29. J. A. Desor and G. K. Beauchamp, "Longitudinal Changes in Sweet Preferences in Humans," *Physiology and Behavior* 39(1987):639–641.

30. A. Drewnowski, "Sensory Preferences for Fat and Sugar in Adolescent and Adult Life," in *Nutrition and the Chemical Senses in Aging: Recent Advances and Current Research Needs*, eds. C. Murphy, W. S. Cain, and D. M. Hegsted, New York: New York Academy of Sciences, 1989.

31. Desor et al., "Preferences for Sweet and Salty."

32. B. K. Giza and T. R. Scott, "Blood Glucose Selectively Affects Taste-Evoked Activity in Rat Nucleus Tractus Solitarius," *Physiology and Behavior* 31(1983):643–650.

33. R. E. Nisbett and S. B. Gurwitz, "Weight, Sex and the Eating Behavior of Human Newborns," *Journal of Comparative and Physiological Psychology* 73(1970):245–253.

34. Desor et al., "Taste in Acceptance of Sugars by Human Infants."

J. Dubignon, D. Campbell, M. Curtis, and M. W. Partington, "The Relation between Laboratory Measures of Sucking, Food Intake, and Perinatal Factors During the Newborn Period," *Child Development* 40(1969):1107–1120.

35. Logue and Smith, "Predictors of Food Preferences in Humans."

36. L. S. Greene, J. A. Desor, and O. Maller, "Heredity and Experience: Their Relative Importance in the Development of Taste Preference in Man," *Journal of Comparative and Physiological Psychology* 89(1975):279–284.

37. M. T. Conner and D. A. Booth, "Preferred Sweetness of a Lime Drink and Preference for Sweet over Non-Sweet Foods, Related to Sex and Reported Age and Body Weight," *Appetite* 10(1988):25–35.

H. Tuorila-Ollikainen and S. Mahlamaki-Kultanen, "The Relationship of Attitudes and Experiences of Finnish Youths to Their Hedonic Responses to Sweetness in Soft Drinks," *Appetite* 6(1985):115–124.

38. Bell et al., "Sucrose, Lactose, and Glucose Tolerance."

R. H. Larson, "Sugar Ingestion and Caries," in *Taste and Development*, ed. J. M. Weiffenbach, Bethesda, MD: U.S. Department of Health, Education, and Welfare, 1977.

39. Meiselman et al., *The 1971 Fort Lewis Food Preference Survey.*

40. Bell et al., "Sucrose, Lactose, and Glucose Tolerance."

41. B. G. Galef, "Mechanisms for the Transmission of Acquired Patterns of Feeding from Adult to Weanling Rats," in *Taste and Development*, ed. J. M. Weiffenbach, Bethesda, MD: U.S. Department of Health, Education, and Welfare, 1977.

B. G. Galef, "Communication of Information concerning Distant Diets in a Social, Central-Place Foraging Species: *Rattus Norvegicus*," in *Social Learning: Psychological and Biological Perspectives*, eds. T. R. Zentall and B. G. Galef, Hillsdale, NJ: Lawrence Erlbaum Associates, 1988.

42. L. L. Birch, "Effects of Peer Models' Food Choices and Eating Behaviors on Preschoolers' Food Preferences," *Child Development* 51(1980):489–496.

L. L. Birch, "Children's Food Preferences: Developmental Patterns and Environmental Influences," in *Annals of Child Development*, ed. R. Vasta, Greenwich, CT: JAI Press, 1987.

L. L. Birch, S. I. Zimmerman, and H. Hind, "The Influence of Social-Affective Context on the Formation of Children's Food Preferences," *Child Development* 51(1980):856–861.

43. J. Yudkin, "Patterns and Trends in Carbohydrate Consumption and Their Relation to Disease," *Nutrition Society Proceedings* 23(1964):149–162.

44. G. K. Beauchamp and B. J. Cowart, "Congenital and Experiential Factors in the Development of Human Flavor Preferences," *Appetite* 6(1985):357–372.

45. Greene et al., "Heredity and Experience."

46. M. Krondl, P. Coleman, J. Wade, and J. Milner, "A Twin Study Examining the Genetic Influence on Food Selection," *Human Nutrition: Applied Nutrition* 37A(1983):189–198.

47. M. Nachman, "The Inheritance of Saccharin Preference," *Journal of Comparative and Physiological Psychology* 52(1959):451–457.

48. M. R. Bloch, "The Social Influence of Salt," in *Human Nutrition*, San Francisco: W. H. Freeman and Company, 1978.

D. Denton, *The Hunger for Salt*, New York: Springer-Verlag, 1982.

49. Bloch, "The Social Influence of Salt."

50. Denton, *The Hunger for Salt.*

51. C. P. Richter, "Salt Appetite of Mammals: Its Dependence on Instinct and Metabolism," in *L'Instinct dans le comportement des animaux et de l'homme*, ed. Fondation Singer-Polignac, Paris: Masson, 1956.

52. Denton, *The Hunger for Salt.*
Richter, "Salt Appetite of Mammals."
53. Richter, "Salt Appetite of Mammals."
54. Denton, *The Hunger for Salt.*
A. N. Epstein, "Hormonal Synergy as the Cause of Salt Appetite," in *The Physiology of Thirst and Sodium Appetite,* eds. G. de Caro, A. N. Epstein, and M. Massi, New York: Plenum, 1986.
55. R. J. Contreras and M. Frank, "Sodium Deprivation Alters Neural Responses to Gustatory Stimuli," *The Journal of General Physiology* 73(1979):569–594.
56. B. G. Galef, "Social Interaction Modifies Learned Aversions, Sodium Appetite, and Both Palatability and Handling-Time Induced Dietary Preference in Rats (*Rattus Norvegicus*)," *Journal of Comparative Psychology* 100(1986):432–439.
57. U. Roze, "How to Select, Climb, and Eat a Tree," *Natural History* (May 1985):63–69.
58. L. Wilkins and C. P. Richter, "A Great Craving for Salt by a Child with Cortico-Adrenal Insufficiency," *Journal of the American Medical Association* 114(1940):866–868.
59. Desor et al., "Preferences for Sweet and Salty."
60. U. S. Department of Health and Human Services, *The Surgeon General's Report on Nutrition and Health.*
61. Denton, *The Hunger for Salt.*
62. Rozin, "The Selection of Foods by Rats, Humans, and Other Animals."
63. G. K. Beauchamp, "The Human Preference for Excess Salt," *American Scientist* 75(1)(1987):27–33.
G. K. Beauchamp, B. J. Cowart, and M. Moran, "Developmental Changes in Salt Acceptability in Human Infants," *Developmental Psychobiology* 19(1986):17–25.
64. G. K. Beauchamp, M. Bertino, and K. Engelman, "Failure to Compensate Decreased Dietary Sodium with Increased Table Salt Usage," *Journal of the American Medical Association* 258(1987):3275–3278.
R. Shepherd, C. A. Farleigh, and S. G. Wharf, "Limited Compensation by Table Salt for Reduced Salt within a Meal," *Appetite* 13(1989):193–200.
65. N. Kretchmer, "Lactose and Lactase," in *Human Nutrition,* San Francisco: W. H. Freeman and Company, 1978.
66. Ibid.
67. Ibid.
F. J. Simoons, "Geography and Genetics as Factors in the Psychobiology of Human Food Selection," in *The Psychobiology of Human Food Selection,* ed. L. M. Barker, Westport, CT: AVI Publishing, 1982.
68. Kretchmer, "Lactose and Lactase."
69. Ibid.
70. "Season, Latitude, and Ability of Sunlight to Promote Synthesis of Vitamin D3 in Skin," *Nutrition Reviews* 47(1989):252–253.
71. Simoons, "Geography and Genetics as Factors."
72. M. L. Pelchat and P. Rozin, "The Special Role of Nausea in the Acquisition of Food Dislikes by Humans," *Appetite* 3(1982):341–351.
Rozin, "Human Food Selection."
73. R. Lewin, "Biology and Culture Meet in Milk," *Science* 211(1980):40.
74. J. Pager, "Nutritional States, Food Odors, and Olfactory Function," in *The Chemical Senses and Nutrition,* eds. M. R. Kare and O. Maller, New York: Academic Press, 1977.
75. G. D. Mower, R. G. Mair, and T. Engen, "Influence of Internal Factors on the Perceived Intensity and Pleasantness of Gustatory and Olfactory Stimuli," in *The Chemical Senses and Nutrition,* eds. M. R. Kare and O. Maller, New York: Academic Press, 1977.
76. J. J. Wurtman, "Neurotransmitter Regulation of Protein and Carbohydrate Consumption," in *Nutrition and Behavior,* ed. S. A. Miller, Philadelphia: Franklin Institute, 1981.
R. J. Wurtman and J. J. Wurtman, "Nutrients, Neurotransmitter Synthesis, and the Control of Food Intake," in *Eating and Its Disorders,* eds. A. J. Stunkard and E. Stellar, New York: Raven Press, 1984.
R. J. Wurtman and J. J. Wurtman, "Do Carbohydrates Affect Food Intake via Neurotransmitter Activity?" *Appetite* 11 Supplement(1988):42–47.
77. J. D. Fernstrom, "Food-Induced Changes in Brain Serotonin Synthesis: Is There a Relationship to Appetite for Specific Macronutrients?" *Appetite* 8(1987):163–182.
S. F. Leibowitz and G. Shor-Posner, "Brain Serotonin and Eating Behavior," *Appetite* 7 (Supplement)(1986):1–14.
78. Steiner, "Facial Expressions of the Neonate," p. 175.
79. Ibid.
80. Steiner, "Facial Expressions of the Neonate."
81. Grill and Norgren, "Chronically Decerebrate Rats Demonstrate Satiation."

82. F. A. Geldard, *The Human Senses*, New York: John Wiley & Sons, 1972.

E. V. Glanville and A. R. Kaplan, "Food Preference and Sensitivity of Taste for Bitter Compounds," *Nature* 205(1965):851–853.

Rozin, "Human Food Selection."

83. S. Y. Babayan, B. Budayr, and H. C. Lindgren, "Age, Sex, and Culture as Variables in Food Aversion," *The Journal of Social Psychology* 68(1966):15–17.

H. C. Lindgren, "Age as a Variable in Aversion," *Journal of Consulting Psychology* 26(1961):101–102.

84. Glanville and Kaplan, "Food Preference and Sensitivity of Taste."

85. Logue and Smith, "Predictors of Food Preferences in Humans."

86. M. Zuckerman, *Sensation Seeking: Beyond the Optimal Level of Arousal*, Hillsdale, NJ: Lawrence Erlbaum Associates, 1979.

87. G. B. Kish and G. V. Donnenwerth, "Sex Differences in the Correlates of Stimulus Seeking," *Journal of Consulting and Clinical Psychology*, 38(1972):42–49.

88. Logue and Smith, "Predictors of Food Preferences in Humans."

89. Zuckerman, *Sensation Seeking*.

M. Zuckerman, ed., *Biological Bases of Sensation Seeking, Impulsivity, and Anxiety*, Hillsdale, NJ: Lawrence Erlbaum Associates, 1983.

M. Zuckerman, M. S. Buchsbaum, and D. L. Murphy, "Sensation Seeking and Its Biological Correlates," *Psychological Bulletin* 88(1980):187–214.

90. B. F. Skinner, "The Phylogeny and Ontogeny of Behavior," *Science* 153(1966):1205–1213.

Chapter 6: Environmental Contributions to Food Preferences

1. N. Hrboticky and M. Krondl, "Acculturation to Canadian Foods by Chinese Immigrant Boys: Changes in the Perceived Flavor, Health Value and Prestige of Foods," *Appetite* 5(1984):117–126.

M. Krondl, N. Hrboticky, and P. Coleman, "Adapting to Cultural Changes in Food Habits," in *Malnutrition: Determinants and Consequences*, eds. P. L. White and N. Selvey, New York: Alan R.

Liss, 1984.

2. W. F. Hill, "Effects of Mere Exposure on Preferences in Nonhuman Animals," *Psychological Bulletin* 85(1978):1177–1198.

3. Hill, "Effects of Mere Exposure on Preferences in Nonhuman Animals."

R. B. Zajonc, "Attitudinal Effects of Mere Exposure," *Journal of Personality and Social Psychology* Monograph Supplement 9 (No. 2, Part 2)(1968):1–27.

4. L. Partridge, "Increased Preferences for Familiar Foods in Small Mammals," *Animal Behaviour* 29(1981):211–216.

5. G. M. Burghardt and E. H. Hess, "Food Imprinting in the Snapping Turtle, *Chelydra serpentina*," *Science* 151(1966):108–109.

6. P. Pliner, "The Effects of Mere Exposure on Liking for Edible Substances," *Appetite* 2(1982):283–290.

7. L. L. Birch, L. McPhee, B. C. Shoba, E. Pirok, and L. Steinberg, "What Kind of Exposure Reduces Children's Food Neophobia," *Appetite* 9(1987):171–178.

8. L. L. Birch and M. Deysher, "Caloric Compensation and Sensory Specific Satiety: Evidence for Self Regulation of Food Intake By Young Children," *Appetite* 7(1986):323–331.

Hill, "Effects of Mere Exposure on Preferences in Nonhuman Animals."

P. Pliner, J. Polivy, and C. P. Herman, "Short-Term Intake of Overweight Individuals and Normal Weight Dieters and Non-Dieters with and without Choice among a Variety of Foods," *Appetite* 1(1980):203–213.

9. D. J. Stang, "When Familiarity Breeds Contempt, Absence Makes the Heart Grow Fonder: Effects of Exposure and Delay on Taste Pleasantness Ratings," *Bulletin of the Psychonomic Society* 6 (1975):273–275.

10. B. J. Rolls, E. T. Rolls, and E. A. Rowe, "The Influence of Variety on Human Food Selection and Intake," in *The Psychobiology of Human Food Selection*, ed. L. M. Barker, Westport, CT: AVI Publishing, 1982.

11. M. Hetherington, B. J. Rolls, and V. J. Burley, "The Time Course of Sensory-Specific Satiety," *Appetite* 12(1989):57–68.

12. B. J. Rolls, "Experimental Analyses of the Effects of Variety in a Meal on Human Feeding," *The American Journal of Clinical Nutrition* 42(1985):932–939.

13. P. Rozin, "Specific Aversions as a Component of Specific Hungers," in *Biological Boun-*

daries of Learning, eds. M. E. P. Seligman and J. L. Hager, New York: Appleton-Century-Crofts, 1972.

P. Rozin, "The Selection of Foods by Rats, Humans, and Other Animals," in *Advances in the Study of Behavior,* vol. 6, eds. J. S. Rosenblatt, R. A. Hinde, E. Shaw, and C. Beer, New York: Academic Press, 1976.

14. Q. R. Rogers and P. M. B. Leung, "The Control of Food Intake: When and How Are Amino Acids Involved?" in *The Chemical Senses and Nutrition,* eds. M. R. Kare and O. Maller, New York: Academic Press, 1977.

15. D. M. Zahorik and K. A. Houpt, "The Concept of Nutritional Wisdom: Applicability of Laboratory Learning Models to Large Herbivores," in *Learning Mechanisms in Food Selection,* eds. L. M. Barker, M. R. Best, and M. Domjan, Waco, TX: Baylor University Press, 1977.

D. M. Zahorik and S. F. Maier, "Appetitive Conditioning with Recovery from Thiamine Deficiency as the Unconditional Stimulus," in *Biological Boundaries of Learning,* eds. M. E. P. Seligman and J. L. Hager, New York: Appleton-Century-Crofts, 1972.

16. *American Psychiatric Association: Diagnostic and Statistical Manual of Mental Disorders,* 3rd ed. rev., Washington, DC: APA, 1987, p. 69.

17. *American Psychiatric Association: Diagnostic and Statistical Manual of Mental Disorders,* 3rd ed. rev.

M. Cooper, *Pica,* Springfield, IL: Charles C. Thomas, 1957.

D. Sanjur and A. D. Scoma, "Food Habits of Low-Income Children in Northern New York," *Journal of Nutrition Education* 2(1971):85–95.

18. Cooper, *Pica.*

Rozin, "The Selection of Foods by Rats, Humans, and Other Animals."

19. R. W. Furness, "Not by Grass Alone," *Natural History* (December 1989):8, 10, 12.

20. Rozin, "The Selection of Foods by Rats, Humans, and Other Animals."

21. C. P. Richter, "Total Self Regulatory Functions in Animals and Human Beings," *The Harvey Lecturers* 38(1942–1943):63–103.

22. C. M. Davis, "Self Selection of Diet by Newly Weaned Infants," *American Journal of Disease of Children* 36(1928):651–679.

C. M. Davis, "Can Babies Choose Their Food?" *The Parents' Magazine* (January 1930):22, 23, 42, 43.

C. M. Davis, "Results of the Self-Selection of Diets by Young Children," *The Canadian Medical Association Journal* (September 1939):257–261.

23. M. A. Einstein and I. Hornstein, "Food Preferences of College Students and Nutritional Implications," *Food Science* 35(1970):429–436.

24. R. C. Bolles, L. Hayward, and C. Crandall, "Conditioned Taste Preferences Based on Caloric Density," *Journal of Experimental Psychology: Animal Behavior Processes* 7(1981):59–69.

25. S. C. Brake, "Suckling Infant Rats Learn a Preference for a Novel Olfactory Stimulus Paired with Milk Delivery," *Science* 211(1981):506–508.

D. H. Campbell, E. D. Capaldi, and D. E. Myers, "Conditioned Flavor Preferences as a Function of Deprivation Level: Preferences or Aversions?" *Animal Learning and Behavior* 15(1987):193–200.

E. D. Capaldi, D. H. Campbell, J. Sheffer, and J. P. Bradford, "Conditioned Flavor Preferences Based on Delayed Caloric Consequences," *Journal of Experimental Psychology: Animal Behavior Processes* 13(1987):150–155.

L. Hayward, "The Role of Oral and Postingestional Cues in the Conditioning of Taste Preferences Based on Differing Caloric Density and Caloric Outcome in Weanling and Mature Rats," *Animal Learning and Behavior* 11(1983):325–331.

J. A. Hogan, "The Ontogeny of Food Preferences in Chicks and Other Animals," in *Learning Mechanisms in Food Selection,* eds. L. M. Barker, M. R. Best, and M. Domjan, Waco, TX: Baylor University Press, 1977.

A. J. Hogan-Warburg and J. A. Hogan, "Feeding Strategies in the Development of Food Recognition in Young Chicks," *Animal Behaviour* 29(1981):143–154.

26. D. A. Booth, "How Nutritional Effects of Foods Can Influence People's Dietary Choices," in *The Psychobiology of Human Food Selection,* ed. L. M. Barker, Westport, CT: AVI Publishing, 1982.

D. A. Booth, P. Mather, and J. Fuller, "Starch Content of Ordinary Foods Associatively Conditions Human Appetite and Satiation, Indexed by Intake and Eating Pleasantness of Starch-Paired Flavours," *Appetite* 3(1982):163–184.

27. L. L. Birch and M. Deysher, "Conditioned and Unconditioned Caloric Compensation: Evidence for Self-Regulation of Food Intake in Young Children," *Learning and Motivation* 16(1985):341–355.

28. U. S. Department of Health and Human Services, *The Surgeon General's Report on Nutrition and Health: Summary and Recommendations* (DHHS Publication No. 88-50211), Washington, DC: U. S. Government Printing Office, 1988.

29. S. R. Overmann, "Dietary Self-Selection by Animals," *Psychological Bulletin* 83(1976):218–235.

30. Rozin, "Specific Aversions as a Component of Specific Hungers."

Rozin, "The Selection of Foods by Rats, Humans, and Other Animals."

31. A. L. Riley and C. M. Clarke, "Conditioned Taste Aversions: A Bibliography," in *Learning Mechanisms in Food Selection*, eds. L. M. Barker, M. R. Best, and M. Domjan, Waco, TX: Baylor University Press, 1977.

32. S. A. Barnett, *The Rat: A Study in Behavior*, Chicago: Aldine, 1963.

33. J. Garcia, D. J. Kimeldorf, and E. L. Hunt, "The Use of Ionizing Radiation as a Motivating Stimulus," *Psychological Review* 68(1961):383–395.

J. Garcia, D. J. Kimeldorf, and R. A. Koelling, "Conditioned Aversion to Saccharin Resulting from Exposure to Gamma Radiation," *Science* 122(1955):157–158.

R. G. Y. Robertson and J. Garcia, "X-Rays and Learned Taste Aversions: Historical and Psychological Ramifications," in *Cancer, Nutrition, and Eating Behavior*, eds. T. G. Burish, S. M. Levy, and B. E. Meyerowitz, Hillsdale, NJ: Lawrence Erlbaum Associates, 1985.

34. M. Nachman and J. H. Ashe, "Learned Taste Aversions in Rats as a Function of Dosage, Concentration, and Route of Administration of LiCl," *Physiology and Behavior* 10(1973):73–78.

35. J. Garcia, B. K. McGowan, and K. F. Green, "Biological Constraints on Conditioning," in *Biological Boundaries of Learning*, eds. M. E. P. Seligman and J. L. Hager, New York: Appleton-Century-Crofts, 1972.

36. J. Garcia and R. A. Koelling, "Relation of Cue to Consequence in Avoidance Learning," *Psychonomic Science* 4(1966):123–124.

37. Garcia et al., "Biological Constraints on Conditioning."

38. F. Etscorn and R. Stephens, "Establishment of Conditioned Taste Aversions with a 24-Hour CS–US Interval," *Physiological Psychology* 1(1973):251–253.

Garcia et al., "Biological Constraints on Conditioning."

39. Garcia et al., "Biological Constraints on Conditioning."

40. J. Garcia, W. G. Hankins, and K. W. Rusiniak, "Behavioral Regulation of the Milieu Interne in Man and Rat," *Science* 185(1974):824–831.

41. K. Clay, "Tresspassers Will Be Poisoned," *Natural History* (September 1989):8, 10, 12, 14.

42. R. C. Bolles, "The Comparative Psychology of Learning: The Selective Association Principle and Some Problems with 'General' Laws of Learning," in *Perspectives on Animal Behavior*, ed. G. Bermant, Glenview, IL: Scott, Foresman, 1973.

P. Rozin and J. W. Kalat, "Specific Hungers and Poison Avoidance as Adaptive Specializations of Learning," *Psychological Review* 78(1971):459–486.

M. E. P. Seligman, "On the Generality of the Laws of Learning," *Psychological Review* 77(1970):406–418.

S. J. Shettleworth, "Constraints on Learning," in *Advances in the Study of Behavior*, vol. 4, eds. D. S. Lehrman, R. A. Hinde, and E. Shaw, New York: Academic Press, 1972.

43. M. Domjan and B. G. Galef, "Biological Constraints on Instrumental and Classical Conditioning: Retrospect and Prospect," *Animal Learning and Behavior* 11(1983):151–161.

A. W. Logue, "Taste Aversion and the Generality of the Laws of Learning," *Psychological Bulletin* 86(1979):276–296.

S. H. Revusky, "Learning as a General Process with an Emphasis on Data from Feeding Experiments," in *Food Aversion Learning*, eds. N. W. Milgram, L. Krames, and T. M. Alloway, New York: Academic Press, 1977.

S. J. Settleworth, "Function and Mechanism in Learning," in *Advances in Analysis of Behaviour: Vol. 3. Biological Factors in Learning*, eds. M. D. Zeiler and P. Harzem, New York: John Wiley & Sons, 1983.

44. H. C. Wilcoxon, W. B. Dragoin, and P. A. Kral, "Illness-Induced Aversions in Rat and Quail: Relative Salience of Visual and Gustatory Cues," *Science* 171(1971):826–828.

45. N. S. Braveman, "Poison-Based Avoidance Learning with Flavored or Colored Water in Guinea Pigs," *Learning and Motivation* 5(1974):182–194.

N. S. Braveman, "Relative Salience of Gustatory and Visual Cues in the Formation of Poison-Based Food Aversions by Guinea Pigs (Cavia porcellus)," *Behavioral Biology* 14(1975):189–199.

46. K. L. Coburn, J. Garcia, S. W. Kiefer, and K. W. Rusiniak, "Taste Potentiation of Poisoned Odor by Temporal Contiguity," *Behavioral Neuroscience* 98(1984):813–819.

P. J. Durlach and R. A. Rescorla, "Potentiation Rather than Overshadowing in Flavor-Aversion Learning: An Analysis in Terms of Within-Compound Associations," *Journal of Experimental Psychology: Animal Behavior Processes* 6(1980):175–187.

B. G. Galef and B. Osborne, "Novel Taste Facilitation of the Association of Visual Cues with Toxicosis in Rats," *Journal of Comparative and Physiological Psychology* 92(1978):907–916.

C. R. Gustavson, "Comparative and Field Aspects of Learned Food Aversions," in *Learning Mechanisms in Food Selection*, eds. L. M. Barker, M. R. Best, and M. Domjan, Waco, TX: Baylor University Press, 1977.

B. T. Lett, "Taste Potentiates Color-Sickness Associations in Pigeons and Quail," *Animal Learning and Behavior* 8(1980):193–198.

47. C. S. Mellor and H. P. White, "Taste Aversions to Alcoholic Beverages Conditioned by Motion Sickness," *American Journal of Psychology* 135(1978):125–126.

48. S. Lamon, G. T. Wilson, and R. C. Leaf, "Human Classical Aversion Conditioning: Nausea versus Electric Shock in the Reduction of Target Beverage Consumption," *Behaviour Research and Therapy* 15(1977):313–320.

49. J. L. Garb and A. J. Stunkard, "Taste Aversions in Man," *American Journal of Psychiatry* 131(1974):1204–1207.

A. W. Logue, I. Ophir, and K. E. Strauss, "The Acquisition of Taste Aversions in Humans," *Behaviour Research and Therapy* 19(1981):319–333.

50. A. W. Logue, "Conditioned Food Aversion Learning in Humans," in *Experimental Assessments and Clinical Applications of Conditioned Food Aversions*, eds. N. S. Braveman and P. Bronstein, New York: New York Academy of Sciences, 1985.

A. W. Logue, "A Comparison of Taste Aversion Learning in Humans and Other Vertebrates: Evolutionary Pressures in Common, in *Evolution and Learning*, eds. R. C. Bolles and M. D. Beecher, Hillsdale, NJ: Lawrence Erlbaum Associates, 1988.

51. M. E. P. Seligman and J. L. Hager, eds., *Biological Boundaries of Learning*, New York: Appleton-Century-Crofts, 1972.

52. Logue et al., "The Acquisition of Taste Aversions in Humans."

53. C. R. Gustavson and J. C. Gustavson, "Predation Control Using Conditioned Food Aversion Methodology: Theory, Practice, and Implications," in *Experimental Assessments and Clinical Applications of Conditioned Food Aversions*, eds. N. S. Braveman and P. Bronstein, New York: New York Academy of Sciences, 1985.

54. J. R. Mason and R. F. Reidinger, "Con-

specific Individual Recognition between Starlings after Toxicant-Induced Sickness," *Animal Learning and Behavior* 11(1983):332–336.

55. L. P. Brower, "Ecological Chemistry," *Scientific American* (February 1969):22–29.

L. P. Brower and L. S. Fink, "A Natural Toxic Defense System: Cardenolides in Butterflies versus Birds," in *Experimental Assessments and Clinical Applications of Conditioned Food Aversions*, eds N. S. Braveman and P. Bronstein, New York: New York Academy of Sciences, 1985.

56. J. Garcia and L. P. Brett, "Conditioned Responses to Food Odor and Taste in Rats and Wild Predators," in *The Chemical Senses and Nutrition*, eds. M. R. Kare and O. Maller, New York: Academic Press, 1977.

Gustavson, "Comparative and Field Aspects of Learned Food Aversions." C. R. Gustavson, L. P. Brett, J. Garcia, and D. J. Kelly, "A Working Model and Experimental Solutions to the Control of Predatory Behavior," in *Behavior of Captive Wild Animals*, eds. H. Markowitz and V. J. Stevens, Chicago: Nelson-Hall, 1978.

C. R. Gustavson, D. J. Kelly, M. Sweeney, and J. Garcia, "Prey-Lithium Aversions. I: Coyotes and Wolves," *Behavioral Biology* 17(1976):61–72.

57. W. Timberlake and T. Melcer, "Effects of Poisoning on Predatory and Ingestive Behavior toward Artificial Prey in Rats (*Rattus norvegicus*)," *Journal of Comparative Psychology* 102(1988):182–187.

58. D. S. Booth, "Commentary on 'Coyote Control and Taste Aversion': Editor's Report," *Appetite* 6(1985):282–283.

R. J. Burns and G. E. Connolly, "A Comment on 'Coyote Control and Taste Aversion,'" *Appetite* 6(1985):276–281.

S. R. Ellins, "Coyote Control and Taste Aversion: A Predation Problem or a People Problem?" *Appetite* 6(1985):272–275.

S. R. Ellins, C. R. Gustavson, and J. Garcia, "Conditioned Taste Aversion in Predators: Response to Sterner and Shumake," *Behavioral Biology* 24(1978):554–556.

D. L. Forthman Quick, C. R. Gustavson, and K. W. Rusiniak, "Coyote Control and Taste Aversion," *Appetite* 6(1985):253–264.

D. L. Forthman Quick, C. R. Gustavson, and K. W. Rusiniak, "Coyotes and Taste Aversion: The Authors' Reply," *Appetite* 6(1985):284–290.

P. N. Lehner and S. W. Horn, "Research on Forms of Conditioned Avoidance in Coyotes," *Appetite* 6(1985):265–267.

R. T. Sterner and S. A. Shumake, "Bait-Induced Prey Aversions in Predators: Some Methodological Issues," *Behavioral Biology* 22(1978):565–566.

D. A. Wade, "Brief Comments on 'Coyote Control and Taste Aversion,'" *Appetite* 6(1985):268–271.

59. M. J. Lavin, "The Establishment of Flavor–Flavor Associations Using a Sensory Preconditioning Procedure," *Learning and Motivation* 7(1976):173–183.

60. M. S. Fanselow and J. Birk, "Flavor–Flavor Associations Induce Hedonic Shifts in Taste Preference," *Animal Learning and Behavior* 10(1982):223–228.

61. R. C. Bolles, "A 'Mixed' Model of Taste Preference," in *Animal Cognition and Behavior,* eds. R. L. Mellgren, New York: North-Holland, 1983.

D. A. Zellner, P. Rozin, M. Aron, and C. Kulish, "Conditioned Enhancement of Human's Liking for Flavor by Pairing with Sweetness," *Learning and Motivation* 14(1983):338–350.

62. Zellner et al., "Conditioned Enhancement of Human's Liking for Flavor."

63. L. L. Birch, D. Birch, D. W. Marlin, and L. Kramer, "Effects of Instrumental Consumption on Children's Food Preference," *Appetite* 3(1982):125–134.

64. L. L. Birch, S. I. Zimmerman, and H. Hind, "The Influence of Social-Affective Context on the Formation of Children's Food Preferences," *Child Development* 51(1980):856–861.

65. C. F. Flaherty, "Incentive Contrast: A Review of Behavioral Changes Following Shifts in Reward," *Animal Learning and Behavior* 10(1982):409–440.

66. R. R. Fabsitz, R. J. Garrison, M. Feinleib, and M. Hjortland, "A Twin Analysis of Dietary Intake: Evidence for a Need to Control for Possible Environmental Differences in MZ and DZ Twins," *Behavior Genetics* 8(1978):15–25.

J. Faust, "A Twin Study of Personal Preferences," *Journal of Biosocial Science* 6(1974):75–91.

A. W. Logue, C. M. Logue, R. G. Uzzo, M. J. McCarty, and M. E. Smith, "Food Prefereneces in Families," *Appetite* 10(1988):169–180.

P. Pliner and M. L. Pelchat, "Similarities in Food Preferences between Children and Their Siblings and Parents," *Appetite* 7(1986):333–342.

P. Rozin and L. Millman, "Family Environment, Not Heredity, Accounts for Family Resemblances in Food Preferences and Attitudes: A Twin Study," *Appetite* 8(1987):125–134.

67. B. G. Galef, "Mechanisms for the Social Transmission of Acquired Food Preferences from Adult to Weanling Rats," in *Learning Mechanisms in Food Selection,* eds. L. M. Barker, M. R. Best, and M. Domjan, Waco, TX: Baylor University Press, 1977.

B. G. Galef, "Mechanisms for the Transmission of Acquired Patterns of Feeding from Adult to Weanling Rats," in *Taste and Development,* ed. J. M. Weiffenbach, Bethesda, MD: U.S. Department of Health, Education, and Welfare, 1977.

B. G. Galef, "Studies of Social Learning in Norway Rats: A Brief Review," *Developmental Psychobiology* 15(1982):279–295.

68. M. Kawai, "Newly-Acquired Pre-Cultural Behavior of the Natural Troop of Japanese Monkeys on Koshima Islet," *Primates* 6(1965):1–30.

M. D. Suboski and C. Bartashunas, "Mechanisms for Social Transmission of Pecking Preferences to Neonatal Chicks," *Journal of Experimental Psychology* 10(1984):182–194.

W. Wyrwicka, *The Development of Food Preferences,* Springfield, IL: Charles C Thomas, 1981.

69. B. G. Galef, D. J. Kennett, and S. W. Wigmore, "Transfer of Information Concerning Distant Foods in Rats: A Robust Phenomenon," *Animal Learning and Behavior* 12(1984):292–296.

B. G. Galef and S. W. Wigmore, "Transfer of Information Concerning Distant Foods: A Laboratory Investigation of the 'Information-Centre' Hypothesis," *Animal Behaviour* 31(1983):748–758.

70. B. G. Galef and M. Stein, "Demonstrator Influence on Observer Diet Preference: Analyses of Critical Social Interactions and Olfactory Signals," *Animal Learning and Behavior* 13(1985):31–38.

71. B. G. Galef, J. R. Mason, G. Preti, N. J. Bean, "Carbon Disulfide: A Semiochemical Mediating Socially-Induced Diet Choice in Rats," *Physiology and Behavior* 42(1988):119–124.

72. B. G. Galef, A. Mischinger, and S. A. Malenfant, "Hungry Rats' Following of Conspecifics to Food Depends on the Diets Eaten by Potential Leaders," *Animal Behaviour* 35(1987):1234–1239.

73. M. Beck and B. G. Galef, "Social Influences on the Selection of a Protein-Sufficient Diet by Norway Rats (*Rattus norvegicus*)," *Journal of Comparative Psychology* 103(1989):132–139.

74. W. J. Carr, J. T. Hirsch, B. E. Campellone, and E. Marasco, "Some Determinants of a Natural Food Aversion in Norway Rats," *Journal of Comparative and Physioiogical Psychology*

93(1979):899–906.

W. J. Carr, M. R. Landauer, R. E. Wiese, and D. H. Thor, "A Natural Food Aversion in Rats," *Journal of Comparative and Physiological Psychology* 93(1979):574–584.

75. W. J. Carr, S. Y. Choi, E. Arnholt, and M. H. Sterling, "The Ontogeny of a Natural Food Aversion in Domestic Rats (*Rattus norvegicus*) and House Mice (*Mus musculus*)," *Journal of Comparative and Physiological Psychology* 97(1983):260–268.

76. B. G. Galef, "Socially Induced Diet Preference Can Partially Reverse a LiCl-Induced Diet Aversion," *Animal Learning and Behavior* 13(1985):415–418.

77. M. J. Lavin, B. Freise, and S. Coombes, "Transferred Flavor Aversions in Adult Rats," *Behavioral and Neural Biology* 28(1980):15–33.

S. Revusky, S. Coombes, and R. W. Pohl, "US Preexposure: Effects on Flavor Aversions Produced by Pairing a Poisoned Partner with Ingestion," *Animal Learning and Behavior* 10(1980):83–90.

78. G. A. Gemberling, "Ingestion of a Novel Flavor before Exposure to Pups Injected with Lithium Chloride Produces a Taste Aversion in Mother Rats (*Rattus norvegicus*)," *Journal of Comparative and Physiological Psychology* 98(1984):285–301.

79. S. K. Escalona, "Feeding Disturbances in Very Young Children," *American Journal of Orthopsychiatry* 15(1945):76–80.

80. Ibid, p. 78.

81. J. E. Steiner, "Facial Expressions of the Neonate Infant Indicating the Hedonics of Food-Related Chemical Stimuli," in *Taste and Development*, ed. J. M. Weiffenbach, Bethesda, MD: U.S. Department of Health, Education, and Welfare, 1977.

82. T. M. Field, R. Woodson, R. Greenberg, and D. Cohen, "Discrimination and Imitation of Facial Expressions by Neonates," *Science* 218(1982):179–181.

83. L. L. Birch, "Generalization of a Modified Food Preference," *Child Development* 52(1981):755–758.

L. L. Birch, "Children's Food Preferences: Developmental Patterns and Environmental Influences," in *Annals of Child Development*, vol. 4, ed. R. Vasta, Greenwich, CT: JAI Press, 1987.

84. L. L. Birch, "Effects of Peer Models' Food Choices and Eating Behaviors on Preschoolers' Food Preferences," *Child Development*

51(1980):489–496.

Birch, "Children's Food Preferences."

85. L. V. Harper and K. M. Sanders, "The Effect of Adults' Eating on Young Children's Acceptance of Unfamiliar Foods," *Journal of Experimental Child Psychology* 20(1975):206–214.

86. Logue et al., "The Acquisition of Taste Aversions in Humans."

87. A. C. Huston, B. A. Watkins, and D. Kunkel, "Public Policy and Children's Television," *American Psychologist* 44(1989):424–433.

88. D. B. Jeffrey, D. Bolin, N. B. Lemnitzer, J. S. Hickey, M. J. Hess, and J. M. Stroud, "The Impact of Television Advertising on Children's Eating Behaviour: An Integrative Review," *Catalog of Selected Documents in Psychology* 10(1980): 11 (MS. No. 2011).

89. J. P. Galst and M. A. White, "The Unhealthy Persuader: The Reinforcing Value of Television and Children's Purchase-Influencing Attempts at the Supermarket," *Child Development* 47(1976):1089–1096.

M. E. Goldberg, G. J. Gorn, and W. Gibson, "TV Messages for Snack and Breakfast Foods: Do They Influence Children's Preferences?" *Journal of Consumer Research* 5(1978):73–81.

90. Jeffrey et al., "The Impact of Television Advertising."

D. B. Jeffrey, R. W. McLellarn, and D. T. Fox, "The Development of Children's Eating Habits: The Role of Television Commercials," *Health Education Quarterly* 9(1982):174–189.

D. B. Jeffrey, R. W. McLellarn, J. S. Hickey, N. B. Lemnitzer, M. J. Hess, and J. M. Stroud, "Television Food Commercials and Children's Eating Behavior: Some Empirical Evidence," *Journal of the University Film Association* 32(1980):41–43.

91. L. L. Birch, J. Billman, and S. S. Richards, "Time of Day Influences Food Acceptability," *Appetite* 5(1984):109–116.

H. Tuorila, "Selection of Milks with Varying Fat Contents and Related Overall Liking, Attitudes, Norms and Intentions," *Appetite* 8(1987):1–14.

D. A. Zellner, W. F. Stewart, P. Rozin, and J. M. Brown, "Effect of Temperature and Expectations on Liking for Beverages," *Physiology and Behavior* 44(1988):61–68.

92. J. Brody, *Jane Brody's Nutrition Book*, New York: W. W. Norton, 1981.

93. M. Krondl and D. Lau, "Social Deter-

minants in Human Food Selection," in *The Psychobiology of Human Food Selection*, ed. L. M. Barker, Westport, CT: AVI Publishing, 1982.

94. P. Rozin and A. Fallon, "The Psychological Categorization of Foods and Non-Foods: A Preliminary Taxonomy of Food Rejections," *Appetite* 1(1980):193–201.

95. P. de Silva and S. Rachman, "Human Food Aversions: Nature and Acquisition," *Behaviour Research and Therapy* 25(1987):457–468.

P. Rozin, "One-Trial Acquired Likes and Dislikes in Humans: Disgust as a US, Food Predominance, and Negative Learning Predominance," *Learning and Motivation* 17(1986):180–189.

96. A. E. Fallon and P. Rozin, "The Psychological Bases of Food Rejections by Humans," *Ecology of Food and Nutrition* 13(1983):15–26.

A. E. Fallon, P. Rozin, and P. Pliner, "The Child's Conception of Food: The Development of Food Rejections with Special Reference to Disgust and Contamination Sensitivity," *Child Development* 55(1984):566–575.

Rozin and Fallon, "The Psychological Categorization of Foods and Non-Foods."

P. Rozin and A. E. Fallon, "A Perspective on Disgust," *Psychological Review* 94(1987):23–41.

P. Rozin, A. Fallon, and R. Mandell, "Family Resemblance in Attitudes to Foods," *Developmental Psychology* 20(1984):309–314.

97. P. Rozin, A. Fallon, and M. Augustoni-Ziskind, "The Child's Conception of Food: The Development of Contamination Sensitivity to 'Disgusting' Substances," *Developmental Psychology* 21(1985):1075–1079.

P. Rozin, A. Fallon, and M. Augustoni-Ziskind, "The Child's Conception of Food: The Development of Categories of Acceptable and Rejected Substances," *Journal of Nutrition Education* 18(1986):75–81.

P. Rozin, L. Hammer, H. Oster, T. Horowitz, and V. Marmora, "The Child's Conception of Food: Differentiation of Categories of Rejected Substances in the 16 months to 5 year age range," *Appetite* 7(1986):141–151.

98. C. Nemeroff and P. Rozin, "Sympathetic Magic in Kosher Practice and Belief at the Limits of the Laws of *Kashrut*," *Jewish Folklore and Ethnology* 9(1987):31–32.

P. Rozin, L. Millman, and C. Nemeroff, "Operation of the Laws of Sympathetic Magic in Disgust and Other Domains," *Journal of Personality and Social Psychology* 50(1986):703–712.

99. M. L. Pelchat, H. J. Grill, P. Rozin, and J. Jacobs, "Quality of Acquired Responses to Tastes by *Rattus norvegicus* Depends on Type of Associated Discomfort," *Journal of Comparative Psychology* 97(1983):140–153.

M. L. Pelchat and P. Rozin, "The Special Role of Nausea in the Acquisition of Food Dislikes by Humans," *Appetite* 3(1982):341–351.

Chapter 7: Choice

1. S. R. Sunday, S. A. Sanders, and G. Collier, "Palatability and Meal Patterns," *Physiology and Behavior* 30(1983):915–918.

2. R. Brown and R. J. Herrnstein, *Psychology*, Boston: Little, Brown, 1975.

3. D. P. Barash, *Sociobiology and Behavior*, New York: Elsevier, 1977.

W. D. Hamilton, "The Genetical Evolution of Social Behaviour. I," *Journal of Theoretical Biology* 7(1964):1–16.

W. D. Hamilton, "The Genetical Evolution of Social Behaviour. II," *Journal of Theoretical Biology* 7(1964):17–52.

J. Maynard Smith, "Optimization Theory in Evolution," *Annual Review of Ecology and Systematics* 9(1978):31–56.

4. G. H. Collier, "Determinants of Choice," in *Nebraska Symposium on Motivation 1981: Response Structure and Organization*, ed. D. J. Bernstein, Lincoln: University of Nebraska Press, 1981.

R. J. Herrnstein and W. Vaughan, "Melioration and Behavioral Allocation," in *Limits to Action*, ed. J. E. R. Staddon, New York: Academic Press, 1980.

A. C. Kamil and T.D. Sargent, "Introduction," in *Foraging Behavior: Ecological, Ethological, and Psychological Approaches*, eds. A. C. Kamil and T. D. Sargent, New York: Garland, 1981.

J. M. Maynard Smith, "Game Theory and the Evolution of Behaviour," *The Behavioral and Brain Sciences* 7(1984):95–125.

G. H. Pyke, H. R. Pulliam, and E. L. Charnov, "Optimal Foraging: A Selective Review of Theory and Tests," *Quarterly Review of Biology* 52(1977):137–154.

H. Rachlin, R. Battalio, J. Kagel, and L. Green, "Maximization Theory in Behavioral Psychology," *The Behavioral and Brain Sciences* 4(1981):371–417.

B. F. Skinner, "The Evolution of Behavior," *Journal of the Experimental Analysis of Behavior* 41(1984):217–221.

J. E. R. Staddon, "Optimality Analyses of Operant Behavior and Their Relation to Optimal Foraging," in *Limits to Action,* ed. J. E. R. Staddon, New York: Academic Press, 1980.

5. R. J. Herrnstein, "Relative and Absolute Strength of Response as a Function of Frequency of Reinforcement," *Journal of the Experimental Analysis of Behavior* 4(1961):267–272.

R. J. Herrnstein, "On the Law of Effect," *Journal of the Experimental Analysis of Behavior* 13(1970):243–266.

6. W. F. Buskist, R. H. Bennett, and H. L. Miller, "Concurrent Operant Performance in Humans: Matching When Food Is the Reinforcer," *The Psychological Record* 35(1981):217–225.

M. Davison and D. McCarthy, *The Matching Law: A Research Review,* Hillsdale, NJ: Lawrence Erlbaum Associates, 1988.

P. de Villiers, "Choice in Concurrent Schedules and a Quantitative Formulation of the Law of Effect," in *Handbook of Operant Behavior,* eds. W. K. Honig and J. E. R. Staddon, Englewood Cliffs, NJ: Prentice-Hall, 1977.

B. A. Williams, "Reinforcement, Choice, and Response Strength," in *Stevens' Handbook of Experimental Psychology,* 2nd ed., vol. 2, eds. R. C. Atkinson, R. J. Herrnstein, G. Lindzey, and R. D. Luce, New York: John Wiley & Sons, 1988.

7. W. M. Baum, "Choice in Free-Ranging Wild Pigeons," *Science* 185(1974):78–79.

8. G. Ainslie and R. J. Herrnstein, "Preference Reversal and Delayed Reinforcement," *Animal Learning and Behavior* 9(1981):476–482.

9. G. W. Ainslie, "Impulse Control in Pigeons," *Journal of the Experimental Analysis of Behavior* 21(1974):485–489.

J. Grosch and A. Neuringer, "Self-Control in Pigeons under the Mischel Paradigm," *Journal of the Experimental Analysis of Behavior* 35(1981):3–21.

A. W. Logue, "Research on Self-Control: An Integrating Framework," *Behavioral and Brain Sciences* 11(1988):665–709.

W. Mischel, "Theory and Research on the Antecedents of Self-Imposed Delay of Reward," in *Progress in Experimental Personality Research,* ed. B. A. Maher, New York: Academic Press, 1966.

H. Rachlin and L. Green, "Commitment, Choice and Self-Control," *Journal of the Experimental Analysis of Behavior* 17(1972):15–22.

10. G. W. Ainslie, "Specious Reward: A Behavioral Theory of Impulsiveness and Impulse Control," *Psychological Bulletin* 82(1975):463–496.

H. Rachlin, "Self-Control," *Behaviorism* 2(1974):94–107.

11. Ainslie, "Specious Reward."
Rachlin, "Self-Control."

12. Ainslie, "Impulse Control in Pigeons."
Rachlin and Green, "Commitment, Choice and Self-Control."

13. J. E. Mazur and A. W. Logue, "Choice in a Self-Control Paradigm: Effects of a Fading Procedure," *Journal of the Experimental Analysis of Behavior* 30(1978):11–17.

14. J. B. Schweitzer and B. Sulzer-Azaroff, "Self-Control: Teaching Tolerance for Delay in Impulsive Children," *Journal of the Experimental Analysis of Behavior* 50(1988):173–186.

15. A. W. Logue and J. E. Mazur, "Maintenance of Self-Control Acquired through a Fading Procedure: Follow-Up on Mazur and Logue (1978)," *Behavior Analysis Letters* 1(1981):131–137.

16. Mischel, "Theory and Research on the Antecedents."

W. Mischel, Y. Shoda, and M. L. Rodriguez, "Delay of Gratification in Children," *Science* 244(1989):933-938.

M. L. Rodriguez, W. Mischel, and Y. Shoda, "Cognitive Person Variables in the Delay of Gratification of Older Children at Risk," *Journal of Personality and Social Psychology* 57(1989):358–367.

17. Grosch and Neuringer, "Self-Control in Pigeons."

A. W. Logue and T. E. Pena-Correal, "Responding during Reinforcement Delay in a Self-Control Paradigm," *Journal of the Experimental Analysis of Behavior* 41(1984):267–277.

18. A. W. Logue, M. L. Rodriguez, T. E. Pena-Correal, and B. C. Mauro, "Choice in a Self-Control Paradigm: Quantification of Experience-Based Differences," *Journal of the Experimental Analysis of Behavior* 41(1984): 53–67.

Logue, "Research on Self-Control."

19. H. L. Miller, "Matching-Based Hedonic Scaling in the Pigeon," *Journal of the Experimental Analysis of Behavior* 26(1976):335–347.

20. G. R. King and A. W. Logue, "Choice in a Self-Control Paradigm: Effects of Reinforcer Quality," *Behavioural Processes* (in press).

21. E. W. Menzel and E. J. Wyers, "Cognitive Aspects of Foraging Behavior," in *Foraging Behavior: Ecological, Ethological, and Psychological Ap-*

proaches, eds. A. C. Kamil and T. D. Sargent, New York: Garland, 1981, p. 355.

22. Kamil and Sargent, "Introduction," pp. 1–2.

23. Menzel and Wyers, "Cognitive Aspects of Foraging Behavior."

24. D. W. Stephens and J. R. Krebs, *Foraging Theory,* Princton, NJ: Princeton University Press, 1986.

25. P. Rozin, "The Selection of Foods by Rats, Humans, and Other Animals," in *Advances in the Study of Behavior,* vol. 6, eds. J. S. Rosenblatt, R. A. Hinde, E. Shaw, and C. Beer, New York: Academic Press, 1976.

26. J. Allison, "Economics and Operant Conditioning," in *Predictability, Correlation, and Contiguity,* eds. P. Harzem and M. D. Zeiler, New York: John Wiley & Sons, 1981.

S. R. Hursh, "Economic Concepts for the Analysis of Behavior," *Journal of the Experimental Analysis of Behavior* 34(1980):219–238.

S. E. G. Lea, "The Psychology and Economics of Demand," *Psychological Bulletin* 85(1978):441–466.

H. Rachlin, "Economics and Behavioral Psychology," in *Limits to Action,* ed. J. E. R. Staddon, New York: Academic Press, 1980.

27. J. Allison, "Behavioral Substitutes and Complements," in *Animal Cognition and Behavior,* ed. R. L. Mellgren, New York: North-Holland, 1983.

B. Burkhard, "Preference and Response Substitutability in the Maximization of Behavioral Value," in *Quantitative Analyses of Behavior: Matching and Maximizing Accounts,* eds. M. L. Commons, R. J. Herrnstein, and H. Rachlin, Cambridge, MA: Ballinger, 1982.

S. R. Hursh, "The Economics of Daily Consumption Controlling Food- and Water-Reinforced Responding," *Journal of the Experimental Analysis of Behavior* 29(1978):475–491.

S. R. Hursh, "Behavioral Economics," *Journal of the Experimental Analysis of Behavior* 42(1984):435–452.

Rachlin, et al., "Maximization Theory."

28. J. E. R. Staddon, *Adaptive Behavior and Learning,* New York: Cambridge University Press, 1983.

29. Collier, "Determinants of Choice."

L. Green, J. H. Kagel, and R. C. Battalio, "Ratio Schedules of Reinforcement and Their Relation to Economic Theories of Labor Supply," in *Quantitative Analyses of Behavior: Matching and Maximizing*

Accounts, eds. M. L. Commons, R. J. Herrnstein, and H. Rachlin, Cambridge, MA: Ballinger, 1982.

J. M. Hinson and J. E. R. Staddon, "Maximizing on Interval Schedules," in *Quantification of Steady-State Operant Behaviour,* eds. C. M. Bradshaw, E. Szabadi, and C. F. Lowe, Amsterdam: Elsevier/North-Holland, 1981.

J. M. McNamara and A. I. Houston, "Optimal Responding on Variable Interval Schedules," *Behaviour Analysis Letters* 3(1983):157–170.

30. G. Collier, "Operant Methodologies for Studying Feeding and Drinking," in *Feeding and Drinking,* eds. F. M. Toates and N. E. Rowland, New York: Elsevier, 1987.

S. M. Dow and S. E. G. Lea, "Foraging in a Changing Environment: Simulations in the Operant Laboratory," in *Quantitative Analyses of Behavior: Vol. 6 Foraging,* eds. M. L. Commons, A. Kacelnik, and S. J. Shettleworth, Hillsdale, NJ: Lawrence Erlbaum Associates, 1987.

E. Fantino and N. Abarca, "Choice, Optimal Foraging, and the Delay-Reduction Hypothesis," *The Behavioral and Brain Sciences* 8 (1985): 315–330.

S. J. Shettleworth, "Animals Foraging in the Lab: Problems and Promises," *Journal of Experimental Psychology: Animal Behavior Processes* 15(1989):81–87.

31. E. L. Charnov, "Optimal Foraging: Attack Strategy of a Mantid," *American Naturalist* 110(1976):141–151.

A. I. Houston and J. M. McNamara, "The Choice of Two Prey Types That Minimises the Probability of Starvation," *Behavioral Ecology and Sociobiology* 17(1985):135–141.

J. R. Krebs, D. W. Stephens, and W. J. Sutherland, "Perspectives in Optimal Foraging," in *Perspectives in Ornithology,* eds. A. H. Brush and G. A. Clark, Cambridge, Great Britain: Cambridge University Press, 1983.

H. R. Pulliam, "On the Theory of Optimal Diets," *American Naturalist* 108:1974:59–74.

32. W. M. Baum, "Random and Systematic Foraging, Experimental Studies of Depletion, and Schedules of Reinforcement," in *Foraging Behavior,* eds A. C. Kamil, J. R. Krebs, and H. R. Pulliam, New York: Plenum, 1987.

S. Engen and N. C. Stenseth, "A General Version of Optimal Foraging Theory: The Effect of Simultaneous Encounters," *Theoretical Population Biology* 26(1984):192–204.

33. C. M. Hodges, "Optimal Foraging in Bumblebees: Hunting by Expectation," *Animal Behaviour* 29(1981):1166–1171.

34. A. T. Pietrewicz and A. C. Kamil, "Search Image Formation in the Blue Jay (*Cyanocitta cristata*), *Science* 204(1979):1332–1333.

35. L. Green, H. Rachlin, and J. Hanson, "Matching and Maximizing with Concurrent Ratio-Interval Schedules," *Journal of the Experimental Analysis of Behavior* 40(1983):217–224.

J. M. Hinson and J. E. R. Staddon, "Hill-Climbing by Pigeons," *Journal of the Experimental Analysis of Behavior* 39(1983):25–47.

36. G. H. Collier and C. K. Rovee-Collier, "A Comparative Analysis of Optimal Foraging Behavior: Laboratory Simulations," in *Foraging Behavior: Ecological, Ethological, and Psychological Approaches*, eds. A. C. Kamil and T. D. Sargent, New York: Garland, 1981.

P. R. Killeen, J. P. Smith, and S. J. Hanson, "Central Place Foraging in *Rattus norvegicus*," *Animal Behaviour* 29(1981):64–70.

37. G. Collier, L. W. Kaufman, R. Kanarek, and J. Fagen, "Optimization of Time and Energy Constraints in the Feeding Behavior of Cats: A Laboratory Simulation," *Carnivore* 1(1978):34–41.

38. Hursh, "The Economics of Daily Consumption Controlling Food- and Water-Reinforced Responding."

39. G. H. Pyke, "Honeyeater Foraging: A Test of Optimal Foraging Theory," *Animal Behaviour* 29(1981):878–888.

G. H. Pyke, "Optimal Foraging in Hummingbirds: Rule of Movement between Inflorescences," *Animal Behaviour* 29 (1981): 889–896.

G. H. Pyke, "Why Hummingbirds Hover and Honeyeaters Perch," *Animal Behaviour* 29(1981):861–867.

40. W. A. Roberts and T. J. Ilersich, "Foraging on the Radial Maze: The Role of Travel Time, Food Accessibility, and the Predictability of Food Location," *Journal of Experimental Psychology: Animal Behavior Processes* 15(1989):274–285.

41. A. I. Houston and J. M. McNamara, "The Variability of Behaviour and Constrained Optimization," *Journal of Theoretical Biology* 112(1985):265–273.

A. C. Lewis, "Memory Constraints and Flower Choice in *Pieris Rapae*," *Science* 232(1986):863–865.

J. M. McNamara and A. I. Houston, "Optimal Foraging and Learning," *Journal of Theoretical Biology* 117(1985):231–249.

J. M. McNamara and A. I. Houston, "Partial Preferences and Foraging," *Animal Behaviour* 35(1987):1084–1099.

A. T. Pietrewicz and J. B. Richards, "Learning to Forage: An Ecological Perspective," in *Issues in the Ecological Study of Learning*, eds T. D. Johnston and A. T. Pietrewicz, Hillsdale, NJ: Lawrence Erlbaum Associates, 1985.

42. D. S. Olton, G. E. Handelmann, and J. A. Walker, "Spatial Memory and Food Searching Strategies," in *Foraging Behavior: Ecological, Ethological, and Psychological Approaches*, eds. A. C. Kamil and T. D. Sargent, New York: Garland, 1981.

43. A. W. Logue and T. E. Pena-Correal, "The Effect of Food Deprivation on Self-Control," *Behavioural Processes* 10(1985):335–368.

G. A. Lucas, D. J. Gawley, and W. Timberlake, "Anticipatory Contrast as a Measure of Time Horizons in the Rat: Some Methodological Determinants," *Animal Learning and Behavior* 16(1988):377–382.

McNamara and Houston, "Partial Preferences and Foraging."

W. Timberlake, "A Temporal Limit on the Effect of Future Food on Current Performance in an Analogue of Foraging and Welfare," *Journal of the Experimental Analysis of Behavior* 41(1984):117–124.

W. Timberlake, D. J. Gawley, and G. A. Lucas, "Time Horizons in Rats: The Effect of Operant Control of Access to Future Food," *Journal of the Experimental Analysis of Behavior* 50(1988):405–417.

44. S. E. G. Lea, "Foraging and Reinforcement Schedules in the Pigeon: Optimal and Non-Optimal Aspects of Choice," *Animal Behaviour* 27(1979):875–886.

Logue and Pena-Correal, "The Effect of Food Deprivation on Self-Control."

H. Rachlin, "Pain and Behavior," *The Behavioral and Brain Sciences* 8(1985):43–83.

45. A. W. Logue, G. R. King, A. Chavarro, and J. S. Volpe, "Matching and Maximizing in a Self-Control Paradigm Using Human Subjects," *Learning and Motivation* 21(1990):340–368.

46. R. G. Jaeger, R. G. Joseph, and D. E. Barnard, "Foraging Tactics of a Terrestrial Salamander: Sustained Yield in Territories," *Animal Behaviour* 29(1981):1100–1105.

47. D. W. Stephens, "The Logic of Risk-Sensitive Foraging Preferences," *Animal Behaviour* 29(1981):628–629.

Stephens and Krebs, *Foraging Theory*.

48. T. Caraco, "White-Crowned Sparrows (*Zonotrichia leucophrys*): Foraging Preferences in a Risky Environment," *Behavioral Ecology and Sociobiology* 12(1983):63–69.

T. Caraco, S. Martindale, and T. S. Whittam,

"An Empirical Demonstration of Risk-Sensitive Foraging Preferences," *Animal Behaviour* 28(1980):820–830.

49. J. H. Kagel, D. N. MacDonald, R. C. Battalio, S. White, and L. Green, "Risk Aversion in Rats (*Rattus norvegicus*) under Varying Levels of Resource Availability," *Journal of Comparative Psychology* 100(1986):95–100.

50. J. H. Kagel, L. Green, and T. Caraco, "When Foragers Discount the Future: Constraint or Adaptation?" *Animal Behaviour* 34(1986):271–283.

J. M. McNamara and A. I. Houston, "A General Framework for Understanding the Effects of Variability and Interruptions on Foraging Behavior," *Acta Biotheoretica* 36(1987):3–22.

J. M. McNamara and A. I. Houston, "Foraging in Patches: There's More to Life than the Marginal Value Theorem," in *Quantitative Analyses of Behavior: Vol. 6. Foraging*, eds. M. L Commons, A. Kacelnik, and S. J. Shettleworth, Hillsdale, NJ: Lawrence Erlbaum Associates, 1987.

Stephens and Krebs, *Foraging Theory.*

51. Logue, "Research on Self-Control."

52. Y. D. Lubin, "Eating Ants is No Picnic," *Natural History* 92(October 1983):54–59.

53. S. E. G. Lea, "The Analysis of Need," in *Animal Cognition and Behavior*, ed. R. L. Mellgren, New York: North-Holland, 1983.

54. J. G. Goode, K. Curtis, and J. Theophano, "Group-Shared Food Patterns as a Unit of Analysis," in *Nutrition and Behavior*, ed. S. A. Miller, Philadelphia: Franklin Institute, 1981.

55. E. S. Wing and A. B. Brown, *Paleonutrition*, New York: Academic Press, 1979.

B. Winterhalder and E. A. Smith, eds. *Hunter-Gatherer Foraging Strategies: Ethnographic and Archeological Analyses*, Chicago: University of Chicago Press, 1981.

56. S. M. Cantor and M. B. Cantor, "Socioeconomic Factors in Fat and Sugar Consumption," in *The Chemical Senses and Nutrition*, eds. M. R. Kare and O. Maller, New York: Academic Press, 1977.

N. S. Scrimshaw and L. Taylor, "Food," *Scientific American* (September 1980):78–88.

57. M. Krondl and D. Lau, "Social Determinants in Human Food Selection," in *The Psychobiology of Human Food Selection*, ed. L. M. Barker, Westport, CT: AVI Publishing, 1982.

Scrimshaw and Taylor, "Food."

J. Yudkin, "Patterns and Trends in Carbohydrate Consumption and Their Relation to Disease," *Nutrition Society Proceedings* 23(1964):149–162.

58. E. A. Smith, "Optimization Theory in Anthropology: Applications and Critiques," in *The Latest on the Best: Essays on Evolution and Optimality*, ed J. Dupre, Cambridge, MA: MIT Press, 1987.

B. Winterhalder, "The Analysis of Hunter-Gatherer Diets: Stalking an Optimal Foraging Model," in *Food and Evolution: Toward a Theory of Human Food Habits*, eds. M. Harris and E. B. Ross, Philadelphia: Temple University Press, 1987.

59. M. P. Ghiglieri, "The Social Ecology of Chimpanzees," *Scientific American* 252(June 1985):102–104, 109–113.

60. K. Hill and A. M. Hurtado, "Hunter-Gatherers of the New World," *American Scientist* (September-October 1989):436–443.

61. W. M. Baum, "Optimization and the Matching Law as Accounts of Instrumental Behavior," *Journal of the Experimental Analysis of Behavior* 36(1981):387–403.

G. M. Heyman and R. J. Herrnstein, "More on Concurrent Interval-Ratio Schedules," *Journal of the Experimental Analysis of Behavior* 46(1986):331–351.

A. I. Houston, "Optimality Theory and Matching," *Behaviour Analysis Letters* 3(1983):1–15.

A. Kacelnik, "Introduction," in *Quantitative Analyses of Behavior: Vol. 6. Foraging*, eds. M. L. Commons, A. Kacelnik, and S. J. Shettleworth, Hillsdale, NJ: Lawrence Erlbaum Associates, 1987.

J. E. Mazur, "Optimization Theory Fails to Predict Performance of Pigeons in a Two-Response Situation," *Science* 214(1981):823–825.

J. E. R. Staddon and J. M. Hinson, "Optimization: A Result or a Mechanism?" *Science* 221(1983):976–977.

B. A. Williams, "Choice Behavior in a Discrete-Trial Concurrent VI-VR: A Test of Maximizing Theories of Matching," *Learning and Motivation* 16(1985):423–443.

M. D. Zeiler, "On Optimal Choice Strategies," *Journal of Experimental Psychology: Animal Behavior Processes* 13(1987):31–39.

J. M. Ziriax and A. Silberberg, "Concurrent Variable-Interval Variable-Ratio Schedules Can Provide Only Weak Evidence for Matching," *Journal of the Experimental Analysis of Behavior* 41(1984):83–100.

62. Staddon, *Adaptive Behavior and Learning*, p. 493.

63. A. I. Houston and J. M. McNamara, "Im-

perfectly Optimal Animals," *Behavioral Ecology and Sociobiology* 15(1984):61–64.

A. C. Janetos and B. J. Cole, "Imperfectly Optimal Animals," *Behavioral Ecology and Sociobiology* 9(1981):203–209.

64. N. Abarca and E. Fantino, "Choice and Foraging," *Journal of the Experimental Analysis of Behavior* 38(1982):117–123.

E. Fantino, "Contiguity, Response Strength, and the Delay-Reduction Hypothesis," in *Predictability, Correlation, and Contiguity*, eds P. Harzem and M. H. Zeiler, New York: John Wiley & Sons, 1981.

E. Fantino and M. Davison, "Choice: Some Quantitative Relations," *Journal of the Experimental Analysis of Behavior* 40(1983):1–13.

65. J. Gibbon, "Scalar Expectancy Theory and Weber's Law in Animal Timing," *Psychological Review* 84(1977):279–325.

66. P. R. Killeen, "Incentive Theory," in *Response Structure and Organization*, ed. D. J. Bernstein, Lincoln: University of Nebraska Press, 1982.

P. R. Killeen, "Incentive Theory: IV. Magnitude of Reward," *Journal of the Experimental Analysis of Behavior* 43(1985):407–417.

Chapter 8: The Effects of Food on Behavior

1. J. D. Fernstrom, "Effects of the Diet on Brain Neurotransmitters," *Metabolism* 26(1977):207–223.

J. D. Fernstrom, "Nutrition, Brain Function and Behavior," in *Nutrition and Behavior*, ed. S. A. Miller, Philadelphia: Franklin Institute, 1981.

J. J. Wurtman, "Neurotransmitter Regulation of Protein and Carbohydrate Consumption," in *Nutrition and Behavior*, ed. S. A. Miller, Philadelphia: Franklin Institute, 1981.

R. J. Wurtman, "Nutrients That Modify Brain Function," *Scientific American* 246(April 1982): 50–59.

R. J. Wurtman and J. D. Fernstrom, "Control of Brain Neurotransmitter Synthesis by Precursor Availability and Nutritional State," *Behavioral Pharmacology* 25(1976):1691–1696.

R. J. Wurtman and J. J. Wurtman, "Nutrients, Neurotransmitter Synthesis, and the Control of Food Intake," in *Eating and Its Disorders*, eds. A. J.

Stunkard and E. Stellar, New York: Raven Press, 1984.

2. M. Sandler and T. Silverstone, eds., *Psychopharmacology and Food*, Oxford, Great Britain: Oxford University Press, 1985.

G. Serban, ed., *Nutrition and Mental Functions*, New York: Plenum, 1975.

B. Spring, J. Chiodo, and D. J. Bowen, "Carbohydrates, Tryptophan, and Behavior: A Methodological Review," *Psychological Bulletin* 102 (1987):234–256.

R. J. Wurtman and J. J. Wurtman, eds., *Nutrition and the Brain: Vol. 7. Food Constituents Affecting Normal and Abnormal Behaviors*, New York: Raven Press, 1986.

3. C. K. Conners, "Artificial Colors in the Diet and Disruptive Behavior: Current Status of Research," in *Nutrition and Behavior*, ed. S. A. Miller, Philadelphia: Franklin Institute, 1981.

P. B. Dews, "Comments on Some Major Methodologic Issues Affecting Analysis of the Behavioral Effects of Foods and Nutrients," *Journal of Psychiatric Research* 17(1982/83):223–225.

D. G. Elmes, B. H. Kantowitz, and H. L. Roediger, *Methods in Experimental Psychology*, Boston: Houghton Mifflin, 1981.

J. P. Harley, "Methodological Issues in Behavioral Nutrition Research," in *Nutrition and Behavior*, ed. S. A. Miller, Philadelphia: Franklin Institute, 1981.

W. L. Hays, *Statistics*, New York: Holt, Rinehart & Winston, 1981.

R. L. Sprague, "Measurement and Methodology of Behavioral Studies: The Other Half of the Nutrition and Behavior Equation," in *Nutrition and Behavior*, ed. S. A. Miller, Philadelphia: Franklin Institute, 1981.

4. C. Cox, "Detection of Treatment Effects When Only a Portion of Subjects Respond," in *Nutrition and Behavior*, ed. S. A. Miller, Philadelphia: Franklin Institute, 1981.

H. G. Birch and J. D. Gussow, *Disadvantaged Children: Health, Nutrition and School Failure*, New York: Harcourt, Brace & World, 1970.

5. J. Brozek, "Nutrition, Malnutrition, and Behavior," *Annual Review of Psychology* 29(1978):157–177.

J. Cravioto and E. DeLicardie, "Longitudinal Study of Language Development in Severely Malnourished Children," in *Nutrition and Mental Functions*, ed. G. Serban, New York: Plenum, 1975.

6. C. K. Conners and A. G. Blouin, "Nutritional Effects on Behavior of Children," *Journal of*

Psychiatric Research 17(1982/83):193–201.

E. Pollitt, N. L. Lewis, C. Garza, and R. J. Shulman, "Fasting and Cognitive Function," *Journal of Psychiatric Research* 17(1982/83):169–174.

7. B. Lozoff, "Nutrition and Behavior," *American Psychologist* 44(1989):231-236.

M. Winick, "Nutrition and Brain Development," in *Nutrition and Mental Functions*, ed. G. Serban, New York: Plenum, 1975.

8. D. A. Levitsky and B. J. Strupp, "Malnutrition and Tests of Brain Function," in *Nutrition and Behavior*, ed. S. A. Miller, Philadelphia: Franklin Institute, 1981.

9. G. Turkewitz, "Learning in Chronically Protein-Deprived Rats," in *Nutrition and Mental Functions*, ed. G. Serban, New York: Plenum, 1975.

R. R. Zimmermann, C. R. Geist, and D. A. Strobel, "Behavioral Deficiencies in Protein-Deprived Monkeys," in *Nutrition and Mental Functions*, ed. G. Serban, New York: Plenum, 1975.

10. Lozoff, "Nutrition and Behavior."

11. R. L. Leibel, E. Pollitt, and D. B. Greenfield, "Methodological Problems in the Assessment of Nutrition–Behavior Interactions: A Study of Effects of Iron Deficiency on Cognitive Function in Children," in *Nutrition and Behavior*, ed. S. A. Miller, Philadelphia: Franklin Institute, 1981.

12. Lozoff, "Nutrition and Behavior."

13. L. Pauling, "Orthomolecular Psychiatry," *Science* 160(1968):265–271.

14. *American Psychiatric Association: Diagnostic and Statistical Manual of Mental Disorders*, 3d ed. rev., Washington, DC: APA, 1987.

15. P. M. Dreyfus, "The Nutritional Management of Neurological Disease," in *Nutrition and Behavior*, ed. S. A. Miller, Philadelphia: Franklin Institute, 1981.

16. Pauling, "Orthomolecular Psychiatry."

17. S. S. Kety, "Nutrition and Psychiatric Illness," in *Nutrition and Mental Functions*, ed. G. Serban, New York: Plenum, 1975.

G. B. Kolata, "Mental Disorders: A New Approach to Treatment?" *Science* 203(1979):36–38.

M. A. Lipton, "Remarks on the Use of Megavitamins in the Treatment of Schizophrenia," in *Nutrition and Mental Functions*, ed. G. Serban, New York: Plenum, 1975.

M. A. Lipton, "Summary," in *Nutrition and Mental Functions*, ed. G. Serban, New York: Plenum, 1975.

18. T. A. Ban, "Megavitamin Therapy in Schizophrenia," in *Nutrition and Behavior*, ed. S. A. Miller, Philadelphia: Franklin Institute, 1981.

19. J. R. Wittenborn, "Premorbid Adjustment and Response to Nicotinic Acid," in *Nutrition and Mental Functions*, ed. G. Serban, New York: Plenum, 1975.

20. A. J. Gelenberg, J. D. Wojcik, C. J. Gibson, and R. J. Wurtman, "Tyrosine for Depression," *Journal of Psychiatric Research* 17(1982/83):175–180.

B. Spring, "Effects of Foods and Nutrients on the Behavior of Normal Individuals," in *Nutrition and the Brain*, vol. 7, eds. R. J. Wurtman & J. J. Wurtman, New York: Raven Press, 1986.

H. M. van Praag and C. Lemus, "Monoamine Precurors in the Treatment of Psychiatric Disorders," in *Nutrition and the Brain*, vol. 7, eds R. J. Wurtman & J. J. Wurtman, New York: Raven Press, 1986.

21. Ban, "Megavitamin Therapy in Schizophrenia."

Kety, "Nutrition and Psychiatric Illness."

L. E. Rosenberg, "Contrast between Vitamin-Responsive Inherited Metabolic Diseases and Vitamin Use in Schizophrenia," in *Nutrition and Mental Functions*, ed. G. Serban, New York: Plenum, 1975.

22. A. S. Boal, S. N. Young, M. Sutherland, F. R. Ervin, and R. Coppinger, "The Effect of Breakfast on Social Behavior and Brain Amine Metabolism in Vervet Monkeys," *Pharmacology, Biochemistry and Behavior* 29(1988):115–123.

J. Danguir, "Cafeteria Diet Promotes Sleep in Rats," *Appetite* 8(1987):49–53.

W. H. Meck and R. M. Church, "Nutrients That Modify the Speed of Internal Clock and Memory Storage Processes," *Behavioral Neuroscience* 101(1987):467–475.

A. Smith and S. Leekam, "The Influence of Meal Composition on Post-Lunch Changes in Performance Efficiency and Mood," *Appetite* 10(1988):195–203.

Spring, "Effects of Foods and Nutrients."

S. H. Zeisel, "Dietary Influences on Neorotransmission," *Advances in Pediatrics* 33(1986):23–48.

23. E. Hartman, "Effects of L-Tryptophan on Sleepiness and on Sleep," *Journal of Psychiatric Research* 17(1982/83):107–113.

P. D. Leathwood and P. Pollet, "Diet-Induced Mood Changes in Normal Populations," *Journal of Psychiatric Research* 17(1982/83):147–154.

H. R. Lieberman, S. Corkin, B. J. Spring, J. H. Growdon, and R. J. Wurtman, "Mood, Performance, and Pain Sensitivity: Changes Induced by Food Constituents," *Journal of Psychiatric Research*

17(1982/83):135–145.

Spring, et al., "Carbohydrates, Tryptophan, and Behavior."

Wurtman, "Nutrients That Modify Brain Function."

Wurtman and Fernstrom, "Control of Brain Neurotransmitter Synthesis."

M. W. Yogman, S. H. Zeisel, and C. Roberts, "Assessing Effects of Serotonin Precursors on Newborn Behavior," *Journal of Psychiatric Research* 17(1982/83):123–133.

24. R. F. Thompson, *Foundations of Physiological Psychology*, New York: Harper & Row, 1967.

25. J. D. Fernstrom, "Role of Precursor Availability in Control of Monoamine Biosynthesis in Brain," *Physiological Reviews* 63(1983):484–546.

Lieberman et al., "Mood, Performance, and Pain Sensitivity."

Wurtman, "Nutrients That Modify Brain Function."

S. N. Young, "The Clinical Psychopharmacology of Tryptophan," in *Nutrition and the Brain*, vol. 7, eds. R. J. Wurtman & J. J. Wurtman, New York: Raven Press, 1986.

26. B. Spring, J. Chiodo, M. Harden, M. J. Bourgeois, J. D. Mason, and L. Lutherer, "Psychobiological Effects of Carbohydrates," *Journal of Clinical Psychiatry* 50 Supplement(1980):27–33.

27. B. Spring, O. Maller, J. Wurtman, L. Digman, and L. Cozolino, "Effects of Protein and Carbohydrate Meals on Mood and Performance: Interactions with Sex and Age," *Journal of Psychiatric Research* 17(1982/83):155–167.

28. J. L. Rapoport, "Effects of Dietary Substances in Children," *Journal of Psychiatric Research* 17(1982/83):187–191.

29. Spring, "Effects of Foods and Nutrients."

30. Fernstrom, "Effects of the Diet on Brain Neurotransmitters."

Fernstrom, "Nutrition, Brain Function and Behavior."

Wurtman, "Nutrients That Modify Brain Function."

Wurtman and Fernstrom, "Control of Brain Neurotransmitter Synthesis."

31. Spring, "Effects of Food and Nutrients."

32. L. M. Bartoshuk, "Taste," in *Stevens' Handbook of Experimental Psychology*, 2nd ed., vol. 1., eds. R. C. Atkinson, R. J. Herrnstein, G. Lindzey, and R. D. Luce, New York: John Wiley & Sons, 1988.

33. G. O. Kermode, "Food Additives," in *Human Nutrition*, San Francisco: W. H. Freeman

and Company, 1978.

C. B. Nemeroff, "Monosodium Glutamate-Induced Neurotoxicity: Review of the Literature and Call for Further Research," in *Nutrition and Behavior*, ed. S. A. Miller, Philadelphia: Franklin Institute, 1981.

34. M. Barinaga, "Amino Acids: How Much Excitement Is Too Much?" *Science* 247(1990):20–22.

35. Nemeroff, "Monosodium Glutamate-Induced Neurotoxicity."

36. Barinaga, "Amino Acids."

M. Barinaga, "MSG: A 20-Year Debate Continues," *Science* 247(1990):21.

37. M. E. Rubini, "The Many-Faceted Mystique of Monosodium Glutamate," *The American Journal of Clinical Nutrition* 24(1971):171.

38. L. D. Dickey, *Clinical Ecology*, Springfield, IL: Charles C Thomas, 1976.

39. G. Guroff, "Inborn Errors of Amino Acid Metabolism in Relation to Diet," in *Nutrition and Behavior*, ed. S. A. Miller: Philadelphia: Franklin Institute, 1981.

39. G. Guroff, "Inborn Errors of Amino Acid Metabolism in Relation to Diet," in *Nutrition and Behavior*, ed. S. A. Miller: Philadelphia, 1981.

40. D. S. King, "Food and Chemical Sensitivities Can Produce Cognitive-Emotional Symptoms," in *Nutrition and Behavior*, ed. S. A. Miller, Philadelphia: Franklin Institute, 1981.

41. R. M. Gilbert, "Caffeine: Overview and Anthology," in *Nutrition and Behavior*, ed. S. A. Miller, Philadelphia: Franklin Institute, 1981.

R. R. Grifiths and P. P. Woodson, "Caffeine Physical Dependence: A Review of Human and Laboratory Animal Studies," *Psychopharmacology* 94(1988):437–451.

42. J. Brody, *Jane Brody's Nutrition Book*, New York: W. W. Norton, 1981.

43. R. Elkins, J. L. Rapoport, T. Zahn, M. S. Buchsbaum, H. Weingartner, I. J. Kopin, D. Langer, and C. Johnson, "Acute Effects of Caffeine in Normal Prepubertal Boys," in *Nutrition and Behavior*, ed. S. A. Miller, Philadelphia: Franklin Institute, 1981.

Gilbert, "Caffeine."

Leathwood and Pollet, "Diet-Induced Mood Changes." Rapoport, "Effects of Dietary Substances in Children."

P. Rozin and B. M. Cines, "Ethnic Differences in Coffee Use and Attitudes to Coffee," *Ecology of Food and Nutrition* 12(1982):79–88.

44. Rapoport, "Effects of Dietary Substances in Children."

45. R. R. Giffiths, G. E. Bigelow, and I. A. Liebson, "Reinforcing Effects of Caffeine in Coffee and Capsules," *Journal of the Experimental Analysis of Behavior* 52(1989):127–140.

46. *American Psychiatric Association: Diagnostic and Statistical Manual of Mental Disorders,* 3d ed. rev., p. 138.

47. L. R. Caporael, "Ergotism: The Satan Loosed in Salem," *Science* 192(1976):21–26.

M. K. Matossian, "Ergot and the Salem Witchcraft Affair," *American Scientist* 70(July/August 1982):355–357.

48. R. Tannahill, *Food in History,* New York: Stein and Day, 1974.

49. W. N. Arnold, "Absinthe," *Scientific American* 260(June 1989):112–117.

50. R. E. Bowman, "Behavioral Teratology of Dietary Constituents: The Vulnerability of the Developing Organism to Toxic Insult," in *Nutrition and Behavior,* ed. S. A. Miller, Philadelphia: Franklin Institute, 1981.

51. H. L. Needleman, S. K. Geiger, and R. Frank, "Lead and IQ Scores: A Reanalysis," *Science* 227(1985):701–702, 704.

52. B. Weiss, "Behavior as a Common Focus of Toxicology," in *Nutrition and Behavior,* ed. S. A. Miller, Philadelphia: Franklin Institute, 1981.

53. "Was the Ill-Fated Franklin Expedition a Victim of Lead Poisoning," *Nutrition Reviews* 47(1989):322–323.

54. Weiss, "Behavior as a Common Focus of Toxicology."

55. *American Psychiatric Association: Diagnostic and Statistical Manual of Mental Disorders,* 3rd ed. rev.

56. Ibid.

57. M. A. Stewart, "Hyperactive Children," *Scientific American* 222 (April 1970): 94–99.

58. K. D. O'Leary, "Assessment of Hyperactivity: Observational and Rating Methodologies," in *Nutrition and Behavior,* ed. S. A. Miller, Philadelphia: Franklin Institute, 1981.

59. J. L. Rapoport, M. S. Buchsbaum, T. P. Zahn, H. Weingartner, C. Ludlow, and E. J. Mikkelsen, "Dextroamphetamine: Cognitive and Behavioral Effects in Normal Prepubertal Boys," *Science* 199(1978):560–563.

Stewart, "Hyperactive Children."

60. Officers of Medical Economics Company, *Physician's Desk Reference,* 34th Edition, Oradell, NJ: Medical Economics Company, 1980.

61. K. D. O'Leary, "Pills or Skills for Hyperactive Children," *Journal of Applied Behavior Analysis* 13(1980):191–204.

62. B. F. Feingold, "Dietary Management of Behavior and Learning Disabilities," in *Nutrition and Behavior,* ed. S. A. Miller, Philadelphia: Franklin Institute, 1981.

63. *The Feingold Association of New York, Inc.,* Smithtown, NY: 1982 (pamphlet).

64. G. J. Augustine and H. Levitan, "Neurotransmitter Release from a Vertebrate Neuromuscular Synapse Affected by a Food Dye," *Science* 207(1980):1489–1490.

65. J. R. Goldenring, R. S. Wool, B. A. Shaywitz, D. K. Batter, D. J. Cohen, J. G. Young, and M. H. Teicher, "Effects of Continuous Gastric Infusion of Food Dyes on Developing Rat Pups," *Life Sciences* 27(1980):1897–1904.

66. B. A. Shaywitz, J. R. Goldenring, and R. S. Wool, "Effects of Chronic Administration of Food Colorings on Activity Levels and Cognitive Performance in Developing Rat Pups Treated With 6-Hydroxydopamine," *Neurobehavioral Toxicology* 1(1979): 41–47.

67. J. M. Swanson and M. Kinsbourne, "Food Dyes Impair Performance of Hyperactive Children on a Laboratory Learning Test," *Science* 207(1980):1485–1487.

68. B. J. Kaplan, J. McNicol, R. A. Conte, and H. K. Moghadam, "Dietary Replacement in Preschool-Aged Hyperactive Boys," *Pediatrics* 83(1989):7–17.

69. J. P. Harley, R. S. Ray, L. Tomasi, P. L. Eichman, C. G. Matthews, R. Chun, C. S. Cleeland, and E. Traisman, "Hyperkinesis and Food Additives: Testing the Feingold Hypothesis," *Pediatrics* 61(1978):818–828.

70. C. K. Conners, "Artificial Colors in the Diet and Disruptive Behavior: Current Status of Research," in *Nutrition and Behavior,* ed. S. A. Miller, Philadelphia: Franklin Institute, 1981.

71. B. Weiss, J. H. Williams, S. Margen, B. Abrams, B. Caan, L. J. Citron, C. Cox, J. McKibben, D. Ogar, and S. Schulz, "Behavioral Responses to Artificial Food Colors," *Science* 207(1980):1487–1489.

72. Conners, "Artificial Colors in the Diet."

G. Kolata, "Consensus on Diets and Hyperactivity," *Science* 215(1982):958.

The National Advisory Committee on Hyperkinesis and Food Additives, *Final Report to the Nutrition Foundation,* New York: The Nutrition Foundation, 1980.

73. B. Brecht, *Galileo,* C. Laughton, trans., New York: Grove, 1966, p. 61.

Chapter 9: Anorexia and Bulimia

1. "ILSI Conference Examines Effects of Calorically Restricted Diets onHealth and Aging in Animals," *ILSI News* (March/April 1990):1, 5.

2. R. Andres, "Influence of Obesity on Longevity in the Aged," *Advances in Pathobiology* 7(1980):238–246.

A. Keys, "Overweight, Obesity, Coronary Heart Disease and Mortality," *Nutrition Reviews* 38(1980):297–307.

3. Ibid.

4. N. E. Grunberg, "Specific Taste Preferences: An Alternative Explanation for Eating Changes in Cancer Patients," in *Cancer, Nutrition, and Eating Behavior*, eds. T. G. Burish, S. M. Levy, and B. E. Meyerowitz, Hillsdale, NJ: Lawrence Erlbaum Associates, 1985.

B. E. Meyerowitz, T. G. Burish, and S. M. Levy, "Cancer, Nutrition, and Eating Behavior: Introduction and Overview," in *Cancer, Nutrition, and Eating Behavior*, eds. T. G. Burish, S. M. Levy, and B. E. Meyerowitz, Hillsdale, NJ: Lawrence Erlbaum Associates, 1985.

U. S. Department of Health and Human Services, *The Surgeon General's Report on Nutrition and Health: Summary and Recommendations* (DHHS Publication No. 88-50211), Washington, DC: U. S. Government Printing Office, 1988.

5. L. E. Carrell, D. S. Cannon, M. R. Best, and M. J. Stone, "Nausea and Radiation-Induced Taste Aversions in Cancer Patients," *Appetite* 7(1986):203–208.

W. DeWys, "Nutritional Problems in Cancer Patients: Overview and Perspective," in *Cancer, Nutrition, and Eating Behavior*, eds. T. G. Burish, S. M. Levy, and B. E. Meyerowitz, Hillsdale, NJ: Lawrence Erlbaum Associates, 1985.

Grunberg, "Specific Taste Preferences."

R. A. Hoerr and V. R. Young, "Alterations in Nutrient Intake and Utilization Caused by Disease," in *Human Obesity*, eds. R. J. Wurtman and J. J. Wurtman, New York: New York Academy of Sciences, 1987.

6. I. L. Bernstein, "Learned Taste Aversions in Children Receiving Chemotherapy," *Science* 200 (1978):1302–1303.

I. L. Berstein and S. Borson, "Learned Food Aversion: A Component of Anorexia Syndromes," *Psychological Review* 93(1986):462–472.

I. L. Bernstein and M. M. Webster, "Learned Taste Aversions in Humans," *Physiology and Behavior* 25(1980):363–366.

I. L Bernstein and M. M. Webster, "Learned Food Aversions: A Consequence of Cancer Chemotherapy," in *Cancer, Nutrition, and Eating Behavior*, eds. T. G. Burish, S. M. Levy, and B. E. Meyerowitz, Hillsdale, NJ: Lawrence Erlbaum Associates, 1985.

7. J. C. Smith, J. T. Blumsack, and F. S. Bilek, "Radiation-Induced Taste Aversions in Rats and Humans," in *Cancer, Nutrition and Eating Behavior*, eds. T. G. Burish, S. M. Levy, and B. E. Meyerowitz, Hillsdale, NJ: Lawrence Erlbaum Associates, 1985.

8. G. R. Morrow and P. L. Dobkin, "Anticipatory Nausea and Vomiting in Cancer Patients Undergoing Chemotherapy Treatment: Prevalence, Etiology, and Behavioral Interventions," *Clinical Psychology Review* 8(1988):517–556.

M. Olafsdottir, P. O. Sjoden, and B. Westling, "Prevalence and Prediction of Chemotherapy-Related Anxiety, Nausea and Vomiting in Cancer Patients," *Behaviour Research and Therapy* 24(1986):59–66.

9. G. R. Morrow and C. Morrell, "Behavioral Treatment for the Anticipatory Nausea and Vomiting Induced by Cancer Chemotherapy," *The New England Journal of Medicine* 307(1982):1476–1480.

10. A. W. Logue, "Taste Aversion and the Generality of the Laws of Learning," *Psychological Bulletin* 86(1979):276–296.

11. T. G. Burish, W. H. Redd, and M. P. Carey, "Conditioned Nausea and Vomiting in Cancer Chemotherapy: Treatment Approaches," in *Cancer, Nutrition, and Eating Behavior*, eds T. G. Burish, S. M. Levy, and B. E. Meyerowitz, Hillsdale, NJ: Lawrence Erlbaum Associates, 1985.

12. Burish et al., "Conditioned Nausea and Vomiting."

M. P. Carey and T. G. Burish, "Etiology and Treatment of the Psychological Side Effects Associated with Cancer Chemotherapy: A Critical Review and Discussion," *Psychological Bulletin* 104(1988):307–325.

Morrow and Dobkin, "Anticipatory Nausea and Vomiting."

Morrow and Morrell, "Behavioral Treatment for the Anticipatory Nausea."

13. I. L. Bernstein and D. P. Fenner, "Learned Food Aversions: Heterogeneity of Animal Models of Tumor-Induced Anorexia," *Appetite*,

4(1983):79–86.

I. L. Bernstein and L. E. Goehler, "Chronic Lithium Chloride Infusions: Conditioned Suppression of Food Intake and Preference," *Behavioral Neuroscience* 97(1983):290–298.

I. L. Bernstein and C. M. Treneer, "Learned Food Aversions and Tumor Anorexia," in *Cancer, Nutrition, and Eating Behavior*, eds. T. G. Burish, S. M. Levy, and B. E. Meyerowitz, Hillsdale, NJ: Lawrence Erlbaum Associates, 1985.

14. J. E. Blundell, "Systems and Interactions: An Approach to the Pharmacology of Eating and Hunger," in *Eating and Its Disorders*, eds. A. J. Stunkard and E. Stellar, New York: Raven Press, 1984.

T. Silverstone and M. Kyriakides, "Clinical Pharmacology of Appetite," in *Drugs and Appetite*, ed. T. Silverstone, London: Academic Press, 1982.

15. Silverstone and Kyriakides, "Clinical Pharmacology of Appetite."

16. J. E. Blundell and C. J. Latham, "Behavioural Pharmacology of Feeding," in *Drugs and Appetite*, ed. T. Silverstone, London: Academic Press, 1982.

17. Blundell, "Systems and Interactions." Blundell and Latham, "Behavioural Pharmacology of Feeding."

S. F. Leibowitz and G. Shor-Posner, "Brain Serotonin and Eating Behavior," *Appetite* 7 Supplement (1986):1–14.

Silverstone and Kyriakides, "Clinical Pharmacology of Appetite."

18. S. M. Paul, B. Hulihan-Giblin, and P. Skolnick, "(+)-Amphetamine Binding to Rat Hypothalamus: Relation to Anorexic Potency of Phenylethylamines," *Science* 218(1982):487–490.

19. Blundell, "Systems and Interactions." Blundell and Latham, "Behavioural Pharmacology of Feeding."

20. M. H. Fernstrom and D. J. Kupfer, "Imipramine Treatment and Preference for Sweets," *Appetite* 10(1988):149–155.

E. Goodall and T. Silverstone, "The Effect of the 5-HT Releasing Drug d-Fenfluramine and the 5-HT Receptor Blocker, Metergoline, on Food Intake in Human Subjects," in *Human Obesity*, eds. R. J. Wurtman and J. J. Wurtman, New York: New York Academy of Sciences, 1987.

M. J. Russ and S. H. Ackerman, "Antidepressants and Weight Gain," *Appetite* 10(1988):103–117.

21. Blundell, "Systems and Interactions."

Silverstone and Kyriakides, "Clinical Pharmacology of Appetite."

22. Blundell, "Systems and Interactions."

23. Ibid.

24. Ibid.

Blundell and Latham, "Behavioural Pharmacology of Feeding."

25. *American Psychiatric Association: Diagnostic and Statistical Manual of Mental Disorders*, 3d ed. rev., Washington, DC: APA, 1987.

J. Slochower, S. P. Kaplan, and L. Mann, "The Effects of Life Stress and Weight on Mood and Eating," *Appetite* 2 (1981): 115–125.

G. I. Szmukler, "Drug Treatment of Anorexic States," in *Drugs and Appetite*, ed. T. Silverstone, London: Academic Press, 1982.

26. D. H. Baucom and P. A. Aiken, "Effect of Depressed Mood on Eating Among Obese and Nonobese Dieting and Nondieting Persons," *Journal of Personality and Social Psychology* 41(1981):577–585.

J. Polivy and C. P. Herman, "Clinical Depression and Weight Change: A Complex Relation," *Journal of Abnormal Psychology* 85(1976):338–340.

27. M. J. Russ and S. H. Ackerman, "Salivation and Depression: A Role for Appetitive Factors," *Appetite* 8(1987):37–47.

28. Blundell, "Systems and Interactions." Szmukler, "Drug Treatment of Anorexic States."

29. E. Fonberg, "The Relation between Alimentary and Emotional Amygdalar Regulation," in *Hunger: Basic Mechanisms and Clinical Implications*, eds. D. Novin, W. Wyrwicka, and G. Bray, New York: Raven Press, 1976.

30. Szmukler, "Drug Treatment of Anorexic States."

31. H. Bruch, *Eating Disorders*, New York: Basic Books, 1973, p. 4.

32. W. S. Agras, *Eating Disorders: Management of Obesity, Bulimia, and Anorexia Nervosa*, New York: Pergamon, 1987.

Bruch, *Eating Disorders*.

H. Bruch, *The Golden Cage*, Cambridge, MA: Harvard University Press, 1978.

A. H. Crisp, *Anorexia Nervosa: Let Me Be*, New York: Grune & Stratton, 1980.

P. E. Garfinkel and D. M. Garner, *Anorexia Nervosa*, New York: Brunner/Mazel, 1982.

B. P. Kinoy, *When Will We Laugh Again?*, New York: Columbia University Press, 1984.

G. R. Leon, *Treating Eating Disorders*, Lexington, MA: Lewis Publishing, 1983.

M. S. Palazzoli, *Self-Starvation*, London: Human Context Books, 1974.

R. L. Palmer, *Anorexia Nervosa*, New York: Penguin, 1980.

33. *American Psychiatric Association: Diagnostic and Statistical Manual of Mental Disorders*, 3rd ed. rev.

Garfinkel and Garner, *Anorexia Nervosa*.

34. A. H. Crisp, R. L. Palmer, and R. S. Kalucy, "How Common Is Anorexia Nervosa? A Prevalence Study," *British Journal of Psychiatry* 128(1976):549–554.

35. *American Psychiatric Association: Diagnostic and Statistical Manual of Mental Disorders*, 3rd ed. rev.

36. K. M. Bemis, "Current Approaches to the Etiology and Treatment of Anorexia Nervosa," *Psychological Bulletin* 85(1978):593–617.

Garfinkel and Garner, *Anorexia Nervosa*.

Palmer, *Anorexia Nervosa*.

G. Szmukler, C. McCance, L. McCrone, and D. Hunter, "Anorexia Nervosa: A Psychiatric Case Register Study from Aberdeen," *Psychological Medicine* 16(1986):49–58.

J. Willi and S. Grossman, "Epidemiology of Anorexia Nervosa in a Defined Region of Switzerland," *American Journal of Psychiatry* 140(1983):564–567.

37. Bruch, *The Golden Cage*, p. 3.

38. *American Psychiatric Association: Diagnostic and Statistical Manual of Mental Disorders*, 3rd ed. rev.

39. Garfinkel and Garner, *Anorexia Nervosa*.

40. *American Psychiatric Association: Diagnostic and Statistical Manual of Mental Disorders* 3rd ed. rev.

41. R. E. Frisch, "Fatness and Fertility," *Scientific American* (March 1988):88–95.

R. E. Frisch, "Food Intake, Fatness, and Reproductive Ability," in *Anorexia Nervosa*, ed. R. A. Vigersky, New York: Raven Press, 1977.

42. *American Psychiatric Association: Diagnostic and Statistical Manual of Mental Disorders*, 3rd ed. rev.

43. Ibid.

44. Ibid.

45. Bruch, *Eating Disorders*.

Bruch, *The Golden Cage*.

Crisp, *Anorexia Nervosa: Let Me Be*.

46. *American Psychiatric Association: Diagnostic and Statistical Manual of Mental Disorders*, 3rd ed. rev.

47. Garfinkel and Garner, *Anorexia Nervosa*.

D. M. Garner, P. E. Garfinkel, H. C. Stancer, and H. Moldofsky, "Body Image Disturbances in Anorexia Nervosa," *Psychosomatic Medicine* 38(1976):327–336.

48. G. I. Szmukler, "Anorexia Nervosa: A Clinical Review," in *Eating Habits: Food, Physiology and Learned Behavior*, eds. R. A. Boakes, D. A. Popplewell, and M. J. Burton, Chichester, Great Britain: John Wiley & Sons, 1987.

49. W. Bennett and J. Gurin, *The Dieter's Dilemma*, New York: Basic Books, 1982.

Bruch, *Eating Disorders*.

Garfinkel and Garner, *Anorexia Nervosa*.

J. Polivy and L. Thomsen, "Dieting and Other Eating Disorders," in *Handbook of Behavioral Medicine for Women*, eds. E. A. Blechman and K. D. Brownell, New York: Pergamon, 1988.

50. A. Drewnowski and D. K. Yee, "Men and Body Image: Are Males Satisfied with Their Body Weight?" *Psychosomatic Medicine* 49(1987):626–634.

A. E. Fallon and P. Rozin, "Sex Differences in Perceptions of Desirable Body Shape," *Journal of Abnormal Psychology* 94(1985):102–105.

P. Rozin and A. Fallon, "Body Image, Attitudes to Weight, and Misperceptions of Figure Preferences of the Opposite Sex: A Comparison of Men and Women in Two Generations," *Journal of Abnormal Psychology* 97(1988):342–345.

J. Wardle and S. Beales, "Restraint, Body Image and Food Attitudes in Children from 12 to 18 Years," *Appetite* 7(1986):209–217.

51. Fallon and Rozin, "Sex Differences in Perceptions of Desirable Body Shape."

52. Bruch, *Eating Disorders*.

53. H. Fries, "Studies on Secondary Amenorrhea, Anorectic Behavior, and Body-Image Perception: Importance for the Early Recognition of Anorexia Nervosa," in *Anorexia Nervosa*, ed. R. A. Vigersky, New York: Raven Press, 1977.

54. Garfinkel and Garner, *Anorexia Nervosa*.

R. S. Mecklenburg, D. L. Loriaux, R. H. Thompson, A. E. Andersen, and M. B. Lipsett, "Hypothalamic Dysfunction in Patients with Anorexia Nervosa," *Medicine* 53(1974):147–157.

Palmer, *Anorexia Nervosa*.

G. Russell, "The Present Status of Anorexia Nervosa," *Psychological Medicine* 7(1977):363–367.

55. Garfinkel and Garner, *Anorexia Nervosa*.

Palmer, *Anorexia Nervosa*.

56. S. F. Leibowitz, "Hypothalamic Neurotransmitters in Relation to Normal and Disturbed Eating Patterns," in *Human Obesity*, eds.

R. J. Wurtman and J. J. Wurtman, New York: New York Academy of Sciences, 1987.

R. Pasquali, E. Strocchi, P. Malini, F. Casimirri, E. Ambrosioni, N. Melchionda, and G. Labo, "Altered Erythrocyte Na-K Pump in Anorectic Patients," *Metabolism* 34(1985):670–674.

K. M. Pirk and D. Ploog, "Psychobiology of Anorexia Nervosa," in *Nutrition and the Brain*, vol. 7, eds. R. J. Wurtman and J. J. Wurtman, New York: Raven Press, 1986.

R. A. Vigersky, A. E. Andersen, R. H. Thompson, and D. L. Loriaux, "Hypothalamic Dysfunction in Secondary Amenorrhea Associated with Simple Weight Loss," *The New England Journal of Medicine* 297(1977):1141–1145.

57. Bemis, "Current Approaches to the Etiology and Treatment."

Bruch, *The Golden Cage.*

J. A. Dinsmoor, "The Effect of Hunger on Discriminated Responding," *Journal of Abnormal and Social Psychology* 47(1952):67–72.

W. F. Epling, W. D. Pierce, and L. Stefan, "A Theory of Activity-Based Anorexia," *The International Journal of Eating Disorders* 3(1983):27–46.

Palmer, *Anorexia Nervosa.*

58. Bruch, *The Golden Cage*, p. 62.

59. Palmer, *Anorexia Nervosa*, p. 20.

60. Bruch, *The Golden Cage*, p. 61.

61. S. S. Van Buskirk, "A Two-Phase Perspective on the Treatment of Anorexia Nervosa," *Psychological Bulletin*, 84(1977):529–538.

62. Garfinkel and Garner, *Anorexia Nervosa.*

63. W. S. Agras and H. C. Kraemer, "The Treatment of Anorexia Nervosa: Do Different Treatments Have Different Outcomes?" in *Eating and Its Disorders*, eds. A. J. Stunkard and E. Stellar, New York: Raven Press, 1984.

Garfinkel and Garner, *Anorexia Nervosa.*

64. Garfinkel and Garner, *Anorexia Nervosa.*

65. H. I. Kalish, *From Behavioral Science to Behavior Modification*, New York: McGraw-Hill, 1981, p. 3.

66. Van Buskirk, "A Two-Phase Perspective on the Treatment."

67. Agras and Kraemer, "The Treatment of Anorexia Nervosa."

G. R. Leon, *Treating Eating Disorders*, Brattleboro, VT: Lewis Publishing, 1983.

68. Leon, *Treating Eating Disorders.*

69. Garfinkel and Garner, *Anorexia Nervosa.*

70. Agras and Kraemer, "The Treatment of Anorexia Nervosa."

71. Garfinkel and Garner, *Anorexia Nervosa.*

72. Ibid.

73. H. Bruch, "Anorexia Nervosa: Therapy and Theory," *American Journal of Psychiatry* 139(1982):1531–1538.

74. Agras and Kraemer, "The Treatment of Anorexia Nervosa."

Agras, *Eating Disorders.*

Van Buskirk, "A Two-Phase Perspective on the Treatment."

75. Agras and Kraemer, "The Treatment of Anorexia Nervosa."

76. Bemis, "Current Approaches to the Etiology and Treatment."

Garfinkel and Garner, *Anorexia Nervosa.*

77. Garfinkel and Garner, *Anorexia Nervosa.*

78. M. K. Jacobs and G. Goodman, "Psychology and Self-Help Groups," *American Psychologist* 44(1989):536–545.

79. Bruch, *Eating Disorders.*

Garfinkel and Garner, *Anorexia Nervosa.*

H. G. Morgan and G. F. M. Russell, "Value of Family Background and Clinical Features as Predictors of Long-Term Outcome in Anorexia Nervosa: Four-Year Follow-Up Study of 41 Patients," *Psychological Medicine* 5(1975):355–371.

80. *American Psychiatric Association: Diagnostic and Statistical Manual of Mental Disorders*, 3rd ed. rev., p. 67.

81. C. L. Johnson, M. K. Stuckey, L. D. Lewis, and D. M. Schwartz, "Bulimia: A Descriptive Survey of 316 Cases," *International Journal of Eating Disorders* 2(1982):3–15.

82. G. Russell, "Bulimia Nervosa: An Ominous Variant of Anorexia Nervosa," *Psychological Medicine* 9(1979):429–448.

83. Logue, "Taste Aversion and the Generality of the Laws of Learning."

A. W. Logue, K. R. Logue, and K. E. Strauss, "The Acquisition of Taste Aversions in Humans with Eating and Drinking Disorders," *Behaviour Research and Therapy* 21(1983):275–289.

84. *American Psychiatric Association: Diagnostic and Statistical Manual of Mental Disorders*, 3rd ed. rev.

C. Johnson and R. Larson, "Bulimia: An Analysis of Moods and Behavior," *Psychosomatic Medicine* 44(1982):341–351.

B. Schlesier-Stropp, "Bulimia: A Review of the Literature," *Psychological Bulletin* 95 (1984): 247–257.

85. C. G. Fairburn, "Bulimia: Its Epidemiology and Management," in *Eating and Its Disorders*, eds. A. J. Stunkard and E. Stellar, New York:

Raven Press, 1984.

R. L. Pyle, J. E. Mitchell, and E. D. Eckert, "Bulimia: A Report of 34 Cases," *The Journal of Clinical Psychiatry* 42(1981):60–64.

Russell, "Bulimia Nervosa."

Schlesier-Stropp, "Bulimia."

86. "Energy Expenditure and the Control of Body Weight," *Nutrition Reviews* 47(1989):249–252.

H. E. Gwirtsman, W. H. Kaye, E. Obarzanek, D. T. George, D. C. Jimerson, and M. H. Ebert, "Decreased Caloric Intake in Normal-Weight Patients with Bulimia: Comparison with Female Volunteers," *American Journal of Clinical Nutrition* 49(1989):86–92.

87. D. J. Broberg and I. L. Bernstein, "Preabsorptive Insulin Release in Bulimic Women and Chronic Dieters," *Appetite* 13(1989):161–169.

J. Russell, L. Storlien, and P. Beumont, "A Proposed Model of Bulimic Behavior: Effect on Plasma Insulin, Noradrenalin, and Cortisol Levels," *International Journal of Eating Disorders* 6(1987):609–614.

U. Schweiger, J. Poellinger, R. Laessle, G. Wolfram, M. M. Fichter, K.-M. Pirke, "Altered Insulin Response to a Balanced Test Meal in Bulimic Patients," *International Journal of Eating Disorders* 6 (1987):551–556.

H. P. Weingarten, R. Hendler, and J. Rodin, "Metabolism and Endocrine Secretion in Response to a Test Meal in Normal-Weight Bulimic Women," *Psychosomatic Medicine* 50(1988):273–285.

88. H. R. Kissileff, B. T. Walsh, J. G. Kral, and S. M. Cassidy, "Laboratory Studies of Eating Behavior in Women with Bulimia," *Physiology and Behavior* 38(1986):563–570.

B. T. Walsh, H. R. Kissileff, S. M. Cassidy, and S. Dantzic, "Eating Behavior of Women with Bulimia," *Archives of General Psychiatry* 46(1989): 54–58.

89. Schlesier-Stropp, "Bulimia."

90. Ibid.

91. A. Drewnowski, S. A. Hopkins, and R. C. Kessler, "The Prevalence of Bulimia Nervosa in the US College Student Population," *American Journal of Public Health* 78(1988):1322–1325.

K. A. Halmi, J. R. Falk, and E. Schwartz, "Binge-Eating and Vomiting: A Survey of a College Population," *Psychological Medicine* 11(1981):697–706.

D. E. Schotte and A. J. Stunkard, "Bulimia vs. Bulimic Behaviors on a College Campus," *Journal*

of the *American Medical Association* 258(1987):1213–1215.

R. H. Striegel, L. R. Silberstein, P. Frensch, and J. Rodin, "A Prospective Study of Disordered Eating among College Students," *International Journal of Eating Disorders* 8(1989):499–509.

92. G. Kolata, "Epidemic of Dangerous Eating Disorders May Be False Alarm," *The New York Times* (August 25, 1988):B16.

93. C. G. Fairburn, "Bulimia: Its Epidemiology and Management," in *Eating and Its Disorders*, eds. A. J. Stunkard and E. Stellar, New York: Raven Press, 1984.

94. Garfinkel and Garner, *Anorexia Nervosa*, p. 5.

95. Leon, *Treating Eating Disorders.*

Russell, "Bulimia Nervosa."

96. Russell, "Bulimia Nervosa."

97. Leon, *Treating Eating Disorders.*

98. M. R. Lowe, "Dieting and Binging: Some Unanswered Questions," *American Psychologist* 41(1986):326–327.

J. Polivy and C. P. Herman, "Dieting and Binging," *American Psychologist* 40(1985):193–201.

J. Polivy and C. P. Herman, "Dieting and Binging Reexamined: A Response to Lowe," *American Psychologist* 41(1986):327–328.

99. Johnson and Larson, "Bulimia."

R. G. Laessle, S. Kittl, U. Schweiger, M. M. Fichter, and K. M. Pirke, "The Major Affective Disorder in Anorexia Nervosa and Bulimia," in *Human Obesity*, eds R. J. Wurtman and J. J. Wurtman, New York: New York Academy of Sciences, 1987.

Leon, *Treating Eating Disorders.*

100. J. I. Hudson, P. S. Laffer, and H. G. Pope, "Bulimia Related to Affective Disorder by Family History and Response to the Dexamethasone Suppression Test," *American Journal of Psychiatry* 139(1982):685–687.

M. Strober, B. Salkin, J. Burroughs, and W. Morrell, "Validity of the Bulimia-Restricter Distinction in Anorexia Nervosa: Parental Personality Characteristics and Family Psychiatric Morbidity," *The Journal of Nervous and Mental Disease* 170(1982):345–351.

101. H. G. Pope and J. I. Hudson, *New Hope for Binge Eaters*, New York: Harper & Row, 1984.

102. L. D. Hinz and D. A. Williamson, "Bulimia and Depression: A Review of the Affective Variant Hypothesis," *Psychologiacal Bulletin* 102(1987): 150–158.

N. E. Rosenthal and M. M. Heffernan,

"Bulimia, Carbohydrate Craving, and Depression: A Central Connection?" in *Nutrition and the Brain*, vol. 7, eds. R. J. Wurtman and J. J. Wurtman, New York: Raven Press, 1986.

B. T. Walsh, M. Gladis, and S. P. Roose, "Food Intake and Mood in Anorexia Nervosa and Bulimia," in *Human Obesity*, eds. R. J. Wurtman and J. J. Wurtman, New York: New York Academy of Sciences, 1987.

103. C. Fairburn, "A Cognitive Behavioural Approach to the Treatment of Bulimia," *Psychological Medicine* 11(1981):707–711.

P. M. Monti, B. S. McCrady, and D. H. Barlow, "Effect of Positive Reinforcement, Informational Feedback, and Contingency Contracting on a Bulimic Anorexic Female," *Behavior Therapy* 8(1977):258–263.

104. W. G. Johnson, D. G. Schlundt, M. L. Kelley, and L. Ruggiero, "Exposure with Response Prevention and Energy Regulation in the Treatment of Bulimia," *International Journal of Eating Disorders* 3(1984):37–46.

J. C. Rosen and H. Leitenberg, "Bulimia Nervosa: Treatment with Exposure and Response Prevention," *Behavior Therapy* 13(1982):117–124.

105. G. T. Wilson, E. Rossiter, E. I. Kleifield, and L. Lindholm, "Cognitive-Behavioral Treatment of Bulimia Nervosa: A Controlled Evaluation," *Behaviour Research and Therapy* 24(1986):277–288.

106. S. Dalvit-McPhillips, "A Dietary Approach to Bulimia Treatment," *Physiology and Behavior* 33(1984):769–775.

107. Agras, *Eating Disorders.*

J. I. Hudson, H. G. Pope, and J. M. Jonas, "Treatment of Bulimia with Antidepressants: Theoretical Considerations and Clinical Findings," in *Eating and Its Disorders*, eds. A. J. Stunkard and E. Stellar, New York: Raven Press, 1984.

E. M. Rossiter, W. S. Agras, and M. Losch, "Changes in Self-Reported Food Intake in Bulimics as a Consequence of Antidepressant Treatment," *International Journal of Eating Disorders* 7(1988):779–783.

B. T. Walsh, J. W. Stewart, L. Wright, W. Harrison, S. P. Roose, and A. H. Glassman, "Treatment of Bulimia with Monoamine Oxidase Inhibitors," *The American Journal of Psychiatry* 139(1982):1629–1630.

108. H. G. Pope, J. I. Hudson, J. M. Jonas, and D. Yurgelun-Todd, "Bulimia Treated with Imipramine: A Placebo-Controlled, Double-Blind Study," *American Journal of Psychiatry* 140(1983):554–558.

109. Russell, "Bulimia Nervosa."

110. E. M. Rossiter, W. S. Agras, M. Losch, and C. F. Telch, "Dietary Restraint of Bulimic Subjects Following Cognitive-Behavioral or Pharmacological Treatment," *Behaviour Research and Therapy* 26(1988):495–498.

111. Agras, *Eating Disorders.*

Chapter 10:
Overeating and Obesity

1. G. A. Bray, "Overweight is Risking Fate: Definition, Classification, Prevalence, and Risks," in *Human Obesity*, eds. R. J. Wurtman and J. J. Wurtman, New York: New York Academy of Sciences, 1987.

2. H. A. Guthrie, *Introductory Nutrition*, St. Louis: C. V. Mosby, 1975.

3. A. P. Simopoulos, "Characteristics of Obesity: An Overview," in *Human Obesity*, eds. R. J. Wurtman and J. J. Wurtman, New York: New York Academy of Sciences, 1987.

4. G. Kolata, "Obese Children: A Growing Problem," *Science* 232(1986):20–21.

5. Simopoulos, "Characteristics of Obesity." R. B. Stuart and B. Davis, *Slim Chance in a Fat World*, Champaign, IL: Research Press, 1972.

6. J. Sobal and A. J. Stunkard, "Socioeconomic Status and Obesity: A Review of the Literature," *Psychological Bulletin* 105(1989):260–275.

7. L. Spitzer and J. Rodin, "Human Eating Behavior: A Critical Review of Studies in Normal Weight and Overweight Individuals," *Appetite* 2(1981):293–329.

8. W. Kulesza, "Dietary Intake in Obese Women," *Appetite* 3(1982):61–68.

9. J. M. Slattery and R. M. Potter, "Hyperphagia: A Necessary Precondition to Obesity?" *Appetite* 6(1985):133–142.

10. J. Gormally, S. Black, S. Daston, and D. Rardin, "The Assessment of Binge Eating Severity among Obese Persons," *Addictive Behaviors* 7(1982):47–55.

11. R. Plutchik, "Emotions and Attitudes Related to Being Overweight," *Journal of Clinical Psychology* 32(1976):21–24.

12. J. Slochower and S. P. Kaplan, "Anxiety, Perceived Control, and Eating in Obese and Normal Weight Persons," *Appetite* 1(1980):75–83.

13. J. Slochower, S. P. Kaplan, and L. Mann, "The Effects of Life Stress and Weight on Mood and Eating," *Appetite* 2(1981):115–125.

14. A. J. Ruderman, "Dietary Restraint: A Theoretical and Empirical Review," *Psychological Bulletin* 99(1986):247–262.

15. R. J. Wurtman and J. J. Wurtman, "Carbohydrates and Depression," *Scientific American* 260(January 1989):68–75.

16. R. Gurney, "The Hereditary Factor in Obesity," *Archives of Internal Medicine* 57(1936):557–561.

17. G. A. Bray and D. A. York, "Genetically Transmitted Obesity in Rodents," *Physiological Reviews* 51(1971): 598–646.

J. F. Hayes and J. C. McCarthy, "The Effects of Selection at Different Ages for High and Low Body Weight on the Pattern of Fat Deposition in Mice," *Genetical Research* 27(1976):389–433.

C. E. Hunt, J. R. Linsey, and S. U. Walkey, "Animal Models of Diabetes and Obesity, Including the PBB/Ld Mouse," *Federation Proceedings* 35(1976):1206-1217.

18. T. T. Foch and G. E. McClearn, "Genetics, Body Weight, and Obesity," in *Obesity*, ed. A. J. Stunkard, Philadelphia: W. B. Saunders, 1980.

A. J. Stunkard, T. T. Foch, and Z. Hrubec, "A Twin Study of Human Obesity," *The Journal of the American Medical Association* 256 (1986):51–54.

A. J. Stunkard, T. I. A. Sorensen, C. Hanis, T. W. Teasdale, R. Chakraborty, W. J. Schull, and F. Schulsinger, "An Adoption Study of Human Obesity," *The New England Journal of Medicine* 314(1986):193–198.

19. Foch and McClearn, "Genetics, Body Weight, and Obesity."

20. L. Sjöström, "The Contribution of Fat Cells to the Determination of Body Weight," in *Symposium on Obesity: Basic Mechanisms and Treatment*, ed. A. J. Stunkard, Philadelphia: W. B. Saunders, 1978.

L. Sjöström, "Fat Cells and Body Weight," in *Obesity*, ed. A. J. Stunkard, Philadelphia: W. B. Saunders, 1980.

21. P. Björntorp, "Fat Cell Distribution and Metabolism," in *Human Obesity*, eds. R. J. Wurtman and J. J. Wurtman, New York: New York Academy of Sciences, 1987.

22. Sjöström, "The Contribution of Fat Cells." Sjöström, "Fat Cells and Body Weight."

23. E. Jéquier, "Energy Utilization in Human Obesity," in *Human Obesity*, eds. R. J. Wurtman and J. J. Wurtman, New York: New York

Academy of Sciences, 1987.

G. A. Bray, *The Obese Patient*, Philadelphia: W. B. Saunders, 1976.

24. C. Geissler, "Genetic Differences in Metabolic Rate," in *Low-Calorie Products*, eds. G. G. Birch and M. G. Lindley, New York: Elsevier, 1988.

E. Ravussin, S. Lillioja, W. C. Knowler, L. Christin, D. Freymond, W. G. H. Abbott, V. Boyce, B. V. Howard, and C. Bogardus, "Reduced Rate of Energy Expenditure as a Risk Factor for Body-Weight Gain," *The New England Journal of Medicine* 318(1988):467–472.

25. W. H. Dietz, "Childhood Obesity," in *Human Obesity*, eds. R. J. Wurtman and J. J. Wurtman, New York:New York Academy of Sciences, 1987.

N. Finer, "Consequences of Obesity," in *Low-Calorie Products*, eds. G. G. Birch and M. G. Lindley, New York: Elsevier, 1988.

Jéquier, "Energy Utilization in Human Obesity."

26. R. E. Keesey and S. W. Corbett, "Metabolic Defense of the Body Weight Set-Point," in *Eating and Its Disorders*, eds. A. J. Stunkard and E. Stellar, New York: Raven Press, 1984.

S. N. Steen, R. A. Oppliger, and K. D. Brownell, "Metabolic Effects of Repeated Weight Loss and Regain in Adolescent Wrestlers," *The Journal of the American Medical Association* 260(1988):1–50.

27. D. L. Elliot, L. Goldberg, K. S. Kuehl, and W. M. Bennett, "Sustained Depression of the Resting Metabolic Rate After Massive Weight Loss," *American Journal of Clinical Nutrition* 49(1989): 93–96.

28. H. T. Edwards, A. Thorndike, and D. B. Dill, "The Energy Requirements in Strenuous Muscular Exercise," *The New England Journal of Medicine* 213(1935):532–535.

E. T. Poehlman and E. S. Horton, "The Impact of Food Intake and Exercise on Energy Expenditure," *Nutrition Reviews* 47(1989):129–137.

29. S. A. Bingham, G. R. Goldberg, W. A. Coward, A. M. Prentice, and J. H. Cummings, "The Effect of Exercise and Improved Physical Fitness on Basal Metabolic Rate," *British Journal of Nutrition* 61(1989):155–173.

30. D. van Dale and W. H. M. Saris, "Repetitive Weight Loss and Weight Regain: Effects on Weight Reduction, Resting Metabolic Rate, and Lipolytic Activity before and after Exercise and/or Diet Treatment," *American Journal of Clini-*

cal Nutrition 49(1989):409–416.

31. J. Brener, "Behavioural Energetics: Some Effects of Uncertainty on the Mobilization and Distribution of Energy," *Psychophysiology* 24(1987):499–512.

J. Brener and S. Mitchell, "Changes in Energy Expenditure and Work during Response Acquisition in Rats," *Journal of Experimantal Psychology: Animal Behavior Processes* 15(1989):166–175.

32. K. D. Brownell and A. J. Stunkard, "Physical Activity in the Development and Control of Obesity," in *Obesity,* ed. A. J. Stunkard, Philadelphia: W. B. Saunders, 1980.

Dietz, "Childhood Obesity."

J. K. Thompson, G. J. Jarvie, B. B. Lahey, and K. J. Cureton, "Exercise and Obesity: Etiology, Physiology, and Intervention," *Psychological Bulletin* 91(1982):55–79.

33. Jéquier, "Energy Utilization in Human Obesity."

34. Dietz, "Childhood Obesity."

35. R. S. Schwartz, E. Ravussin, M. Massari, M. O'Connell, and D. C. Robbins, "The Thermic Effect of Carbohydrate versus Fat Feeding in Man," *Metabolism* 34(1985):285–293.

36. Jéquier, "Energy Utilization in Human Obesity."

37. Keesey and Corbett, "Metabolic Defense of the Body Weight Set-Point."

38. "Lean Body Mass and Food-Induced Thermogenesis in Obesity," *Nutrition Reviews* 45(1987):264–265.

Schwartz et al., "The Thermic Effect of Carbohydrate versus Fat."

39. E. T. Poehlman, A. Tremblay, E. Fontaine, J. P. Depres, A. Nadeau, J. Dussault, and C. Bouchard, "Genotype Dependency of the Thermic Effect of a Meal and Associated Hormonal Changes Following Short-Term Overfeeding," *Metabolism* 35(1986):30–36.

40. T. Silverstone, "Mood and Food: A Psychopharmacological Enquiry," in *Human Obesity,* eds. R. J. Wurtman and J. J. Wurtman, New York: New York Academy of Sciences, 1987.

J. J. Wurtman, "Disorders of Food Intake: Excessive Carbohydrate Snack Intake among a Class of Obese People," in *Human Obesity,* eds. R. J. Wurtman and J. J. Wurtman, New York: New York Academy of Sciences, 1987.

R. J. Wurtman and J. J. Wurtman, "Carbohydrates and Depression."

41. E. M. Bobroff and H. R. Kissileff, "Effects of Changes in Palatability on Food Intake and the Cumulative Food Intake Curve in Man," *Appetite* 7(1986):85–96.

H. A. Jordan and T. A. Spiegel, "Palatability and Oral Factors and Their Role in Obesity," in *The Chemical Senses and Nutrition,* eds. M. R. Kare and O. Maller, New York: Academic Press, 1977.

A. Sclafani, "Dietary Obesity," in *Obesity,* ed. A. J. Stunkard, Philadelphia: W. B. Saunders, 1980.

A. Sclafani and D. Springer, "Dietary Obesity in Adult Rats: Similarities to Hypothalamic and Human Obesity Syndromes," *Physiology and Behavior* 17(1976):461–471.

42. P. G. Clifton, M. J. Burton, and C. Sharp, "Rapid Loss of Stimulus-Specific Satiety after Consumption of a Second Food," *Appetite* 9(1987):149–156.

B. J. Rolls, E. A. Rowe, E. T. Rolls, B. Kingston, A. Megson, and R. Gunary, "Variety in a Meal Enhances Food Intake in Man," *Physiology and Behavior* 26(1981):215–221.

43. J. E. Blundell and A. J. Hill, "Paradoxical Effects of an Intense Sweetener (Aspartame) on Appetite," *The Lancet* (May 10, 1986):1092–1093.

P. M. Brala and R. L. Hagen, "Effects of Sweetness Perception and Caloric Value of a Preload on Short Term Intake," *Physiology and Behavior* 30(1983):1–9.

K. P. Porikos and H. S. Koopmans, "The Effect of Non-Nutritive Sweeteners on Body Weight in Rats," *Appetite* 11 Supplement(1988):12–15.

M. G. Tordoff and M. I. Friedman, "Drinking Saccharin Increases Food Intake and Preference—I. Comparison with Other Drinks," *Appetite* 12(1989):1–10.

44. D. G. Bruce, L. H. Storlien, S. M. Furler, and D. J. Chisholm, "Cephalic Phase Metabolic Responses in Normal Weight Adults," *Metabolism* 36(1987):721–725.

P. J. Geiselman, "Sugar-Induced Hyperphagia: Is Hyperinsulinemia, Hypoglycemia, or Any Other Factor a 'Necessary' Condition?" *Appetite* 11 Supplement(1988):26–34.

J. Rodin, "Insulin Levels, Hunger, and Food Intake: An Example of Feedback Loops in Body Weight Regulation," *Health Psychology* 4(1985):1–24.

J. Rodin, J. Wack, E. Ferrannini, and R. A. DeFronzo, "Effect of Insulin and Glucose on Feeding Behavior," *Metabolism* 34(1985):826–831.

C. Simon, J. L. Schlienger, R. Sapin, and M. Imler, "Cephalic Phase Insulin Secretion in Relation to Food Presentation in Normal and Overweight Subjects," *Physiology and Behavior* 36(1986):465–469.

M. G. Tordoff and M. I. Friedman, "Drinking Saccharin Increases Food Intake and Preference—IV. Cephalic Phase and Metabolic Factors," *Appetite* 12(1989):37–56.

D. A. VanderWeele, "Hyperinsulinism and Feeding; Not All Sequences Lead to the Same Behavioral Outcome or Conclusions," *Appetite* 6(1985):47–52.

J. R. Vasselli, "Carbohydrate Ingestion, Hypoglycemia, and Obesity," *Appetite* 6(1985):53–59.

45. S. Schachter, "Some Extraordinary Facts about Obese Humans and Rats," *American Psychologist* 26(1971):129–144.

46. J. Rodin, "Obesity: Why the Losing Battle?" *JSAS: Catalog of Selected Documents in Psychology* 9(2, 1979):17 (ms. no. 1839).

J. Rodin, "The Externality Theory Today," in *Obesity,* ed. A. J. Stunkard, Philadelphia: W. B. Saunders, 1980.

J. Rodin, "Current Status of the Internal-External Hypothesis for Obesity," *American Psychologist* 36(1981):361–372.

47. R. Deutsch, "Conditioned Hypoglycemia: A Mechanism for Saccharin-Induced Sensitivity to Insulin in the Rat," *Journal of Comparative and Physiological Psychology* 86(1974):350–358.

48. N. E. Rowland and S. M. Antelman, "Stress-Induced Hyperphagia and Obesity in Rats: A Possible Model for Understanding Human Obesity," *Science* 191(1976):310–312.

49. S. M. Antelman and A. R. Caggiula, "Tails of Stress-Related Behavior: A Neuropharmacological Model," in *Animal Models in Psychiatry and Neurology,* eds. I. Hanin and E. Usdin, New York: Pergamon, 1977.

D. M. Marques, A. E. Fisher, M. S. Okrutny, and N. E. Rowland, "Tail Pinch Induced Fluid Ingestion: Interactions of Taste and Deprivation," *Physiology and Behavior* 22(1979):37–41.

50. M. B. Cantor, "Bad Habits: Models of Induced Ingestion in Satiated Rats and People," in *Nutrition and Behavior,* ed. S. A. Miller, Philadelphia: Franklin Institute, 1981.

51. J. F. Wilson and M. B. Cantor, "An Animal Model of Excessive Eating: Schedule-Induced Hyperphagia in Food-Satiated Rats," *Journal of the Experimental Analysis of Behavior* 47(1987):335–346.

52. M. B. Cantor, S. E. Smith, and B. R. Bryan, "Induced Bad Habits: Adjunctive Ingestion and Grooming in Human Subjects," *Appetite* 3(1982):1–12.

53. Ibid.

M. B. Cantor and J. F. Wilson, "Feeding the Face: New Directions in Adjunctive Behavior Research," in *Affect, Conditioning, and Cognition: Essays on the Determinants of Behavior,* eds. F. R. Brush and J. B. Overmier, Hillsdale, NJ: Lawrence Erlbaum Associates, 1985.

54. C. Ferber and M. Cabanac, "Influence of Noise on Gustatory Affective Ratings and Preference for Sweet or Salt," *Appetite* 8(1987):229–235.

A. McCarron and K. J. Tierney, "The Effect of Auditory Stimulation on the Consumption of Soft Drinks," *Appetite* 13(1989):155–159.

T. C. Roballey, C. McGreevy, R. R. Rongo, M. L. Schwantes, P. J. Steger, M. A. Wininger, and E. B. Gardner, "The Effect of Music on Eating Behavior," *Bulletin of the Psychonomic Society* 23(1985):221–222.

55. T. W. Robbins and P. J. Fray, "Stress-Induced Eating: Fact, Fiction or Misunderstanding?" *Appetite* 1(1980):103–133.

56. H. Bruch, *Eating Disorders,* New York: Basic Books, 1973.

57. Cantor et al., "Induced Bad Habits."

Robbins and Fray, "Stress-Induced Eating: Fact, Fiction or Misunderstanding?"

58. S. M. Antelman and N. Rowland, "Endogenous Opiates and Stress-Induced Eating," *Science* 214(1981):1149–1150.

R. C. Bolles, "Stress-Induced Overeating? A Response to Robbins and Fray," *Appetite* 1(1980):229–230.

P. J. Fray and T. W. Robbins, "Stress-Induced Eating: Rejoinder," *Appetite* 1(1980):349–353.

C. P. Herman and J. Polivy, "Stress-Induced Eating and Eating-Induced Stress (Reduction?): A Response to Robbins and Fray," *Appetite* 1(1980):135–139.

J. E. Morley and A. S. Levine, "Stress-Induced Eating is Mediated through Endogenous Opiates," *Science* 209(1980):1259–1261.

J. E. Morley and A. S. Levine, "Endogenous Opiates and Stress-Induced Eating," *Science* 214(1981):1150–1151.

Robbins and Fray, "Stress-Induced Eating: Fact, Fiction or Misunderstanding?"

T. W. Robbins and P. J. Fray, "Stress-Induced Eating: Reply to Bolles, Rowland and Marques, and Herman and Polivy," *Appetite* 1(1980):231–239.

N. Rowland and D. M. Marques, "Stress-Induced Eating: Misrepresentation?" *Appetite* 1(1980):225–228.

L. Spitzer, J. Marcus, and J. Rodin, "Arousal-Induced Eating: A Response to Robbins and Fray," *Appetite* 1(1980):343–348.

59. Bruch, *Eating Disorders.*

60. H. P. Weingarten, "Conditioned Cues Elicit Feeding in Sated Rats: A Role for Learning in Meal Initiation," *Science* 220(1983):431–433.

61. L. L. Birch, L. McPhee, S. Sullivan, and S. Johnson, "Conditioned Meal Initiation in Young Children," *Appetite* 13(1989):105–113.

62. M. G. Lowe, "The Role of Anticipated Deprivation in Overeating," *Addictive Behaviors* 7(1982):103–112.

63. D. A. Booth, "Acquired Behavior Controlling Energy Intake and Output," in *Obesity*, ed. A. J. Stunkard, Philadelphia: W. B. Saunders, 1980.

R. C. Hawkins, "Learning to Initiate and Terminate Meals: Theoretical Clinical and Developmental Aspects," in *Learning Mechanisms in Food Selection*, eds. L. M. Barker, M. Best, and M. Domjan, Waco, TX: Baylor University Press, 1977.

64. S. L. Berry, W. W. Beatty, and R. C. Klesges, "Sensory and Social Influences on Ice Cream Consumption by Males and Females in a Laboratory Setting," *Appetite* 6(1985):41–45.

65. B. Edelman, D. Engell, P. Bronstein, and E. Hirsh, "Environmental Effects on the Intake of Overweight and Normal-Weight Men," *Appetite* 7(1986):71–83.

66. J. Polivy, C. P. Herman, J. C. Younger, and B. Erskine, "Effects of a Model on Eating Behavior: The Induction of a Restrained Eating Style," Journal of Personality 47(1979):100–117.

67. D. B. Jeffrey, "Treatment Evaluation Issues in Research on Addictive Behaviors," *Addictive Behaviors* 1(1975):23–26.

G. T. Wilson, "Methodological Considerations in Treatment Outcome Research on Obesity," *Journal of Consulting and Clinical Psychology* 46(1978):687–702.

68. K. D. Brownell, G. A. Marlatt, E. Lichtenstein, and G. T. Wilson, "Understanding and Preventing Relapse," *American Psychologist* 41(1986):765–782.

69. G. A. Bray, "Intestinal Bypass Surgery for Obese Patients," in *Symposium on Obesity: Basic Mechanisms and Treatment*, ed. A. J. Stunkard, Philadelphia: W. B. Saunders, 1978.

D. Halmi, "Gastric Bypass for Massive Obesity," in *Obesity*, ed. A. J. Stunkard, Philadelphia: W. B. Saunders, 1980.

70. G. A. Bray and D. S. Gray, "Obesity. Part II—Treatment," *Western Journal of Medicine* 149(1988):555–571.

71. Ibid.

72. Ibid.

P. Castelnuovo-Tedesco and D. Schiebel, "Studies of Superobesity II. Psychiatric Appraisal of Surgery for Superobesity," in *Hunger*, eds. D. Novin, W. Wyrwicka, and G. A. Bray, New York: Raven Press, 1976.

73. Bray and Gray, "Obesity. Part II—Treatment."

74. Ibid.

J. F. Munro, I. C. Stewart, P. H. Seidelin, H. S. Mackenzie, and N. G. Dewhurst, "Mechanical Treatment for Obesity," in *Human Obesity*, eds. R. J. Wurtman and J. J. Wurtman, New York: New York Academy of Sciences, 1987.

75. Bray and Gray, "Obesity. Part II—Treatment."

76. Munro et al., "Mechanical Treatment for Obesity."

77. J. E. Brody, "Stomach Balloon for Obesity Gains Favor amid Concerns," *The New York Times* (April 29, 1986):C1, C6.

78. R. B. Hogan, J. H. Johnston, B. W. Long, J. Q. Sones, L. A. Hinton, J. Burge, S. A. Corrigan, "A Double-Blind, Randomized, Sham-Controlled Trial of the Gastric Bubble for Obesity," *Gastrointestinal Endoscopy* 35(1989):381–385.

79. J. E. Blundell and P. J. Rogers, "Pharmocologic Approaches to the Understanding of Obesity," in *Symposium on Obesity: Basic Mechanisms and Treatment*, ed. A. J. Stunkard, Philadelphia: W. B. Saunders, 1978.

B. J. Vernace, "Controlled Comparative Investigation of Mazindol, D-Amphetamine, and Placebo," *Obesity and Bariatric Medicine* 3(1974):124–129.

80. Blundell and Rogers, "Pharmacologic Approaches."

Bray and Gray, "Obesity. Part II—Treatment."

J. F. Munro and M. J. Ford, "Drug Treatment of Obesity," in *Drugs and Appetite*, ed. T. Silverstone, London: Academic Press, 1982.

81. Bray and Gray, "Obesity. Part II—Treatment."

A. C. Sullivan, S. Hogan, and J. Triscari, "New Developments in Pharmacological Treatments for Obesity," in *Human Obesity*, eds. R. J. Wurtman and J. J. Wurtman, New York: New York Acacemy of Sciences, 1987.

82. A. S. Levine, "Centrally Active Peptides: Are They Useful Agents in the Treatment of Obesity?" in *Human Obesity*, eds. R. J. Wurtman and J. J. Wurtman, New York: New York Academy of Sciences, 1987.

G. P Smith and J. Gibbs, "The Effect of Gut Peptides on Hunger, Satiety, and Food Intake in Humans," in *Human Obesity*, eds. R. J. Wurtman and J. J. Wurtman, New York: New York Academy of Sciences, 1987.

83. Wurtman and Wurtman, "Carbohydrates and Depression."

84. Sullivan et al., "New Developments in Pharmacological Treatments."

85. C. H. Folkins and W. E. Sime, "Physical Fitness Training and Mental Health," *American Psychologist* 36(1981):373–389.

86. P. M. Dubbert and J. E. Martin, "Exercise," in *Handbook of Behavioral Medicine for Women*, eds. E. A. Blechman and K. D. Brownell, New York: Pergamon, 1988.

87. K. D. Brownell, P. S. Bachorik, and R. S. Ayerle, "Changes in Plasma Lipid and Lipoprotein Levels in Men and Women after a Program of Moderate Exercise," *Circulation* 65(1982):477–484.

R. M. Lampman, J. T. Santinga, P. J. Savage, D. R. Bassett, C. R. Hydrick, J. D. Flora, and W. D. Block, "Effect of Exercise Training on Glucose Tolerance, in Vivo Insulin Sensitivity, Lipid and Lripopotein Concentrations in Middle-Aged Men with Mild Hypertriglyceridemia," *Metabolism* 34 (1985): 205–211.

G. Sopko, A. S. Leon, D. R. Jacobs, N. Foster, J. Hoy, K. Kuba, J. T. Anderson, D. Casal, C. Mc-Nally, and I. Frantz, "The Effects of Exercise and Weight Loss on Plasma Lipids in Young Obese Men," *Metabolism* 34(1985):227–236.

88. Brownell and Stunkard, "Physical Activity in the Development and Control of Obesity."

J. S. Stern, "Is Obesity a Disease of Inactivity?" in *Eating and Its Disorders*, eds. A. J. Stunkard and E. Stellar, New York: Raven Press, 1984.

89. C. R. McGowan, L. H. Epstein, D. J. Kupfer, C. M. Bulik, and R. J. Robertson, "The Effect of Exercise on Non-Restricted Caloric Intake in Male Joggers," *Appetite* 7(1986):97–105.

F. X. Pi-Sunyer, "Exercise Effects on Calorie Intake," in *Human Obesity*, eds. R. J. Wurtman and J. J. Wurtman, New York: New York Academy of Sciences, 1987.

Stern, "Is Obesity a Disease of Inactivity?"

90. Stern, "Is Obesity a Disease of Inactivity?" p. 134.

91. J. Dwyer, "Sixteen Popular Diets: Brief Nutritional Analyses," in *Obesity*, ed. A. J. Stunkard, Philadelphia: W. B. Saunders, 1980.

92. Guthrie, *Introductory Nutrition*.

93. W. Bennett, "Dietary Treatments of Obesity," in *Human Obesity*, eds. R. J. Wurtman and J. J. Wurtman, New York: New York Academy of Sciences, 1987.

Guthrie, *Introductory Nutrition*.

T. B. van Itallie. "Dietary Approaches to the Treatment of Obesity," in *Symposium on Obesity: Basic Mechanisms and Treatment*, ed. A. J. Stunkard, Philadelphia: W. B. Saunders, 1978.

94. D. A. Booth, "Mechanisms from Models—Actual Effects From Real Life: The Zero-Calorie Drink-Break Option," *Appetite* 11 Supplement(1988):94–102.

E. S. Parham and A. R. Parham, "Saccharin Use and Sugar Intake By College Students," *Journal of the American Dietetic Association* 76(1980):560–563.

S. D. Stellman and L. Garfinkel, "Patterns of Artificial Sweetener Use and Weight Change in an American Cancer Society Prospective Study," *Appetite* 11 Supplement(1988):85–91.

95. B. S. Kanders, P.T. Lavin, M. B. Kowalchuk, I. Greenberg, and G. L. Blackburn, "An Evaluation of the Effect of Aspartame on Weight Loss, *Appetite* 11 Supplement(1988):73–84.

B. J. Rolls, L. J. Laster, and A. Summerfelt, "Hunger and Food Intake Following Consumption of Low-Caloric Foods," *Appetite* 13(1989):115–127.

M. G. Tordoff, "Saccharin and Food Intake," in *Low-Calorie Products*, eds, G. G. Birch and M. G. Lindley, New York: Elsevier, 1988.

T. B. Van Itallie, M.-U. Yang, and K. P. Porikos, "Use of Aspartame to Test the 'Body Weight Set Point' Hypothesis," *Appetite* 11 Supplement(1988):68–72.

96. R. W. Foltin, M. W. Fischman, C. S. Emurian, and J. J. Rachlinski, "Compensation for Caloric Dilution in Humans Given Unrestricted Access to Food in a Residential Laboratory," *Appetite* 10(1988):13–24.

97. G. A. Leveille, "Adipose Tissue Metabolism: Influence of Periodicity of Eating and Diet Composition," *Federation Proceedings* 29(1970):1294–1301.

98. D. J. A. Jenkins, T. M. S. Wolever, V. Vuksan, F. Brighenti, S. C. Cunnane, A. V. Rao, A. L.

Jenkins, G. Buckley, R. Patten, W. Singer, P. Corey, and R. G. Josse, "Nibbling versus Gorging: Metabolic Advantages of Increased Meal Frequency," *The New England Journal of Medicine* 321(1989):929–934.

99. K. D. Brownell and A. J. Stunkard, "Differential Changes in Plasma High-Density Lipoprotein-Cholesterol Levels in obese Men and Women during Weight Reduction," *Archives of Internal Medicine* 141(1981):1142–1146.

100. P. Hamm, R. B. Shekelle, and J. Stamler, "Large Fluctuations in Body Weight during Young Adulthood and Twenty-Five-Year Risk of Coronary Death in Men," *American Journal of Epidemiology* 129(1989):312–318.

101. D. B. Legoff and M. N. Spigelman, "Salivary Response to Olfactory Food Stimuli as a Function of Dietary Restraint and Body Weight," *Appetite* 8(1987):29–35.

T. J. Yost and R. H. Eckel, "Fat Calories May Be Preferentially Stored in Reduced-Obese Women: A Permissive Pathway for Resumption of the Obese State," *Journal of Clinical Endocrinology and Metabolism* 67(1988):259–264.

102. G. L. Blackburn, G. T. Wilson, B. S. Kanders, L. J. Stein, P. T. Lavin, J. Adler, and K. D. Brownell, "Weight Cycling: The Experience of Human Dieters," *American Journal of Clinical Nutrition* 49(1989):1105–1109.

K. D. Brownell, M. R. C. Greenwood, E. Stellar, and E. E. Shrager, "The Effects of Repeated Cycles of Weight Loss and Regain in Rats," *Physiology and Behavior* 38(1986):459–464.

103. C. P. Herman, "Restrained Eating," in *Symposium on Obesity: Basic Mechanisms and Treatment*, ed. A. J. Stunkard, Philadelphia: W. B. Saunders, 1978.

Ruderman, "Dietary Restraint."

A. J. Stunkard and S. Messick, "The Three-Factor Eating Questionnaire to Measure Dietary Restraint, Disinhibition and Hunger," *Journal of Psychosomatic Research* 29(1985):71–83.

104. H. Gleitman, *Psychology*, New York: W. W. Norton, 1981.

105. J. D. Nash and J. W. Farquhar, "Community Approaches to Dietary Modification and Obesity," in *Symposium on Obesity: Basic Mechanisms and Treatment*, ed. A. J. Standard, Philadelphia: W. B. Saunders, 1978.

R. B. Stuart and C. Mitchell, "Self-Help Groups in the Control of Body Weight," in *Obesity*, ed. A. J. Stunkard, Philadelphia: W. B. Saunders, 1980.

A. Stunkard, "The Social Environment and the Control of Obesity," in *Obesity*, ed. A. J. Stunkard, Philadelphia: W. B. Saunders, 1980.

106. Nash and Farquhar, "Community Approaches to Dietary Modification."

107. K. D. Brownell, R. Y. Cohen, A. J. Stunkard, M. R. J. Felix, and N. B. Cooley, "Weight Loss Competitions at the Work Site: Impact on Weight, Morale and Cost-Effectiveness," *American Journal of Public Health* 74(1984):1283–1285.

108. J. R. Garb and A. J. Stunkard, "Effectiveness of a Self-Help Group in Obesity Control," *Archives of Internal Medicine* 134(1974):716–720.

109. A. Stunkard, H. Levine, and S. Fox, "The Management of Obesity: Patient Self-Help and Medical Treatment," *Archives of Internal Medicine* 125(1970):1067–1072.

110. Stuart and Mitchell, "Self-Help Groups."

111. Ibid, p. 349.

112. Bruch, *Eating Disorders*.

113. C. S. W. Rand, "Treatment of Obese Patients in Psychoanalysis," in *Symposium on Obesity: Basic Mechanisms and Treatment*, ed. A. J. Stunkard, Philadelphia: W. B. Saunders, 1978.

A. J. Stunkard, "Psychoanalysis and Psychotherapy," in *Obesity*, ed. A. J. Stunkard, Philadelphia: W. B. Saunders, 1980.

114. Rand, "Treatment of Obese Patients in Psychoanalysis," p.671.

115. Stunkard, "Psychoanalysis and Psychotherapy."

116. T. A. Wadden and A. J. Stunkard, "Psychopathology and Obesity," in *Human Obesity*, eds. R. J. Wurtman and J. J. Wurtman, New York: New York Academy of Sciences, 1987.

117. E. E. Abramson, "A Review of Behavioral Approaches to Weight Control," *Behaviour Research and Therapy* 11(1973):547–556.

E. E. Abramson, "Behavioral Approaches to Weight Control: An Updated Review," *Behaviour Research and Therapy* 15(1977):355–363.

G. A. Bennett, "Behaviour Therapy in the Treatment of Obesity," in *Eating Habits: Food, Physiology and Learned Behavior*, eds. R. A. Boakes, D. A. Popplewell, and M. J. Burton, Chichester, Great Britain: John Wiley & Sons, 1987.

L. H. Epstein and R. R. Wing, "Behavioral Treatment of Childhood Obesity," *Psychological Bulletin* 101 (1987): 331–342.

M. J. Mahoney, "Behavior Modification in the Treatment of Obesity," in *Symposium on Obesity: Basic Mechanisms and Treatment*, ed. A. J. Stunkard, Philadelphia: W. B. Saunders, 1978.

G. T. Wilson, "Behavior Modification and the Treatment of Obesity," in *Obesity*, ed. A. J. Stunkard, Philadelphia: W. B. Saunders, 1980.

118. G. R. Leon, "Cognitive-Behavior Therapy for Eating Disturbances," in *Cognitive-Behavioral Interventions*, eds. P. C. Kendall and S. D. Hollon, New York: Academic Press, 1979.

G. R. Leon, *Treating Eating Disorders*, Lexington, MA: Lewis Publishing, 1983.

119. Abramson, "A Review of Behavioral Approaches to Weight Control."

Abramson, "Behavioral Approaches to Weight Control: An Updated Review."

Mahoney, "Behavior Modification in the Treatment of Obesity."

120. Abramson, "A Review of Behavioral Approaches to Weight Control."

Abramson, "Behavioral Approaches to Weight Control: An Updated Review."

K. D. Brownell, "Obesity: Understanding a Serious, Prevalent, and Refractory Disorder," *Journal of Consulting and Clinical Psychology* 50(1982):820–840.

P. M. Dubbert and G. T. Wilson, "Goal-Setting and Spouse Involvement in the Treatment of Obesity," *Behaviour Research and Therapy* 22(1984):227–242.

D. B. Jeffrey, "Self-Control Techniques in the Management of Obesity," in *Behavior Modification Approaches to Obesity*, ed. J. P. Foreyt, New York: Pergamon, 1977.

G. T. Wilson, "Behavioral Treatment of Obesity: Maintenance Strategies and Long-Term Efficacy," in *Trends in Behavior Therapy*, eds. P.-O. Sjoden, S. Bates, and W. S. Dockens, New York: Academic Press, 1979.

Wilson, "Behavior Modification and the Treatment of Obesity."

S. C. Wooley, O. W. Wooley, and S. R. Dyrenforth, "Theoretical, Practical, and Social Issues in Behavioral Treatments of Obesity," *Journal of Applied Behavior Analysis* 12(1979):3–25.

121. Jeffrey, "Self-Control Techniques in the Management of Obesity."

122. Wooley et al., "Theoretical, Practical, and Social Issues."

123. Wilson, "Behavioral Treatment of Obesity."

124. J. Hirsch and R. L. Leibel, "What Constitutes a Sufficient Psychobiologic Explanation for Obesity?" in *Eating and Its Disorders*, eds. A. J. Stunkard and E. Stellar, New York: Raven Press, 1984.

D. B. Jeffrey and M. R. Knauss, "The Etiologies, Treatments, and Assessments of Obesity," in *Psychosomatic Disorders: A Psychophysiological Approach to Etiology and Treatment*, eds. S. N. Haynes and L. Gannon, New York: Praeger, 1981.

R. J. Wurtman and J. J. Wurtman, "Introduction," in *Human Obesity*, ed R. J. Wurtman and J. J. Wurtman, New York: New York Academy of Sciences, 1987.

125. A. J. Stunkard, "The Current Status of Treatment for Obesity in Adults," in *Eating and Its Disorders*, eds. A. J. Stunkard and E. Stellar, New York: Raven Press, 1984.

126. T. S. Van Itallie, "The Enduring Storage Capacity for Fat: Implications for Treatment of Obesity," in *Eating and its Disorders*, eds. A. J. Stunkard and E. Stellar, New York: Raven Press, 1984.

S. C. Wooley and O. W. Wooley, "Should Obesity Be Treated at All?" in *Eating and Its Disorders*, eds. A. J. Stunkard and E. Stellar, New York: Raven Press, 1984.

127. Bennett, "Behaviour Therapy in the Treatment of Obesity."

128. S. M. Garn and W. R. Leonard, "What Did Our Ancestors Eat?" *Nutrition Reviews* 47(1989):337–345.

129. M. Konner, "What Our Ancestors Ate," *The New York Times Magazine* (June 5, 1988):54–55.

130. S. C. Wooley and O. W. Wooley. "Should Obesity Be Treated at All?"

Chapter 11: Alcohol Use and Abuse

1. *American Psychiatric Association: Diagnostic and Statistical Manual of Mental Disorders*, 3rd ed. rev., Washington, DC: APA, 1987.

2. D. B. Goldstein, *Pharmacology of Alcohol*, New York: Oxford University Press, 1983.

R. E. LaPorte, J. A. Cauley, L. H. Kuller, K. Flegal, J. S. Gavaler, and D. Van Thiel, "Alcohol, Coronary Heart Disease, and Total Mortality," in *Recent Developments in Alcoholism*, vol. 3, ed. M. Galanter, New York: Plenum, 1985.

3. P. Hudson, "The Medical Examiner Looks at Drinking," in *Drinking*, eds. J. A. Ewing and B. A. Rouse, Chicago: Nelson-Hall, 1978.

4. D. E. Koshland, "Drunk Driving and Statistical Mortality," *Science* 244 (1989):513.

5. Hudson, "The Medical Examiner Looks at Drinking."

6. W. Mayer, "Alcohol Abuse and Alcoholism," *American Psychologist* 38(1983):1116–1121.

7. B. S. McCrady, "Alcoholism," in *Handbook of Behavioral Medicine for Women*, eds. E. A. Blechman and K. D. Brownell, New York: Pergamon, 1988.

U.S. Department of Health and Human Services, *The Surgeon General's Report on Nutrition and Health: Summary and Recommendations* (DHHS Publication No. 88-50211), Washington, DC: U.S. Government Printing Office, 1988.

M. O. West and R. J. Prinz: "Parental Alcoholism and Childhood Psychopathology," *Psychological Bulletin* 102(1987):204-218.

8. Z. Ingalls, "Higher Education's Drinking Problem," *The Chronicle of Higher Education* (July 21, 1982):1, 6, 7.

9. C. Holden, "Is Alcoholism Treatment Effective?" *Science* 236(1987):20–22.

10. D. M. Barnes, "Drugs: Running the Numbers," *Science* 240(1988):1729–1731.

11. G. R. Jacobson, "Detection, Assessment, and Diagnosis of Alcoholism: Current Techniques," in *Recent Developments in Alcoholism*, vol. 1, ed. M. Galanter, New York: Plenum, 1983.

12. E. M. Jellinek, "Phases of Alcohol Addiction," *Quarterly Journal of Studies on Alcohol* 13(1952):673–684.

13. W. Mandell, "Types and Phases of Alcohol Dependence Illness," in *Recent Developments in Alcoholism*, vol. 1, ed. M. Galanter, New York: Plenum, 1983.

14. K. W. Wanberg and J. L. Horn, "Assessment of Alcohol Use with Multidimensional Concepts and Measures," *American Psychologist* 38(1983):1055–1069.

15. *American Psychiatric Association: Diagnostic and Statistical Manual of Mental Disorders*, 3d ed. rev., p. 173.

16. Barnes, "Drugs: Running the Numbers."

C. J. Furst, "Estimating Alcoholic Prevalence," in *Recent Developments in Alcoholism*, vol. 1, ed. M. Galanter, New York: Plenum, 1983.

M. Keller, "Problems of Epidemiology in Alcohol Problems," *Journal of Studies on Alcohol* 36(1975):1442–1451.

17. *American Psychiatric Association: Diagnostic and Statistical Manual of Mental-Disorders*, 3d ed. rev.

18. G. Chu, "Drinking Patterns and Attitudes of Rooming-House Chinese in San Francisco," *Quarterly Journal of Studies on Alcohol*, Supplement 6(1972):58–68.

19. S. Encel, K. C. Kotowicz, and H. E. Resler, "Drinking Patterns in Sydney, Australia," *Quarterly Journal of Studies* on Alcohol, Supplement 6(1972):1–27.

20. Ibid, p. 7.

21. D. Cahalan, "Subcultural Differences in Drinking Behavior in U.S. National Surveys and Selected European Studies," in *Alcoholism: New Directions in Behavioral Research and Treatment*, eds. P. E. Nathan, G. A. Marlatt, and T. Loberg, New York: Plenum, 1978.

22. R. Hannon, C. P. Butler, C. L. Day, S. A. Khan, L. A. Quitoriano, A. M. Butler, and L. A. Meredith, "Alcohol Use and Cognitive Functioning in Men and Women College Students," in *Recent Developments in Alcoholism*, vol. 3, ed. M. Galanter, New York: Plenum, 1985.

23. W. H. George and G. A. Marlatt, "Alcoholism: The Evolution of a Behavioral Perspective," in *Recent Developments in Alcoholism*, vol. 1, ed. M. Galanter, New York: Plenum, 1983.

G. A. Marlatt, B. Demming, and J. B. Reid, "Loss of Control Drinking in Alcoholics: An Experimental Analogue," *Journal of Abnormal Psychology* 81(1973):233–241.

24. J. G. Hull and C. F. Bond, "Social and Behavioral Consequences of Alcohol Consumption and Expectancy: A Meta-Analysis," *Psychological Bulletin* 99(1986):347–360.

25. B. Critchlow, "The Powers of John Barleycorn: Beliefs about the Effects of Alcohol on Social Behavior," *American Psychologist* 41(1986):751-764.

26. C. S. Lieber, "The Metabolism of Alcohol," *Scientific American* 234(March 1976):25–33.

27. N. K. Mello, "Some Aspects of the Behavioral Pharmacology of Alcohol," in *Psychopharmacology: A Review of Progress, 1957-1967*, ed. D. H. Efron, Washington, DC: U.S. Government Printing Office, 1968.

28. V. C. Taasan, A. J. Block, P. G. Boyson, J. W. Wynne, C. White, and S. Lindsey, "Alcohol Increases Sleep Apnea and Oxygen Desaturation in Asymptomatic Men," *The American Journal of Medicine* 71(1981):240–245.

29. J. B. Knowles, S. G. Laverty, and H. A. Kuechler, "Effects of Alcohol on REM Sleep," *Quarterly Journal of Studies on Alcohol* 29(1968):342–349.

R. B. Yules, D. X. Freedman, and K. A. Chandler, "The Effect of Ethyl Alcohol on Man's Electroencephalographic Sleep Cycle," *Electroen-*

cephalography and Clinical Neurophysiology
20(1966):109–111.

30. D. Goldberg, "Red Head," *The Lancet*
1(May 2, 1981):1003.

31. D. E. Johnston, Y.-B. Chiao, J. S. Gavaler,
and D. H. Van Thiel, "Inhibition of Testosterone
Synthesis by Ethanol and Acetaldehyde,"
Biochemical Pharmacology 30(1981):1827–1831.

32. D. M. Lovinger, G. White, and F. F.
Weight, "Ethanol Inhibits NMDA -Activated Ion
Current in Hippocampal Neurons," *Science*
243(1989):1721–1724.

33. Hull and Bond, "Social and Behavioral
Consequences."

J. R. Tinklenberg, "Alcohol and Violence," in
Alcoholism: Progress in Research and Treatment, ed.
P. G. Bourne, New York: Academic Press, 1973.

34. A. R. Lang, D. J. Goeckner, V. J. Adesso,
and G. A. Marlatt, "Effects of Alcohol on Aggression in Male Social Drinkers," *Journal of Abnormal
Psychology* 84(1975):508–518.

35. H. Moskowitz and J. T. Murray, "Decrease
of Iconic Memory after Alcohol," *Journal of
Studies on Alcohol* 37(1976):278–283.

R. S. Ryback, "The Continuum and Specificity
of the Effects of Alcohol on Memory," *Quarterly
Journal of Studies on Alcohol* 32(1971):995–1016.

R. E. Tarter, N. Buonpane, and C. Wynant, "Intellectual Competence of Alcoholics," *Journal of
Studies on Alcohol* 36(1975):381–386.

36. I. M. Birnbaum, M. K. Johnson, J. T.
Hartley, and T. H. Taylor, "Alcohol and Elabora-
tive Schemas for Sentences," *Journal of Experimental Psychology* 6(1980):293–300.

37. M. K. Jones and B. M. Jones, "The
Relationship of Age and Drinking Habits to the
Effects of Alcohol on Memory in Women," *Jour-
nal of Studies on Alcohol* 41(1980):179–186.

38. J. Polivy and C. P. Herman, "Effects of Al-
cohol on Eating Behavior: Influence of Mood and
Perceived Intoxication," *Journal of Abnormal
Psychology* 85(1976):601–606.

39. LaPorte et al., "Alcohol, Coronary Heart
Disease, and Total Mortality."

D. H. Van Thiel and J. S. Gavaler, "Myocardial
Effects of Alcohol Abuse: Clinical and
Physiologic Consequences," in *Recent Develop-
ments in Alcoholism*, vol. 3, ed. M. Galanter, New
York: Plenum, 1985.

D. H. Van Thiel, J. S. Gavaler, and D. C.
Lehotay, "Biochemical Mechanisms Responsible
for Alcohol-Associated Myocardiopathy," in
Recent Developments in Alcoholism, vol. 3, ed. M.

Galanter, New York: Plenum, 1985.

40. K. M. Flegal and J. A. Cauley, "Alcohol
Consumption and Cardiovascular Risk Factors,"
in *Recent Developments in Alcoholism*, vol. 3, ed. M.
Galanter, New York: Plenum, 1985.

41. Lieber, "The Metabolism of Alcohol."

42. T. R. Stockwell, R. J. Hodgson, H. C.
Rankin, and C. Taylor, "Alcohol Dependence,
Beliefs and the Priming Effect," *Behaviour Re-
search and Therapy* 20(1982):513–522.

43. *American Psychiatric Association: Diagnostic
and Statistical Manual of Mental Disorders*, 3d ed.
rev.

44. S. Siegel, "Morphine Analgesic Tolerance:
Its Situation Specificity Supports a Pavlovian
Conditioning," *Science* 193(1976):323–325.

S. Siegel, R. E. Hinson, M. D. Krank, and J. Mc-
Cully, "Heroin 'Overdose' Death: Contribution of
Drug-Associated Environmental Cues," *Science*
216(1982):436–437.

45. R. L. Solomon, "The Opponent-Process
Theory of Acquired Motivation," *American
Psychologist* 35(1980):691–712.

46. A. D. Lê, C. X. Poulos, and H. Cappell,
"Conditioned Tolerance of the Hypothermic Effect of Ethyl Alcohol," *Science* 206(1979):1109–
1110.

47. J. R. Wenger. T. M. Tiffany, C. Bombarier,
K. Nicholls, and S. C. Woods, "Ethanol Tolerance
in the Rat is Learned," *Science* 213(1981):575–577.

48. B. Tabakoff, C. L. Melchior, and P. Hof-
fman, "Factors in Ethanol Tolerance," *Science*
224(1984):523–524.

J. R. Wenger and S. C. Woods, "Factors in
Ethanol Tolerance," *Science* 224 (1984): 524.

49. Lieber, "The Metabolism of Alcohol."

C. S. Lieber, "The Influence of Alcohol on
Nutritional Status," *Nutrition Reviews*
46(1988):241–254.

50. Lieber, "The Metabolism of Alcohol."

51. G. Freund, "Neurobiological Relation-
ships Between Aging and Alcohol Abuse," in
Recent Developments in Alcoholism, vol. 2, ed. M.
Galanter, New York: Plenum, 1984.

G. Goldstein and C. Shelly, "A Multivariate
Neuropsychological Approach to Brain Lesion
Localization in Alcoholism," *Addictive Behaviors*
7(1982):165–175.

C. J. Golden, B. Graber, I. Blose, R. Berg, J. Cof-
fman, and S. Bloch, "Difference in Brain Densities
between Chronic Alcoholic and Normal Control
Patients, *Science* 211(1981):508–510.

R. E. Tarter and C. M. Ryan, "Neuropsychology of Alcoholism: Etiology, Phenomenology, Process, and Outcome," in *Recent Developments in Alcoholism*, vol. 1, ed. M. Galanter, New York: Plenum, 1983.

52. M. S. Goldman, "Cognitive Impairment in Chronic Alcoholics," *American Psychologist* 38(1983):1045–1054.

G. Goldstein and C. H. Shelly, "Field Dependence and Cognitive, Perceptual and Motor Skills in Alcoholics," *Quarterly Journal of Studies on Alcohol* 32(1971):29–40.

A. B. Heilbrun, A. R. Tarbox, and J. K. Madison, "Cognitive Structure and Behavioral Regulation in Alcoholics," *Journal of Studies on Alcohol* 40(1979):387–400.

C.-O. Jonsson, B. Cronholm, and S. Izikowitz, "Intellectual Changes in Alcoholics," *Quarterly Journal of Studies on Alcohol* 23(1962):221–242.

G. B. Kish and T. M. Cheney, "Impaired Abilities in Alcoholism Measured by the General Aptitude Test Battery," *Quarterly Journal of Studies on Alcohol* 30(1969):384–388.

T. Løberg and W. R. Miller, "Personality, Cognitive, and Neuropsychological Correlates of Harmful Alcohol Consumption: A Cross-National Comparison of Clinical Samples," in *Alcohol and Culture: Comparative Perspectives from Europe and America*, ed. T. F. Babor, New York: New York Academy of Sciences, 1986.

J. W. Smith, D. W. Burt, and R. F. Chapman, "Intelligence and Brain Damage in Alcoholics: A Study in Patients of Middle and Upper Social Class," *Quarterly Journal of Studies on Alcohol* 34(1973):414–422.

Tarter and Ryan, "Neuropsychology of Alcoholism."

53. R. K. Hester, J. W. Smith, and T. R. Jackson, "Recovery of Cognitive Skills in Alcoholics," *Journal of Studies on Alcohol* 41(1980):363–367.

J. A. Long and J. F. C. McLachlan, "Abstract Reasoning and Perceptual Motor Efficiency in Alcoholics: Impairment and Reversibility," *Quarterly Journal of Studies on Alcohol* 35(1974):1220–1229.

R. D. Page and J. D. Linden, "'Reversible' Organic Brain Syndrome in Alcoholics," *Quarterly Journal of Studies on Alcohol* 35(1974):98–107.

R. D. Page and L. H. Schaub, "Intellectual Functioning in Alcoholics during Six Months Abstinence," *Journal of Studies on Alcohol* 38(1977):1240–1246.

54. S. Y. Hill and C. Ryan, "Brain Damage in Social Drinkers? Reasons for Caution," in *Recent Developments in Alcoholism*, vol. 3, ed. M.

Galanter, New York: Plenum, 1985.

55. M. S. Albert, N. Butters, and J. Brandt, "Memory for Remote Events in Alcoholics," *Journal of Studies on Alcohol* 41(1980):1071–1081.

H. Weingartner, L. A. Faillance, and H. G. Markley, "Verbal Information Retention in Alcoholics," *Quarterly Journal of Studies on Alcohol* 32(1971):293–303.

56. C. Ryan, "Learning and Memory Deficits in Alcoholics," *Journal of Studies on Alcohol* 41(1980):437–447.

57. J. Curlee, "Alcoholic Blackouts: Some Conflicting Evidence," *Quarterly Journal of Studies on Alcohol* 34(1973):409–413.

58. *American Psychiatric Association: Diagnostic and Statistical Manual of Mental Disorders*, 3d ed. rev.

D. Kohl and J. Brandt, "An Automatic Encoding Deficit in the Amnesia of Korsakoff's Syndrome," in *Memory Dysfunctions: An Integration of Animal and Human Research from Preclinical and Clinical Perspectives*, eds. D. S. Olton, E. Gamzu, and S. Corkin, New York: New York Academy of Sciences, 1985.

59. L. S. Cermak, "Improving Retention in Alcoholic Korsakoff Patients," *Journal of Studies on Alcohol* 41(1980):159–169.

H. Weingartner, J. Grafman, W. Boutelle, W. Kaye, and P. R. Martin, "Forms of Memory Failure," *Science* 221(1983):380–382.

60. U.S. Department of Health and Human Services, *The Surgeon General's Report on Nutrition and Health*.

61. D. R. Petersen, "Pharmacogenetic Approaches to the Neuropharmacology of Ethanol," in *Recent Developments in Alcoholism*, vol. 1, ed. M. Galanter, New York: Plenum, 1983.

62. K. Eriksson and M. Rusi; "Finnish Selection Studies on Alcohol-Related Behaviors: General Outline," in *Development of Animal Models as Pharmacogenetic Tools*, eds. G. E. McClearn, R. A. Dietrich, and V. G. Erwin, Rockville, MD: U.S. Department of Health and Human Services, 1981.

63. J. A. Ewing and B. A. Rouse, "Drinks, Drinkers, and Drinking," in *Drinking: Alcohol in American Society—Issues and Current Research*, eds. J. A. Ewing and B. A. Rouse, Chicago: Nelson-Hall, 1978.

T.-K. Li, L. Lumeng, W. J. McBride, and M. B. Waller, "Indiana Selection Studies on Alcohol-Related Behaviors." in *Development of Animal Models as Pharmacogenetic Tools*, eds. G. E. McClearn, R.

A. Dietrich, and V. G. Erwin, Rockville, MD: U.S. Department of Health and Human Services, 1981.

64. Petersen, "Pharmacogenetic Approaches to the Neuropharmacology of Ethanol."

65. M. B. Waller, W. J. McBride, G. J. Gatto, L. Lumeng, and T.-K. Li, "Intragastric Self-Infusion of Ethanol by Ethanol-Preferring and -Nonpreferring Lines of Rats," *Science* 225(1984):78–80.

66. Ewing and Rouse, "Drinks, Drinkers, and Drinking."

67. Waller et al., "Intragastric Self-Infusion of Ethanol."

68. W. R. Proctor and T. V. Dunwiddie, "Behavioral Sensitivity to Purinergic Drugs Parallels Ethanol Sensitivity in Selectively Bred Mice," *Science* 224(1984):519–521.

L. J. Ryan, J. E. Barr, B. Sanders, and S. K. Sharpless, "Electrophysiological Responses to Ethanol, Pentobarbital, and Nicotine in Mice Genetically Selected for Differential Sensitivity to Ethanol," *Journal of Comparative and Physiological Psychology* 93(1979):1035–1052.

69. G. E. Vaillant and E. S. Milofsky, "The Etiology of Alcoholism: A Prospective Viewpoint," *American Psychologist* 37(1982):494–503.

70. J. A. Ewing, B. A. Rouse, and E. D. Pellizzari, "Alcohol Sensitivity and Ethnic Background," *American Journal of Psychiatry* 131(1974):206–210.

J. J. Park, Y.-H. Huang, C. T. Nagoshi, S. Yuen, R- C. Johnson, C. A. Ching, and K. S. Bowman, "The Flushing Response to Alcohol Use among Koreans and Taiwanese," *Journal of Studies on Alcohol* 45 (1984): 481–485.

71. M. A. Schuckit and V. Rayses, "Ethanol Ingestion: Differences in Blood Acetaldehyde Concentrations in Relatives of Alcoholics and Controls," *Science* 203(1979):54–55.

72. M. A. Korsten, S. Matsuzaki, L. Feinman, and C. S. Lieber, "High Blood Acetaldehyde Levels after Ethanol Administration: Difference between Alcoholic and Nonalcoholic Subjects," *The New England Journal of Medicine* 292(8)(1975):386–389.

73. H. Begleiter, B. Porjesz, B. Bihari, and B. Kissin, "Event-Related Brain Potentials in Boys at Risk for Alcoholism," *Science* 225(1984):1493–1496.

74. M. A. Schuckit, "Behavioral Effects of Alcohol in Sons of Alcoholics," in *Recent Developments in Alcoholism,* vol. 3, ed. M. Galanter, New York: Plenum, 1985.

J. Volavka, V. Pollock, W. F. Gabrielli, and S. A. Mednick, "The EEG in Persons at Risk for Al-coholism," in *Recent Developments in Alcoholism,* vol. 3, ed. M. Galanter, New York: Plenum, 1985.

75. C. R. Cloninger, M. Bohman, S. Sigvardsson, and A.-L. Von Knorring, "Psychopathology in Adopted-Out Children of Alcoholics: The Stockholm Adoption Study," in *Recent Developments in Alcoholism,* vol. 3, ed. M. Galanter, New York: Plenum, 1985.

R. M. Murray, C. A. Clifford, and H. M. D. Gurling, "Twin and Adoption Studies: How Good Is the Evidence for a Genetic Role?" in *Recent Developments in Alcoholism,* vol. 1, ed. M. Galanter, New York: Plenum, 1983.

76. K. Blum, E. P. Noble, P. J. Sheridan, A. Montgomery, T. Ritchie, P. Jagadeeswaran, H. Nogami, A. H. Briggs, and J. B. Cohn, "Allelic Association of Human Dopamine D_2 Receptor Gene in Alcoholism," *The Journal of the American Medical Association* 263(1990):2055–2060.

T. Adler, "Alcoholism Gene Study Is Controversial," *APA Monitor* (July 1990):8.

77. D. M. Barnes, "The Biological Tangle of Drug Addiction," *Science* 241(1988):415–417.

C. R. Cloninger, "Neurogenetic Adaptive Mechanisms in Alcoholism," *Science* 236(1987):410–416.

78. G. A. Marlatt, "Behavioral Assessment of Social Drinking and Alcoholism," in *Behavioral Approaches to Alcoholism,* eds. G. A. Marlatt and P. E. Nathan, New Brunswick, NJ: Rutgers Center of Alcohol Studies, 1978.

P. E. Nathan, "Behavioral Theory and Behavioral Theories of Alcoholism," in *Behavioral Approaches to Alcoholism,* eds. G. A. Marlatt and P. E. Nathan, New Brunswick, NJ: Rutgers Center of Alcohol Studies, 1978.

G. T. Wilson, "Booze, Beliefs, and Behavior: Cognitive Processes in Alcohol Use and Abuse," in *Alcoholism: New Directions in Behavioral Research and Treatment,* eds. P. E. Nathan, G. A. Marlatt, and T. Loberg, New York: Plenum, 1978.

79. G. A. Marlatt, "Alcohol Use and Problem Drinking: A Cognitive-Behavioral Analysis," in *Cognitive-Behavioral Interventions,* eds. P. C. Kendall and S. D. Hollon, New York: Academic Press, 1979.

Nathan, "Behavioral Theory and Behavioral Theories of Alcoholism."

Wilson, "Booze, Beliefs, and Behavior."

80. P. M. Miller and R. M. Eisler, "Alcohol and Drug Abuse," in *Behavior Modification: Principles, Issues, and Applications,* eds. W. E. Craighead, A. E. Kazdin, and M. J. Mahoney, Boston: Houghton

Mifflin, 1976, p. 380.

81. Marlatt, "Behavioral Assessment of Social Drinking and Alcoholism."

82. S. A. Maisto, L. C. Sobell, A. M. Cooper, and M. B. Sobell, "Comparison of Two Techniques to Obtain Retrospective Reports of Drinking Behavior from Alcohol Abusers," *Addictive Behaviors* 7(1982):33–38.

J. M. Polich, "The Validity of Self-Reports in Alcoholism Research," *Addictive Behaviors* 7(1982):123–132.

83. George and Marlatt, "Alcoholism: The Evolution of a Behavioral Perspective."

84. Ibid.

85. A. L. Riley and C. L. Wetherington, "Schedule-Induced Polydipsia: Is the Rat a Small Furry Human? (An Analysis of an Animal Model of Human Alcoholism)," in *Contemporary Learning Theories: Instrumental Conditioning Theory and the Impact of Biological Constraints on Learning*, eds. S. B. Klein and R. R. Mowrer, Hillsdale, NJ: Lawrence Erlbaum Associates, 1989.

86. J. L. Falk and H. H. Samson, "Schedule-Induced Physical Dependence on Ethanol," *Pharmacological Reviews* 27(1976):449–464.

J. L. Falk and M. Tang, "Schedule Induction and Overindulgence," *Alcoholism: Clinical and Experimental Research* 4(1980):266–270.

87. J. L. Falk, "The Nature and Determinants of Adjunctive Behavior," *Physiology and Behavior* 6(1971):577–588.

88. J. L. Falk and M. Tang, "Animal Model of Alcoholism: Critique and Progress," in *Alcohol Intoxication and Withdrawal*, vol. 38, ed. M. M. Gross, New York: Plenum, 1977.

89. G. D. Ellison and A. D. Potthoff, "Social Models of Drinking Behavior in Animals: The Importance of Individual Differences," in *Recent Developments in Alcoholism*, vol. 2, ed. M. Galanter, New York: Plenum, 1984.

90. D. A. Deems, R. L. Oetting, J. E. Sherman, and J. Garcia, "Hungry, But Not Thirsty, Rats Prefer Flavors Paired with Ethanol," *Physiology and Behavior* 36(1986):141–144.

R. Mehiel and R. C. Bolles, "Learned Flavor Preferences Based on Caloric Outcome," *Animal Learning and Behavior* 12(1984):421–427.

J. E. Sherman, C. F. Hickis, A. G. Rice, K. W. Rusiniak, and J. Garcia, "Preferences and Aversions for Stimuli Paired with Ethanol in Hungry Rats," *Animal Learning and Behavior* 11(1983):101–106.

J. Sherman, K. W. Rusiniak, and J. Garcia, "Alcohol-Ingestive Habits: The Role of Flavor and Ef-

fect," in *Recent Developments in Alcoholism*, vol. 2, New York: Plenum, 1984.

91. W. J. Darby, "The Nutrient Contributions of Fermented Beverages," in *Fermented Food Beverages in Nutrition*, eds. C. F. Gastineau, W. J. Darby, and T. B. Turner, New York: Academic Press, 1979.

H. A. Guthrie, *Nutrition*, St. Louis: C. V. Mosby, 1975.

C. D. Leake and M. Silverman, *Alcoholic Beverages in Clinical Medicine*, Cleveland: World Publishing, 1966.

R. Passmore, "The Energy Value of Alcohol," in *Fermented Food Beverages in Nutrition*, eds. C. F. Gastineau, W. J. Darby, and T. B. Turner, New York: Academic Press, 1979.

92. H. Cappell, "An Evaluation of Tension Models of Alcohol Consumption," in *Research Advances in Alcohol and Drug Problems*, vol. 2, eds. R. J. Gibbins, Y. Israel, H. Kalant, R. E. Popham, W. Schmidt, and R. G. Smart, New York: Wiley, 1975.

George and Marlatt, "Alcoholism: The Evolution of a Behavioral Perspective."

G. T. Wilson, "Alcohol and Anxiety: Recent Evidence on the Tension Reduction Theory of Alcohol Use and Abuse," in *Self-Control and Self-Modification*, eds. K. R. Blankstein and J. Polivy, New York: Plenum, 1982.

93. J. B. Reid, "Study of Drinking in Natural Settings," in *Behavioral Approaches to Alcoholism*, eds. G. A. Marlatt and P. E. Nathan, New Brunswick, NJ: Rutgers Center of Alcohol Studies, 1978.

94. D. W. Watson and M. B. Sobell, "Social Influences on Alcohol Consumption by Black and White Males," *Addictive Behaviors* 7(1982):87–91.

95. R. L. Collins and G. A. Marlatt, "Social Modeling as a Determinant of Drinking Behavior: Implications for Prevention and Treatment," *Addictive Behaviors* 6(1981):233–239.

R. L. Collins and G. A. Marlatt, "Psychological Correlates and Explanations of Alcohol Use and Abuse," in *Medical and Social Aspects of Alcohol Abuse*, eds. B. Tabakoff, P. B. Sutker, and C. L. Randall, New York: Plenum, 1983.

96. G. N. Braucht, "How Environments and Persons Combine to Influence Problem Drinking: Current Research Issues," in *Recent Developments in Alcoholism*, vol. 1, ed. M. Galanter, New York: Plenum, 1983.

T. C. Harford, "Drinking Patterns among Black and Nonblack Adolescents: Results of A National Survey," in *Alcohol and Culture: Comparative*

Perspectives from Europe and America, ed. T. F. Babor, New York: New York Academy of Sciences, 1986.

97. S. I. Ornstein and D. Levy, "Price and Income Elasticities of Demand for Alcoholic Beverages," in *Recent Developments in Alcoholism,* vol. 1, ed. M. Galanter, New York: Plenum, 1983.

98. J. Rabow and R. K. Watts, "The Role of Alcohol Availability in Alcohol Consumption and Alcohol Problems," in *Recent Developments in Alcoholism,* vol. 1, ed. M. Galanter, New York: Plenum, 1983.

99. R. E. Vuchinich and J. A. Tucker, "Contributions from Behavioral Theories of Choice to an Analysis of Alcohol Abuse," *Journal of Abnormal Psychology* 97(1988):181–195.

R. E. Vuchinich, J. A. Tucker, and E. J. Rudd, "Preference for Alcohol Consumption as a Function of Amount and Delay of Alternative Reward," *Journal of Abnormal Psychology* 96(1987):259–263.

100. R. Fox, "Treatment of the Problem Drinker by the Private Practitioner," in *Alcoholism: Progress in Research and Treatment,* eds. P. G. Bourne and R. Fox, New York: Academic Press, 1973.

B. Kissin, "Medical Management of the Alcoholic Patient," in *Treatment and Rehabilitation of the Chronic Alcoholic,* eds. B. Kissin and H. Begleiter, New York: Plenum, 1977.

M. Victor and S. M. Wolfe, "Causation and Treatment of the Alcohol Withdrawal Syndrome," in *Alcoholism: Progress in Research and Treatment,* eds. P. B. Bourne and R. Fox, New York: Academic Press, 1973.

101. K. D. Brownell, G. A. Marlatt, E. Lichtenstein, and G. T. Wilson, "Understanding and Preventing Relapse," *American Psychologist* 41(1986):765–782.

George and Marlatt, "Alcoholism: The Evolution of a Behavioral Perspective."

G. A. Marlatt, "Craving for Alcohol, Loss of Control, and Relapse: A Cognitive-Behavioral Analysis," in *Alcoholism: New Directions in Behavioral Research and Treatment,* eds. P. E. Nathan, G. A. Marlatt, and T. Loberg, New York: Plenum, 1978.

102. J. W. Finney, R. H. Moos, and C. R. Mewborn, "Posttreatment Experiences and Treatment Outcome of Alcoholic Patients Six Months and Two Years after Hospitalization," *Journal of Consulting and Clinical Psychology* 48(1980):17–29.

103. S. E. Gitlow, "Alcoholism: A Disease," in *Alcoholism: Progress in Research and Treatment,* eds.

P. G. Bourne and R. Fox, New York: Academic Press, 1973.

Marlatt, "Craving for Alcohol, Loss of Control, and Relapse."

104. George and Marlatt, "Alcoholism: The Evolution of a Behavioral Perspective."

Marlatt, "Craving for Alcohol, Loss of Control, and Relapse."

Marlatt, "Alcohol Use and Problem Drinking."

105. Holden, "Is Alcoholism Treatment Effective?"

W. R. Miller and R. K. Hester, "Inpatient Alcoholism Treatment: Who Benefits?" *American Psychologist* 41(1986):794–805.

106. Miller and Hester, "Inpatient Alcoholism Treatment."

107. Gitlow, "Alcoholism: A Disease."

M. L. Pendery, I. M. Maltzman, and L. J. West, "Controlled Drinking by Alcoholics?: New Findings and a Reevaluation of a Major Affirmative Study," *Science* 217(1982):169–175.

108. B. Leach and J. L. Norris, "Factors in the Development of Alcoholics Anonymous (A.A.)," in *Treatment and Rehabilitation of the Chronic Alcoholic,* eds. B. Kissin and H. Begleiter, New York: Plenum, 1977.

109. C. B. De Soto, W. E. O'Donnell, and J. L. De Soto, "Long-Term Recovery in Alcoholics," *Alcoholism: Clinical and Experimental Research* 13(1989):693–697.

110. G. A. Marlatt, "The Controlled-Drinking Controversy," *American Psychologist* 38(1983):1097–1110.

M. B. Sobell and L. C. Sobell, *Behavioral Treatment of Alcohol Problems: Individualized Therapy and Controlled Drinking,* New York: Plenum, 1978.

M. B. Sobell and L. C. Sobell, "Controlled Drinking: A Concept Coming of Age," in *Self-Control and Self-Modification of Emotional Behavior,* eds. K. R. Blankstein and J. Polivy, New York: Plenum, 1982.

111. Sobell and Sobell, *Behavioral Treatment of Alcohol Problems.*

112. J. L. Chase, H. C. Salzberg, and A. M. Palotai, "Controlled Drinking Revisited: A Review," in *Progress in Behavior Modification,* vol. 18, eds. M. Hersen, R. M. Eisler, and P. M. Miller, New York: Academic Press, 1984.

R. W. Lloyd and H. C. Salzberg, "Controlled Social Drinking: An Alternative to Abstinence as a Treatment Goal for Some Alcohol Abusers," *Psychological Bulletin* 82(1975):815–842.

113. J. M. Polich, D. J. Armor, and H. B.

Braiker, *The Course of Alcoholism: Four Years after Treatment,* Santa Monica, CA: Rand, 1980.

114. Pendery et al., "Controlled Drinking by Alcoholics?"

115. K. Fisher, "Debate Rages on 1973 Sobell Study," *APA Monitor* (November 1982):8–9.

116. P. H. Abelson, "Alcoholism Studies," *Science* 220(1983):554, 556.

D. H. Barlow, A. S. Bellack, A. M. Buchwald, S. L. Garfield, D. P. Hartmann, C. P. Herman, M. Hersen, P. M. Miller, S. Rachman, and J. Wolpe, "Alcoholism Studies," *Science* 220(1983):554.

Fisher, "Debate Rages on 1973 Sobell Study."

K. A. McDonald, "Rutgers Journal Forced to Publish Paper Despite Threats of Libel Lawsuit," *The Chronicle of Higher Education* (September 13, 1989):A5, A12.

Marlatt, "The Controlled-Drinking Controversy."

117. P. M Boffey, "Showdown Nears in Feud over Alcohol Studies," *The New York Times* (November 2, 1982):C1–C2.

118. C. Norman, "No Fraud Found in Alcoholism Study," *Science* 218(1982):771.

119. K. Fisher, "'Incomplete' Report Clears Sobells," *APA Monitor* (November 1984):2.

120. M. B. Sobell and L. C. Sobell, "The Aftermath of Heresy: A Response to Pendery et al.'s (1982) Critique of 'Individualized Behavior Therapy for Alcoholics,'" *Behaviour Research and Therapy* 22(1984):413–440.

121. S. Peele, "The Cultural Context to Psychological Approaches to Alcoholism: Can We Control the Effects of Alcohol?" *American Psychologist* 39 (1984): 1337–1351.

122. G. R. Caddy, "Blood Alcohol Concentration Discrimination Training: Development and Current Status," in *Behavioral Approaches to Alcoholism,* eds. G. A. Marlatt and P. E. Nathan, New Brunswick, NJ: Rutgers Center of Alcohol Studies, 1978.

P. E. Nathan, "Studies in Blood Alcohol Level Discrimination," in *Alcoholism: New Directions in Behavioral Research and Treatment,* eds. P. E. Nathan, G. A. Marlatt, and T. Loberg, New York: Plenum, 1978.

123. P. M. Miller, "Behavior Therapy in the Treatment of Alcoholism," in *Behavioral Approaches to Alcoholism,* eds. G. A. Marlatt and P. E. Nathan, New Brunswick, NJ: Rutgers Center of Alcohol Studies, 1978.

Sobell and Sobell, *Behavioral Treatment of Alcohol Problems.*

124. S. L. Jones, R. Kanfer, and R. I. Lanyon, "Skill Training with Alcoholics: A Clinical Extension," *Addictive Behaviors* 7(1982):285–290.

125. Ibid, p. 287.

126. Ibid.

127. A. W. Logue, "Research on Self-Control: An Integrating Framework," *Behavioral and Brain Sciences* 11(1988):665–709.

128. G. Ainslie, "The Application of Economic Concepts to the Motivational Conflict in Alcoholism," in *Matching Patient Needs and Treatment Methods,* New York: Pergamon, 1981.

129. G. R. Caddy and T. Block, "Behavioral Treatment Methods for Alcoholism," in *Recent Developments in Alcoholism,* vol. 1, ed. M. Galanter, New York: Plenum, 1983.

130. M. D. Vogel-Sprott and R. K. Banks, "The Effect of Delayed Punishment on an Immediately Rewarded Response in Alcoholics and Nonalcoholics," *Behaviour Research and Therapy* 3(1965):69–73.

131. R. L. Elkins, "Aversion Therapy for Alcoholism: Chemical, Electrical or Imaginary?" *International Journal of the Addictions* 10(1975):157–209.

C. M. Franks, "Conditioning and Conditioned Aversion Therapies in the Treatment of the Alcoholic," *International Journal of the Addictions* 1(1966):61–98.

G. T. Wilson, "Alcoholism and Aversion Therapy: Issues, Ethics and Evidence," in *Behavioral Approaches to Alcoholism,* eds. G. A. Marlatt and P. E. Nathan, New Brunswick, NJ: Rutgers Center of Alcohol Studies, 1978.

132. C. S. Mellor and H. P. White, "Taste Aversions to Alcoholic Beverages Conditioned by Motion Sickness," *American Journal of Psychiatry* 135(1978):125–126.

133. S. Lamon, G. T. Wilson, and R. C. Leaf, "Human Classical Aversion Conditioning: Nausea versus Electric Shock in the Reduction of Target Beverage Consumption," *Behaviour Research and Therapy* 15(1977):313–320.

134. F. J. Soland, C. S. Mellor, and S. Revusky, "Chemical Aversion Treatment of Alcoholism: Lithium as the Aversive Agent," *Behavior Research and Therapy* 16(1978):401–409.

135. A. W. Logue, K. R. Logue, and K. E. Strauss, "The Acquisition of Taste Aversions in Humans with Eating and Drinking Disorders," *Behaviour Research and Therapy* 21(1983):275–289.

136. A. W. Logue, I. Ophir, and K. E. Strauss, "The Acquisition of Taste Aversions in Humans,"

Behavior Research and Therapy 19(1981):319–333.

137. T. B. Baker and D. S. Cannon, "Taste Aversion Therapy with Alcoholics: Techniques and Evidence of a Conditioned Response," *Behaviour Research and Therapy* 17(1979):229–242.

O. W. Neubuerger, J. D. Matarazzo, R. E. Schmitz, and H. H. Pratt, "One Year Follow-Up of Total Abstinence in Chronic Alcoholic Patients Following Emetic Counterconditioning," *Alcoholism: Clinical and Experimental Research* 4(1980):306–312.

A. N. Wiens, J. R. Montague, T. S. Manaugh, and C. J. English, "Pharmacological Aversive Counterconditioning to Alcohol in a Private Hospital; One-Year Follow-Up," *Journal of Studies on Alcohol* 37(1976):1320–1324.

138. R. L. Elkins, "Conditioned Flavor Aversions to Familiar Tap Water in Rats: An Adjustment with Implications for Aversion Therapy Treatment of Alcoholism and Obesity," *Journal of Abnormal Psychology* 83(1974):411–417.

139. A. N. Wiens and C. E. Menustik, "Treatment Outcome and Patient Characteristics in an Aversion Therapy Program for Alcoholism," *American Psychologist* 38(1983):1089–1096.

140. Mellor and White, "Taste Aversions to Alcoholic Beverages."

J. Quinn and R. Henbest, "Partial Failure of Generalization in Alcoholism Following Aversion Therapy," *Quarterly Journal of Studies on Alcohol* 28(1967):70–75.

141. Logue, Logue, and Strauss, "The Acquisition of Taste Aversions in Humans with Eating and Drinking Disorders."

142. Elkins, "Aversion Therapy for Alcoholism."

R. L. Elkins and R. P. Murdock, "The Contribution of Successful Conditioning to Abstinence Maintenance Following Covert Sensitization (Verbal Aversion) Treatment of Alcoholism," *IRCS Medical Science: Psychology and Psychiatry: Social and Occupational Medicine* 5(1977):167.

143. R. L. Elkins, "Aversion Therapy for Alcoholism."

Elkins and Murdock, "The Contribution of Successful Conditioning to Abstinence Maintenance."

144. J. J. Franchina and A. B. Dyer, "Congener Characteristics Influence Aversion Conditioning to Alcoholic Beverages in Rats," *Behaviour Research and Therapy* 24(1986):299–306.

J. J. Franchina, A. B. Dyer, D. W. Gilley, J. Ness, and M. Dodd, "Role of Ethanol in Conditioning Aversion to Alcoholic Beverages in Rats," *Be-*

haviour Research and Therapy 23(1985):521-529.

145. D. S. Cannon and T. B. Baker, "Emetic and Electric Shock Alcohol Aversion Therapy: Assessment of Conditioning," *Journal of Consulting and Clinical Psychology* 49(1981):20-33.

D. S. Cannon, T. B. Baker, and C. K. Wehl, "Emetic and Electric Shock Alcohol Aversion Therapy: Six- and Twelve-Month Follow-Up," *Journal of Consulting and Clinical Psychology* 49(1981):360-368.

Lamon et al., "Human Classical Aversion Conditioning."

P. E. Nathan, "Aversion Therapy in the Treatment of Alcoholism: Success and Failure," in *Experimental Assessments and Clinical Applications of Conditioned Food Aversions*, eds. N. S. Braveman and P. Bronstein, New York: New York Academy of Sciences, 1985.

146. Ayerst Laboratories Inc., *Antabuse^R Brand of Disulfiram in Alcoholism*, New York: Author, 1986.

147. G. K. Litman and A. Topham, "Outcome Studies on Techniques in Alcoholism Treatment," in *Recent Developments in Alcoholism*, vol. 1, ed. M. Galanter, New York: Plenum, 1983, p. 172.

148. Ayerst Laboratories Inc., *Antabuse^R Brand of Disulfiram in Alcoholism*.

149. Litman and Topham, "Outcome Studies on Techniques in Alcoholism Treatment."

150. G. Bigelow, D. Strickler, I. Liebson, and R. Griffiths, "Maintaining Disulfiram Ingestion among Outpatient Alcoholics: A Security-Deposit Contingency Contracting Procedure," *Behaviour Research and Therapy* 14(1976):378–381.

151. G. Kolata, "New Drug Counters Alcohol Intoxication," *Science* 234(1986):1198–1199.

P. D. Suzdak, J. R. Glowa, J. N. Crawley, R. D. Schwartz, P. Skolnick, and S. M. Paul, "A Selective Imidazobenzodiazepine Antagonist of Ethanol in the Rat," *Science* 234(1986):1243–1247.

152. P. D. Suzdak, J. R. Glowa, J. M. Crawley, P. Skolnick, and P. M. Paul, "Is Ethanol Antagonist Ro15-4513 Selective for Ethanol?" *Science* 239(1988):649–650.

153. Kolata, "New Drug Counters Alcohol Intoxication."

154. Personal communication from Alcoholics Anonymous Information Office, August 1990.

155. Finney et al., "Posttreatment Experiences and Treatment Outcome."

156. F. Baekeland, L. Lundwall, and B. Kissin, "Methods for the Treatment of Chronic Alcoholism: A Critical Appraisal," in *Research Ad-*

vances in Alcohol and Drug Problems, vol. 2, eds. R. J. Gibbins, Y. Israel, H. Kalant, R. E. Popham, W. Schmidt, and R. G. Smart, New York: John Wiley & Sons, 1975.

157. Ibid.

158. E. Rubington, "The Role of the Halfway House in the Rehabilitation of Alcoholics," in *Treatment and Rehabilitation of the Chronic Alcoholic*, eds. B. Kissin and H. Begleiter, New York: Plenum, 1977, p. 352.

159. Ibid.

160. T. B. Baker, M. B. Sobell, L. C. Sobell, and D. S. Cannon, "Halfway Houses for Alcoholics: A Review, Analysis and Comparison with Other Halfway House Facilities," *International Journal of Social Psychiatry* 22(1976):130–139.

161. P. E. Nathan, "Failures in Prevention: Why We Can't Prevent the Devastating Effect of Alcoholism and Drug Abuse," *American Psychologist* 38(1983):459–467.

162. W. R. Miller, "Motivation for Treatment: A Review with Special Emphasis on Alcoholism," *Psychological Bulletin* 98(1985):84–107.

R. A. Moore, "Current Status of the Field: Contrasting Perspectives. C. A Medical Clinician's Perspective," in *Recent Developments in Alcoholism*, vol. 1, ed. M. Galanter, New York: Plenum, 1983.

Chapter 12: Eating, Drinking, and Female Reproduction

1. P. J. Brown and M. Konner, "An Anthropological Perspective on Obesity," in *Human Obesity*, eds. R. J. Wurtman and J. J. Wurtman, New York: New York Academy of Sciences, 1987.

2. J. Bancroft, A. Cook, and L. Williamson, "Food Craving, Mood and the Menstrual Cycle," *Psychological Medicine* 18(1988):855–860.

S. T. St. Jeor, M. R. Sutnick, and B. J. Scott, "Nutrition," in *Handbook of Behavioral Medicine for Women*, eds. E. A. Blechman and K. D. Brownell, New York: Pergamon, 1988.

3. *American Psychiatric Association: Diagnostic and Statistical Manual of Mental Disorders*, 3rd ed. rev., Washington, DC: APA, 1987.

C. M. Logue and R. H. Moos, "Perimenstrual Symptoms: Prevalence and Risk Factors," *Psychosomatic Medicine* 48(1986):388–414.

4. "Energy Expenditure during the Menstrual Cycle," *Nutrition Reviews* 45(1987):102–103.

L. A. Leiter, N. Hrboticky, and G. H. Anderson, "Effects of L-Tryptophan on Food Intake and Selection in Lean Men and Women," *Human Obesity*, eds. R. J. Wurtman and J. J. Wurtman, New York: New York Academy of Sciences, 1987.

St. Jeor et al., "Nutrition."

5. "Energy Expenditure during the Menstrual Cycle."

Leiter et al., "Effects of L-Tryptophan on Food Intake."

St. Jeor et al., "Nutrition."

6. R. J. Wurtman and J. J. Wurtman, "Carbohydrates and Depression," *Scientific American* 260(January 1989):68–75.

7. T. Engen, *The Perception of Odors*, New York: Academic Press, 1982.

R. G. Mair, J. A. Bouffard, and T. Engen, "Olfactory Sensitivity During the Menstrual Cycle," *Sensory Processes* 2(1978):90–98.

8. R. E. Frisch, "Fatness and Fertility," *Scientific American* 258(March 1988):88–95.

9. Ibid.

10. J. E. Schneider and G. N. Wade, "Availability of Metabolic Fuels Controls Estrous Cyclicity of Syrian Hamsters," *Science* 244(1989):1326–1328.

11. P. M. Dubbert and J. E. Martin, "Exercise," in *Handbook of Behavioral Medicine for Women*, eds. E. A. Blechman and K. D. Brownell, New York: Pergamon, 1988.

P. Ellison, "American Scientist Interviews," *American Scientist* 75(1987):622–627.

Logue and Moos, "Perimenstrual Symptoms."

12. Frisch, "Fatness and Fertility."

Dubbert and Martin, "Exercise."

13. L. P. Morin, "Effects of Various Feeding Regimens and Photoperiod or Pinealectomy on Ovulation in the Hamster," *Biology of Reproduction* 13(1975):99–103.

14. K. Brownell, "The Yo-Yo Trap," *American Health* (March 1988):78, 80–82, 84.

St. Jeor et al., "Nutrition."

15. P. Rosso, "Regulation of Food Intake during Pregnancy and Lactation," in *Human Obesity*, eds. R. J. Wurtman and J. J. Wurtman, New York: New York Academy of Sciences, 1987.

16. "Tenth Edition of the RDA," *Nutrition Reviews* 48(1990):28–30.

17. L. R. Cohen and B. C. Woodside, "Self-Selection of Protein During Pregnancy and Lactation in Rats," *Appetite* 12(1989):119–136.

18. P. M. Di Lorenzo and S. Monroe, "Taste

Responses in the Parabrachial Pons of Male, Female and Pregnant Rats," *Brain Research Bulletin* 23(1989):219–227.

19. E. J. Callahan and L. Desiderato, "Disorders in Pregnancy," in *Handbook of Behavioral Medicine for Women*, eds. E. A. Blechman and K. D. Brownell, New York: Pergamon, 1988.

K. Uvnas-Moberg, "Gastrointestinal Tract in Growth and Reproduction," *Scientific American* 261(July 1989):78–83.

20. H. A. Guthrie, *Introductory Nutrition*, Saint Louis: C. V. Mosby, 1975.

21. Uvnas-Moberg, "Gastrointestinal Tract in Growth and Reproduction."

22. St. Jeor et al., "Nutrition."

23. P. J. Bradley, "Conditions Recalled to Have Been Associated with Weight Gain in Adulthood," *Appetite* 6(1985):235–241.

24. A. P. Sisopoulos, "Characteristics of Obesity: An Overview," in *Human Obesity*, eds. R. J. Wurtman and J. J. Wurtman, New York: New York Academy of Sciences, 1987.

25. Uvnas-Moberg, "Gastrointestinal Tract in Growth and Reproduction."

26. St. Jeor et al., "Nutrition."

27. Ibid.

28. G.-P. Ravelli, Z. A. Stein, and M. W. Susser, "Obesity in Young Men after Famine Exposure in Utero and Early Infancy," *The New England Journal of Medicine* 295(1976):349–353.

29. Columbia University College of Physicians and Surgeons, *Complete Home Medical Guide*, New York: Crown Publishers, 1985.

30. E. L. Abel, "Fetal Alcohol Syndrome: Behavioral Teratology," *Psychological Bulletin* 87(1980):29–50.

A. P. Streissguth, S. Landesman-Dwyer, J. C. Martin, and D. W. Smith, "Teratogenic Effects of Alcohol in Humans and Laboratory Animals," *Science* 209(1980):353–361.

31. Streissguth et al., "Teratogenic Effects of Alcohol."

32. G. B. Kolata, "Fetal Alcohol Advisory Debated," *Science* 214(1981):642, 643, 645.

Streissguth et al., "Teratogenic Effects of Alcohol."

33. E. L. Abel, "Behavioral Teratology of Alcohol," *Psychological Bulletin* 90(1981):564–581.

34. A. B. Mukherjee and G. D. Hodgen, "Maternal Ethanol Exposure Induces Transient Impairment of Umbilical Circulation and Fetal Hypoxia in Monkeys," *Science* 218(1982):700–702.

35. K. K. Sulik, M. C. Johnston, and M. A.

Webb, "Fetal Alcohol Syndrome: Embryogenesis in a Mouse Model," *Science* 214(1981):936–938.

36. A. W. Kimball, "Alcohol and Pregnancy," *Science* 221(1983):1245.

37. Sulik et al., "Fetal Alcohol Syndrome."

38. B. M. Altura, B. T. Altura, A. Carella, M. Chatterjee, S. Halevy, and N. Tejani, "Alcohol Produces Spasms of Human Umbilical Blood Vessels: Relationship to Fetal Alcohol Syndrome (FAS)," *European Journal of Pharmacology* 86(1983):311–312.

39. Kolata, "Fetal Alcohol Advisory Debated."

U.S. Department of Health and Human Services, *The Surgeon General's Report on Nutrition and Health: Summary and Recommendations* (DHHS Publication No. 88-50211), Washington, DC: U.S. Government Printing Office, 1988.

40. J. M. Joffe, "Alcohol and Pregnancy," *Science* 221(1983):1244–1245.

Kolata, "Fetal Alcohol Advisory Debated."

A. B. Mukherjee and G. D. Hodgen, "Alcohol and Pregnancy," *Science* 221(1983):1245.

41. M. Frezza, C. Di Padova, G. Pozzato, M. Terpin, E. Baraona, and C. S. Lieber, "High Blood Alcohol Levels in Women: The Role of Decreased Gastric Alcohol Dehydrogenase Activity and First-Pass Metabolism," *The New England Journal of Medicine* 322(1990):95–99.

42. R. M. Gilbert, "Caffeine: Overview and Anthology," in *Nutrition and Behavior*, ed. S. A. Miller, Philadelphia: Franklin Institute, 1981.

43. P. Wright, "Hunger, Satiety and Feeding Behavior in Early Infancy," in *Eating Habits: Food, Physiology and Learned Behavior*, eds. R. A. Boakes, D. A. Popplewell, and M. J. Burton, Chichester, Great Britain: John Wiley & Sons, 1987, p. 75.

44. Gilbert, "Caffeine."

St. Jeor et al., "Nutrition.

45. Wright, "Hunger, Satiety and Feeding Behavior in Early Infancy."

46. S. B. Roberts, J. Savage, W. A. Coward, B. Chew, and A. Lucas, "Energy Expenditure and Intake in Infants Born to Lean and Overweight Mothers," *The New England Journal of Medicine* 318(1988):461–466.

47. Uvnas-Moberg, "Gastrointestinal Tract in Growth and Reproduction."

48. P. Rozin and M. L. Pelchat, "Memories of Mammaries: Adaptations to Weaning from Milk," *Progress in Psychobiology and Physiological Psychology* 13(1988):1–29.

49. St. Jeor et al., "Nutrition."

50. Rosso, "Regulation of Food Intake during Pregnancy and Lactation."

51. Cohen and Woodside, "Self-Selection of Protein."

52. Uvnas-Moberg, "Gastrointestinal Tract in Growth and Reproduction."

Chapter 13: Smoking and Weight Loss and Weight Gain

1. *American Psychiatric Association: Diagnostic and Statistical Manual of Mental Disorders*, 3rd ed. rev., Washington, DC: APA, 1987.

P. O. Russell and L. H. Epstein, "Smoking," in *Handbook of Behavioral Medicine for Women*, eds. E. A. Blechman and K. D. Brownell, New York: Pergamon, 1988.

2. R. C. Klesges and L. M. Klesges, "Cigarette Smoking as a Dieting Strategy in a University Population," *International Journal of Eating Disorders* 7(1988):413–419.

3. O. Pomerleau, F. Bass, and V. Crown, "Role of Behavior Modification in Preventive Medicine," *The New England Journal of Medicine* 292(1975):1277–1282.

Russell and Epstein, "Smoking."

4. N. E. Grunberg, "Nicotine, Cigarette Smoking, and Body Weight," *British Journal of Addiction* 80(1985):369–377.

5. Grunberg, "Nicotine, Cigarette Smoking, and Body Weight."

R. C. Klesges and A. W. Meyers, "Smoking, Body Weight, and Their Effects on Smoking Behavior: A Comprehensive Review of the Literature," *Psychological Bulletin* 106(1989):204–230.

6. N. E. Grunberg, D. J. Bowen, V. A. Maycock, and S. M. Nespor, "The Importance of Sweet Taste and Caloric Content in the Effects of Nicotine on Specific Food Consumption," *Psychopharmacology* 87(1985):198–203.

7. R. W. Foltin, M. W. Fischman, and M. F. Byrne, "Effects of Smoked Marijuana on Food Intake and Body Weight of Humans Living in a Residential Laboratory," *Appetite* 11(1988):1–14.

8. Grunberg, "Nicotine, Cigarette Smoking, and Body Weight."

9. S. A. Wager-Srdar, A. S. Levine, J. E. Morley, J. R. Hoidal, and D. E. Niewoehner, "Effects of Cigarette Smoke and Nicotine on Feeding and Energy," *Physiology and Behavior* 32(1984):389–395.

10. J. B. Beckwith, "Eating, Drinking, and Smoking and Their Relationship in Adult Women," *Psychological Reports* 59(1986):1075–1089.

11. Grunberg, "Nicotine, Cigarette Smoking, and Body Weight."

12. N. E. Grunberg and D. E. Morse, "Cigarette Smoking and Food Consumption in the United States," *Journal of Applied Social Psychology* 14(1984):310–317.

13. N. E. Grunberg, "The Effects of Nicotine and Cigarette Smoking on Food Consumption and Taste Preferences," *Addictive Behaviors* 7(1982):317–331.

14. A. J. Jaffe and A. G. Glaros, "Taste Dimensions in Cigarette Discrimination: A Multidimensional Scaling Approach," *Addictive Behaviors* 11(1986):407–413.

15. Grunberg, "Nicotine, Cigarette Smoking, and Body Weight."

16. K. A. Perkins, L. H. Epstein, B. L. Marks, R. L. Stiller, and R. G. Jacob, "The Effect of Nicotine on Energy Expenditure during Light Physical Activity," *The New England Journal Of Medicine* 320(1989):898–903.

17. A. Hofstetter, Y. Schutz, E. Jéquier, and J. Wahren, "Increased 24-Hour Energy Expenditure in Cigarette Smokers," *The New England Journal of Medicine* 314(1986):79–82.

18. Wager-Srdar et al., "Effects of Cigarette Smoke and Nicotine on Feeding and Energy."

19. S. M. Hall, R. McGee, C. Tunstall, J. Duffy, and N. Benowitz, "Changes in Food Intake and Activity after Quitting Smoking," *Journal of Consulting and Clinical Psychology* 57(1989):81–86.

20. Grunberg, "Nicotine, Cigarette Smoking, and Body Weight."

Klesges and Meyers, "Smoking, Body Weight, and Their Effects on Smoking Behavior."

J. Rodin, "Weight Change Following Smoking Cessation: The Role of Food Intake and Exercise," *Addictive Behaviors* 12(1987):303–317.

J. Tuomilehto, A. Nissinen, P. Puska, J. T. Salonen, and L. Jalkanen, "Long-Term Effects of Cessation of Smoking on Body Weight, Blood Pressure and Serum Cholesterol in the Middle-Aged Population with High Blood Pressure," *Addictive Behaviors* 11 (1986): 1–9.

21. Klesges and Meyers, "Smoking, Body Weight, and Their Effects on Smoking Behavior."

S. M. Hall, D. Ginsberg, and R. T. Jones, "Smoking Cessation and Weight Gain," *Journal of Consulting and Clinical Psychology* 54(1986): 342–346.

22. Klesges and Meyers, "Smoking, Body Weight, and Their Effects on Smoking Behavior."

J. Gross, M. L. Stitzer, and J. Maldonado, "Nicotine Replacement: Effects on Postcessation Weight Gain," *Journal of Consulting and Clinical Psychology* 57(1989):87–92.

23. Gross et al., "Nicotine Replacement."

24. Hall et al., "Smoking Cessation and Weight Gain."

R. S. Manley and F. J. Boland, "Side-Effects and Weight Gain Following a Smoking Cessation Program," *Addictive Behaviors* 8(1983):375–380.

25. Grunberg, "Nicotine, Cigarette Smoking, and Body Weight."

26. Hall et al., "Changes in Food Intake and Activity after Quitting Smoking."

27. Grunberg et al., "The Importance of Sweet Taste and Caloric Content."

28. B. Spring, J. Wurtman, R. Gleason, R. Wurtman, and K. Kessler, "Weight Gain and Withdrawal Symptoms after Smoking Cessation: A Preventative Intervention Using d-Fenfluramine, *Health Psychology,* in press.

29. K. A. Perkins, C. Denier, J. A. Mayer, R. R. Scott, and P. M. Dubbert, "Weight Gain Associated with Decreases in Smoking Rate and Nicotine Intake," *International Journal of the Addictions* 22(1987):575–581.

30. Rodin, "Weight Change Following Smoking Cessation."

31. M. B. Cantor and J. F. Wilson, "Feeding the Face: New Directions in Adjunctive Behavior Research," in *Affect, Conditioning, and Cognition: Essays on the Determinants of Behavior,* eds. F. R. Brush and J. B. Overmier, Hillsdale, NJ: Lawrence Erlbaum Associates, 1985.

32. J. Green and W. N. Tapp, "Feeding Cycles in Smokers, Exsmokers and Nonsmokers," *Physiology and Behavior* 36(1986):1059–1063.

33. Grunberg, "Nicotine, Cigarette Smoking, and Body Weight."

34. Hall et al., "Smoking Cessation and Weight Gain."

35. Klesges and Meyers, "Smoking, Body Weight, and Their Effects on Smoking Behavior."

36. Grunberg, "Nicotine, Cigarette Smoking, and Body Weight."

37. Hall et al., "Changes in Food Intake and Activity after Quitting Smoking."

38. Rodin, "Weight Change Following Smoking Cessation."

39. Grunberg et al., "The Importance of Sweet Taste and Caloric Content."

40. Grunberg, "Nicotine, Cigarette Smoking, and Body Weight."

41. Hofstetter et al., "Increased 24-hour Energy Expenditure in Cigarette Smokers."

42. Hall et al., "Smoking Cessation and Weight Gain."

43. Perkins et al., "Weight Gain Associated with Decreases in Smoking Rate and Nicotine Intake."

Rodin, "Weight Change Following Smoking Cessation."

Chapter 14: Cuisine and Wine Tasting

1. E. Rozin, "The Structure of Cuisine," in *The Psychobiology of Human Food Selection,* ed. L. M. Barker, Westport, CT: AVI Publishing, 1982.

E. Rozin, *Ethnic Cuisine: The Flavor-Principle Cookbook,* Brattleboro, VT: The Stephen Greene Press, 1983.

2. P. Rozin, "The Acquisition of Food Habits and Preferences," in *Behavioral Health: A Handbook of Health Enhancement and Disease Prevention,* ed. J. D. Matarazzo, New York: John Wiley & Sons, 1984.

3. S. H. Katz, "Fava Bean Consumption: A Case for the Co-Evolution of Genes and Culture," in *Food and Evolution: Toward a Theory of Human Food Habits,* eds. M. Harris and E. B. Ross, Philadelphia: Temple University Press, 1987.

4. R. Sokolov, "Insects, Worms, and Other Tidbits," *Natural History* (September 1989):84, 86–88.

5. S. H. Katz, "Food Behavior and Biocultural Evolution," in *The Psychobiology of Human Food Selection,* ed. L. M. Barker, Westport, CT: AVI Publishing, 1982.

6. L. L. Birch, J. Billman, and S. S. Richards, "Time of Day Influences Food Acceptability," *Appetite* 5(1984):109–116.

7. C. Nemeroff and P. Rozin, "Sympathetic Magic in Kosher Practice and Belief at the Limits of the Laws of *Kashrut,*" *Jewish Folklore and Ethnology* 9(1987):31–32.

8. N. Hrboticky and M. Krondl, "Acculturation to Canadian Foods by Chinese Immigrant Boys: Changes in the Perceived Flavor, Health Value and Prestige of Foods," *Appetite* 5(1984):117–126.

M. Krondl, N. Hrboticky, and P. Coleman, "Adapting to Cultural Changes in Food Habits," in *Malnutrition: Determinants and Consequences,* eds. P. L. White and N. Selvey, New York: Alan R. Liss, 1984.

9. Rozin, "The Structure of Cuisine."

Rozin, *Ethnic Cuisine.*

E. Rozin and P. Rozin, "Culinary Themes and Variations," *Natural History* (February 1981):6, 8, 12, 14.

P. Rozin, "Human Food Selection: The Interaction of Biology, Culture and Individual Experience," in *The Psychobiology of Human Food Selection,* ed. L. M. Barker, Westport, CT: AVI Publishing, 1982

10. Rozin, *Ethnic Cuisine.*

11. C. Claiborne, "Cajun and Creole: French at Heart," *The New York Times* (April 1, 1987):C1, C6.

R. Sokolov, *Fading Feast,* New York: E. P. Dutton, 1983.

12. B. Greene, "Cajun Country," *Cuisine* (September 1979): 42–54.

13. B. Karoff, "Chilies," *Gourmet* (October 1989): 114-117, 250–259.

F. W. Moore, "Food Habits in Non-Industrial Societies," in *Dimensions of Nutrition,* ed. J. Dupont, Boulder, CO: Colorado Associated University Press, 1970.

F. Rosengarten, *The Book of Spices,* Wynnewood, PA: Livingston Publishing, 1969.

P. Rozin, "Psychobiological and Cultural Determinants of Food Choice," in *Appetite and Food Intake,* ed. T. Silverstone, Berlin: Dahlem Konferenzen, 1976.

P. Rozin, "Getting to Like the Burn of Chili Pepper: Biological, Psychological, and Cultural Perspectives," in *Chemical Senses: Vol 2. Irritation,* eds. B. G. Green, J. R. Mason, and M. R. Kare, New York: Marcel Dekker, 1990.

14. A. K. Naj, "Hot Topic: Chilies Cause Pleasant Pain, Even Mild Euphoria," *Wall Street Journal* (November 25, 1986):1, 20.

15. C. E. Martin, "Appalachian House Beautiful," *Natural History* 91 (2) (1982): 4, 6-8, 10, 12, 14-16.

16. B. G. Galef, "Enduring Social Enhancement of Rats' Preferences for the Palatable and the Piquant," *Appetite* 13(1989):81–92.

17. P. Rozin and K. Kennel, "Acquired Preferences for Piquant Foods by Chimpanzees," *Appetite* 4(1983):69–77.

18. Rozin, "Human Food Selection."

Rozin, "Getting to Like the Burn of Chili Pepper."

19. H. Lawless, P. Rozin, and J. Shenker, "Ef-

fects of Oral Capsaicin on Gustatory, Olfactory and Irritant Sensations and Flavor Identification in Humans Who Regularly or Rarely Consume Chili Pepper," *Chemical Senses* 10(1985):579–589.

Rozin, "Getting to Like the Burn of Chili Pepper."

20. P. Rozin, M. Mark, and D. Schiller, "The Role of Desensitization to Capsaicin in Chili Pepper Ingestion and Preference," *Chemical Senses* 6(1981):23–31.

21. Rozin, "Human Food Selection."

Rozin, "Getting to Like the Burn of Chili Pepper."

22. P. Rozin, D. Reff, M. Mark, and J. Schull, "Conditioned Opponent Responses in Human Tolerance to Caffeine," *Bulletin of the Psychonomic Society* 22 (1984):117–120.

23. Rozin, "Getting to Like the Burn of Chili Pepper."

24. Ibid.

25. W. Root, *Food,* New York: Simon & Schuster, 1980.

R. Tannahill, *Food in History,* New York: Crown Publishers, 1988.

26. P. Rozin, "Sweetness, Sensuality, Sin, Safety, and Socialization: Some Speculations," in *Sweetness,* ed. J. Dobbing, New York: Springer-Verlag, 1987.

27. B. L. Gelb, *The Dictionary of Food,* New York: Ballantine Books, 1978.

28. J. E. Brody, *Jane Brody's The New York Times Guide to Personal Health,* New York: Avon, 1982.

29. M. Harris, "India's Sacred Cow," in *Issues in Nutrition for the 1980s: An Ecological Perspective,* eds. A. L. Tobias and P. J. Thompson, Monterey, CA: Wadsworth, 1980.

K. N. Nair, "Animal Protein Consumption and the Sacred Cow Complex in India," in *Food and Evolution: Toward a Theory of Human Food Habits,* eds. M. Harris and E. B. Ross, Philadelphia: Temple University Press, 1987.

30. Harris, "India's Sacred Cow."

31. Ibid, p. 224.

32. Ibid.

S. E. G. Lea, "Correlation and Contiguity in Foraging Behavior," in *Predictability, Correlation, and Contiguity,* eds. P. Harzem and M. D. Zeiler, New York: John Wiley & Sons, 1981.

A. Roosevelt, "The Evolution of Human Subsistence," in *Food and Evolution: Toward a Theory of Human Food Habits,* eds. M. Harris and E. B. Ross, Philadelphia: Temple University Press, 1987.

33. J. E. Cohen, "Big Fish, Little Fish: The

Search for Patterns in Predator –Prey Relationships," *The Sciences* 29(March/April 1989):36–42.

S. L. Pimm, *Food Webs*, New York: Chapman & Hall, 1982.

G. Sugihara, K. Schoenly, A. Trombla, "Scale Invariance in Food Web Properties," *Science* 245(1989):48–52.

34. S. M. Garn and W. R. Leonard, "What Did Our Ancestors Eat?" *Nutrition Reviews* 47 (1989): 337–345.

35. K. Hill and A. M. Hurtado, "Hunter-Gatherers of the New World," *American Scientist* (September/October 1989):436–443.

36. W. Arens, *The Man-Eating Myth: Anthropology and Anthropophagy*, New York: Oxford University Press, 1979.

37. D. R. Harris, "Aboriginal Subsistence in a Tropical Rain Forest Environment: Food Procurement, Cannibalism, and Population Regulation in Northeastern Australia," in *Food and Evolution: Toward a Theory of Human Food Habits*, eds. M. Harris and E. B. Ross, Philadelphia: Temple University Press, 1987.

G. Kolata, "Anthropologists Suggest Cannibalism Is a Myth," *Science* 232(1986):1497–1500.

P. Villa, C. Bouville, J. Courtin, D. Helmer, E. Mahieu, P. Shipman, G. Belluomini, and M. Branca, "Cannibalism in the Neolithic," *Science* 233(1986):431–438.

38. W. K. Powers and M. N. Powers, "Putting on the Dog," *Natural History* 95(February 1986):6, 8, 10, 14–16.

39. M. A. Amerine and E. B. Roessler, *Wines: Their Sensory Evaluation*, San Francisco: W. H. Freeman and Company, 1976.

J. Durac, *Wines and the Art of Tasting*, New York: E. P. Dutton, 1974.

B. Ensrud, *Wine with Food: A Guide to Entertaining through the Seasons*, New York: Congdon & Weed, 1984.

40. Amerine and Roessler, *Wines*.

41. D. M. Green and J. A. Swets, *Signal Detection Theory and Psychophysics*, New York: Robert E. Krieger, 1974.

42. Amerine and Roessler, *Wines*.

43. Ibid.

Durac, *Wines and the Art of Tasting*.

44. Amerine and Roessler, *Wines*.

45. Ibid.

46. Ibid.

47. Ibid.

Durac, *Wines and the Art of Tasting*.

48. Amerine and Roessler, *Wines*.

49. Ibid.

50. D. A. Norman, *Memory and Attention*, New York: John Wiley & Sons, 1969.

51. Amerine and Roessler, *Wines*.

52. Ibid.

53. Ibid.

54. D. Cross, "On Judgments of Magnitude," in *Social Attitudes and Psychophysical Measurement*, ed. B. Wegener, Hillsdale, NJ: Lawrence Erlbaum Associates, 1982.

Name Index

Subject Index

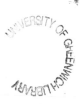

ISBN 0-7167-2232-1

90000>

EAN

9 780716 722328